T0133420

Palliative Care within Mental Health

PRINCIPLES AND PHILOSOPHY

Edited by

DAVID B COOPER

Sigma Theta Tau International: The Honor Society of Nursing Award
Nursing Council on Alcohol: Outstanding Contribution to Nursing Award
Editor-in-Chief, Mental Health and Substance Use
Author/Writer/Editor

and

JO COOPER

Macmillan Clinical Nurse Specialist in Palliative Care
Media Review Editor: Mental Health and Substance Use

Radcliffe Publishing
London • New York

Radcliffe Publishing Ltd
33–41 Dallington Street
London
EC1V 0BB
United Kingdom

www.radcliffehealth.com

British Library Cataloguing in Publication Data

A catalogue record for this book is available from the British Library.

ISBN-13: 978 184619 537 2

The paper used for the text pages of this book is FSC® certified. FSC (The Forest Stewardship Council®) is an international network to promote responsible management of the world's forests.

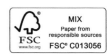

Typeset by Darkriver Design, Auckland, New Zealand
Printed and bound by TJI Digital, Padstow, Cornwall, UK

Contents

Preface

This book is not about caring for the dying in serious mental illness but about applying the principles and philosophy of palliative care within serious and enduring mental health practice. The book focuses on the similarity in philosophy between palliative care and mental health practice.

The common philosophical meeting ground is an excellent foundation for integrating specialist palliative care, now recognised as best-practice end-of-life care, into serious and enduring mental health service delivery. In short, the shared practice values and vision between these two disciplines provide an optimistic starting point from which to plan to address the lack of palliative care service delivery in mental health practice.

The book came into being when Jo and I (editors) were talking and the discussion led on to the need for more information/direction when it comes to humanness and the issue of palliative care within serious and enduring mental health practice. While it could be assumed that mental health has a lot to offer palliative care, we both felt that palliative care could offer more to mental health practice in that it is a neglected area. There is little or no literature related to palliative care within serious mental health practice, and that which does exist relates to care of the dying in terms of cancer.

What struck us was that several chapters within the mental health–substance use series of books (*see* other books by the editors) could equally apply to palliative care within serious and enduring mental health care and practice. In the time it took us to drink our coffee, we had developed a contents list! As the title, *Palliative Care within Mental Health*, suggests, the whole approach would be on the humanistic aspects of care.

Is there a place for palliative care within mental health? At the mention of palliative care, there is a general assumption that:

a. the person has a cancer diagnosis and . . .
b. the person is dying.

However, this is not the true meaning of palliation. A simple understanding might be that if a person has ill-health that is serious and enduring (even with periods of respite) then that person needs careful and continuous symptom management together with skilled emotional support so that she or he can achieve the best quality of life with managed symptom control as effective as possible – that is, palliative care.

We chose the title as it appeared to indicate that while each could be a separate entity, they could also be co-joined in service application. Jo and I have combined our different skills (Jo – palliative care; David – mental health) to edit this book and a highly qualified team were invited to contribute. We hope we have edited a thought-provoking and informative text on *palliative care within mental health*.

David B Cooper and Jo Cooper
July 2012

About the editors

David B Cooper
Sigma Theta Tau International: Honor Society of Nursing Award
Nursing Council on Alcohol: Outstanding Contribution to Nursing Award
Editor-in-Chief: *Mental Health and Substance Use*
Author/Writer/Editor

David has specialised in mental health and substance use for over 30 years. He has worked as a practitioner, manager, researcher, author, lecturer and consultant. He has served as editor, or editor-in-chief, of several journals, and is currently editor-in-chief of *Mental Health and Substance Use*. He has published widely and is *'credited with enhancing the understanding and development of community detoxification for people experiencing alcohol withdrawal'* (Nursing Council on Alcohol; Sigma Theta Tau International citations). Seminal works include *Alcohol Home Detoxification and Assessment* and *Alcohol Use*, both published by Radcliffe Publishing, Oxford. David recently (2011) edited a series of textbooks with the series title of *Mental Health–Substance Use*.

Jo Cooper
Macmillan Clinical Nurse Specialist in Palliative Care
Media Review Editor: Mental Health and Substance Use
Horsham
West Sussex, England

Jo spent 16 years in Specialist Palliative Care, initially working in a hospice in-patient unit, then 12 years as a Macmillan Clinical Nurse Specialist. She gained a Diploma in Oncology at Addenbrookes Hospital, Cambridge, and a BSc (Hons) in Palliative Nursing at The Royal Marsden, London, and an Award in Specialist Practice. Jo edited *Stepping into Palliative Care* (2000) and the 2nd edition, *Stepping into Palliative Care 1: relationships and responses* (2006) and *Stepping into Palliative Care 2: care and practice* (2006), both published by Radcliffe Publishing. Jo has been involved in teaching for many years to all grades of medical and nursing staff and others. Her specialist subjects include management of complex pain and symptoms, terminal agitation, communication at the end of life, therapeutic relationships, and breaking bad news.

The editors welcome approaches and feedback, positive and/or negative.

List of contributors

CHAPTER 2
Poppy Buchanan-Barker
Director, Clan Unity International Ltd
Newport-on-Tay
Fife, Scotland

Poppy is Director of Clan Unity International – a public limited company offering mental health recovery-focused seminars and workshops, internationally. As a social worker, she spent more than 25 years leading innovative community developments for people with multiple disabilities and their families. Poppy began training as a counsellor in the 1980s, working with individuals and families, in the areas of suicide, alcohol and crisis resolution. She is widely published and has presented her work at many international conferences. In 2008, Poppy was the joint winner of the Thomas Szasz Award for Outstanding Contributions to the Cause of Civil Liberties, in New York.

Professor Phil Barker
Honorary Professor
Faculty of Medicine, Dentistry, and Nursing, University of Dundee
Psychotherapist
Newport-on-Tay, Fife, UK

Phil is a psychotherapist. He was the UK's first Professor of Psychiatric Nursing Practice at the University of Newcastle (1993–2002); elected a Fellow of the Royal College of Nursing in 1995; awarded the Red Gate Award for Distinguished Professors at the University of Tokyo in 2000; awarded an honorary Doctorate of the University at Oxford Brookes University in 2001; and has been Visiting Professor at several international universities. In 2008, Phil was the joint winner of the Thomas S Szasz Award for Outstanding Contributions to the Cause of Civil Liberties, in New York.

CHAPTER 3

Professor Larry D Purnell
Emeritus Professor, University of Delaware, USA
Adjunct Professor, Florida International University, USA,
Consulting Faculty, Excelsior College, USA
Funded Professor, Universita di Modena, Italy
Sudlersville, MD, USA

Larry is Emeritus Professor at the University of Delaware where he co-ordinated the graduate programmes in nursing and health services administration and taught culture. His Model, the Purnell Model for Cultural Competence, has been translated into Arabic, Flemish, Korean, French, German, Portuguese, Spanish and Turkish. His textbook, *Transcultural Health Care: a culturally competent approach*, won the Brandon Hill and American Journal of Nursing Book Awards. Larry is a Fellow in the American Academy of Nursing, a Transcultural Nursing Scholar, Luther Christman Fellow, and is in the Rosa Parks Wall of Fame for Teaching Tolerance.

We would like to thank Dr Geraldine S Pearson, PhD, RN, FAAN for her contribution to Case study 3.3. Geraldine is the Director of the HomeCare Program and Associate Professor, Child and Adolescent Division at the University of Connecticut Health Center School of Medicine. She is also the editor of *Perspectives in Psychiatric Care*.

CHAPTER 4

Dr Cynthia MA Geppert
Chief Consultation Psychiatry and Ethics New Mexico Veterans Affairs Health Care System
Associate Professor Department of Psychiatry
Director of Ethics and Professionalism Education
University of New Mexico School of Medicine
Albuquerque, NM, USA

Cynthia is Chief of Consultation Psychiatry and Ethics and Integrated Ethics Program Officer at the New Mexico Veterans Affairs Health Care System. She is also Associate Professor in the Department of Psychiatry and Director of Ethics Education at the University of New Mexico School of Medicine. Cynthia is board certified in general psychiatry, psychosomatic medicine, hospice and palliative medicine, and addiction medicine and holds credentials in pain management. Cynthia is a fellowship and graduate trained bioethicist with a specialty in religious and clinical ethics and the ethics of addiction.

Dr Philip J Candilis
Associate Professor of Psychiatry
Law and Psychiatry Program

Department of Psychiatry
University of Massachusetts Medical School
Worcester, MA, USA

Philip is an Associate Professor of Psychiatry at the University of Massachusetts Medical School. He began his career as a student-researcher at the National Cancer Institute, trained in psychiatry and ethics in the Harvard system, and now treats persons diagnosed with mental illness. Philip conducts research on individual and group decision making, with a focus on decision-making capacity among medically and mentally ill individuals. As a forensic psychiatrist and medical ethicist, he writes and consults widely on matters of forensic, research and professional ethics.

CHAPTER 5

Dr Alyna Turner
Heart Research Centre
North Melbourne
Victoria, Australia

Alyna is a clinical psychologist who has practised in liaison psychiatry, psychiatric rehabilitation and community chronic illness services over the last 11 years. She is currently Senior Research Fellow at the Heart Research Centre in Melbourne, Victoria, Australia. She has contributed to trials evaluating integrated psychological treatment for mental health–substance use problems and research into assessment and treatment of mental health problems in people with chronic physical illness.

Professor Brian Kelly
Faculty of Health
Centre for Brain and Mental Health Research
The University of Newcastle
Callaghan
New South Wales, Australia

Brian is Professor of Psychiatry, School of Medicine and Public Health, Faculty of Health, University of Newcastle, Australia. He has a long-standing clinical and research interest in Consultation-Liaison Psychiatry, focusing on psycho-oncology and palliative care, and public health aspects of mental illness, including rural mental health.

Professor Amanda L Baker
Faculty of Health
Centre for Brain and Mental Health Research
The University of Newcastle

Callaghan
New South Wales, Australia

Amanda is a National Health and Medical Research Council (NHMRC) Senior Research Fellow at the University of Newcastle, NSW, Australia. She is a senior clinical psychologist who has practised in the United Kingdom and Australia. Her research focuses on the challenging area of the psychological treatment of comorbidity (mental health–substance use problems). She has led numerous trials, funded by competitive national grants, investigating integrated psychological treatments for these problems and has published widely in the field.

CHAPTER 6
Jo Cooper
See About the editors.

CHAPTER 7
Jo Cooper and David B Cooper
See About the editors.

CHAPTER 8
Reverend Doctor Je Kan Adler-Collins
Associate Professor of Nursing, Health Promotion Centre
Research Fellow, Centre of Gender Studies, Khon Kaen University, Thailand
President, Non-Profit Organisation: Integrative Care Education Research Association Japan
Health Promotion Centre
Fukuoka Prefectural University
Tagawa City
Fukuoka Prefecture, Japan

Je Kan qualified as an RN, and REMT in the British Army. He became a Buddhist Monk of Shingon Shu in Japan in 1995. Je Kan was awarded his PGCE(FE) in 1998, MA in education 2000, and PhD in education 2007. Je Kan moved to Japan in 2000 where he built a temple, school, centre and hospice. He is an Associate Professor of Nursing at Fukuoka Prefectural University. In 2009, he became Director of Education for the Japanese Holistic Nursing Association. In 2010, Je Kan became President of a new non-profit organisation, Integrative Care Education and Research Association of Japan.

CHAPTER 9
Professor Agnes Higgins
Professor
Trinity College Dublin School of Nursing and Midwifery
Dublin, Ireland

Agnes is Professor in Mental Health at the School of Nursing and Midwifery, Trinity College Dublin, Ireland. She is a registered psychiatric nurse and general nurse, with more than 30 years' experience of working in the areas of mental health, palliative care and general nursing. One of her research interests is in the area of sexualities and mental health. Agnes has completed and published a number of research studies in this area.

CHAPTER 10

Dr John R Ashcroft
Psychiatry Senior Medical Officer
Mental Health Services
Counties Manukau District Board
Auckland
New Zealand

John is currently working as a Locum Consultant Psychiatrist. He qualified at Imperial College London in 2000 after first completing an undergraduate BSc in Neurosciences. He is a member of the Royal College of Psychiatrists and has special interests in Neuropsychiatry and Addiction Psychiatry. In 2006 he completed a Post Graduate Diploma in Clinical Neuropsychiatry at the University of Birmingham. John is a member of the International Advisory Board for the journal *Mental Health–Substance Use*.

CHAPTER 11

Peter Athanasos
School of Nursing
Royal Adelaide Hospital
The University of Adelaide
Adelaide
South Australia, Australia

Peter is a researcher working in Adelaide, Australia. Peter's main area of research interest is the effect of substance use on co-existing disorders such as mental health, pain and other pathophysiology. He has published a textbook and a number of chapters and articles in these areas. He is currently National Secretary and South Australian Representative for the Australasian Professional Society on Alcohol and Other Drugs (APSAD). Peter is also a member of Drug and Alcohol Nurses of Australasia and the Australian College of Mental Health Nurses.

Trevor W Mitten
Gold Standards Co-ordinator
The Swallowcourt Group
Ponsandane Care Home
Penzance, Cornwall, UK

Trevor has worked for over 18 years in palliative care. After five years at the newly built Exeter Hospice, he moved to North Devon Hospice and spent 11 years as a clinical nurse specialist in palliative care. Following two-and-a-half years as a Macmillan Nurse, he now serves as a gold standards co-ordinator in the independent sector. Trevor has a bachelor's degree with honours in health studies and a postgraduate certificate in enhanced palliative care.

Dr Rose Neild
Senior Consultant
Drug and Alcohol Services of South Australia
Parkside
South Australia, Australia

Rose is the Vice President/President Elect of the Australasian Professional Society on Alcohol and Other Drugs (APSAD) and is also on the scientific programme committee for this organisation. She is a fellow of the Chapter of Addiction Medicine. Rose has experience of working in alcohol and other drug services in New Zealand and Australia. She is completing a Doctorate in Public Health. Rose has a particular interest in working with women with substance-use disorders, especially those who are pregnant or parenting, and this has developed over recent times into a wider interest in inclusive practice – working with families and partners. Other interest areas include physical and psychiatric comorbidities with dependence in both clinical and public health arenas.

Professor Charlotte de Crespigny
Professor of Drug and Alcohol Nursing
University of Adelaide
Adelaide
South Australia, Australia

Charlotte is a registered nurse who has been working in the drug and alcohol field as a clinician, educator and researcher since 1988. Charlotte's current research interests include: systems of care; alcohol, drug and mental health comorbidity; co-ordinated Aboriginal mental health care; Aboriginal people's use of over-the-counter analgesics; women, alcohol and licensed premises; social drinking in context; heat wave and the impact on vulnerable people with mental health and substance-use conditions. Charlotte works in partnership with other researchers, service leaders and practitioners from varying health fields including general healthcare, mental health, alcohol and other drugs, public health and health economics, and Aboriginal health. She is committed to translating research findings into everyday healthcare, including clinical practice, health promotion, and community and professional education – in both government and non-government sectors. Charlotte has authored many journal publications, best-practice guidelines, and chapters in texts.

Dr Lynette Cusack
Research Fellow (Population Health)
School of Nursing and Midwifery
Faculty of Health Science
Flinders University
Adelaide
South Australia, Australia

Lynette holds a postdoctoral research fellow (Population Health) position, and is a member of the Board of the Flinders University Research Centre for Disaster Resilience and Health. Lynette previously worked in the alcohol and other drugs field for over 14 years, in an executive role with the Drug and Alcohol Services SA (DASSA), which is a State Government organisation.

CHAPTER 12

Jo Cooper
See About the editors.

CHAPTER 13

Dr Shiphrah Williams-Evans
Associate Professor
University of South Alabama
Mobile, AL, USA

Shiphrah is an advanced practice nurse with more than 20 years' experience. She is certified as a palliative care nurse and has practised palliative care for seven years and helped establish one of the first palliative care practices in the Green Bay, Wisconsin area. Her work has been embraced by physicians and nurses and she has paved the way for patients and families to receive holistic care for a variety of illnesses. Shiphrah is currently an Associate Professor at the University of South Alabama teaching in Mental Health and Palliative Care in the Masters and Doctor of Nursing Practice Programs. She has a private practice in palliative care, called Expanding Boundaries of Practice.

Professor Barbara Broome
Associate Dean
Chair Community/Mental Health
Professor University of South Alabama
Mobile, AL, USA

Barbara is Associate Dean and Chair of the Community/Mental Health Department at the University of South Alabama. She has a certificate in Palliative Care; and has lectured extensively on end-of-life care and death and dying. Barbara maintains a clinical practice with a focus on the bowel and bladder. She is the author of the Broome Pelvic Muscle Self-efficacy Scale, which has been used in national and international pelvic exercise studies.

CHAPTER 14
Jenny Penson
Nurse, Teacher and Therapist
North Devon, UK

Jenny has worked as a therapist, nurse, teacher and writer. She has specialised in mind/body medicine, cancer and palliative care, and in bringing complementary therapies into orthodox care. She was the first Macmillan Nurse in the UK and, until recently, Head of Education at North Devon Hospice. She currently works as a Hypno-psychotherapist and is an enthusiastic supporter of Integrated Medicine.

CHAPTER 15
Dr Cynthia MA Geppert
See Chapter 4.

Dr April H Volk
Associate Professor of Psychiatry
Medical Director Hospice and Palliative Medicine
New Mexico Veterans Affairs Health Care System
Assistant Professor, Department of Medicine
University of New Mexico School of Medicine
Albuquerque, NM, USA

April is the Medical Director of The Hospice and Palliative Medicine Program at New Mexico Veterans Health Care Center. She is also an Assistant Professor of Medicine in the Department of Medicine, Division of Geriatrics at the University of New Mexico School of Medicine. She holds board certification in Internal Medicine and Hospice and Palliative Medicine. April carries special certification in pain management. She has experience in treating patients with mental health disorders and chronic pain in a psychiatry primary care setting, in addition to the hospice and palliative care setting.

CHAPTER 16
David B Cooper
See About the editors.

Terminology

Whenever possible, the following terminology has been applied. However, in certain instances – when referencing a study and/or specific work, when an author has made a specific request, or for the purpose of additional clarity – it has been necessary to deviate from this applied 'norm.'

PROBLEM(S), CONCERNS AND DILEMMAS OR DISORDERS

The terms *problem(s)*, *concerns and dilemmas* and *disorders* can be used interchangeably, as stated by the author's preference. However, where possible, the terms 'problem(s)' or 'concerns and dilemmas' have been adopted as the preferred choice.

INDIVIDUAL, PERSON, PEOPLE

There seems to be a need to label the individual – as a form of recognition! Sometimes the label becomes more than the person! '*Alan is schizophrenic*' – thus it is Alan, rather than an illness that Alan lives with. We refer to patients, clients, service users, customers, consumers and so on. Yet, we feel affronted when we are addressed as anything other than what we are – individuals! We need to be mindful that every person we see during our professional day is an individual – unique. Symptoms are in many ways similar (e.g. delusions, hallucinations), some interventions and treatments are similar (e.g. specific drugs, psychotherapy techniques), but people are not. Alan may experience an illness labelled 'schizophrenia', and so may John, Beth and Mary, and you or I. However, each will have his or her own unique experiences – and life. None will be the same. To keep this constantly in the mind of the reader, throughout the book we shall refer to the *individual*, *person* or *people* – just like us, but different from us by their uniqueness.

PROFESSIONAL

In the eyes of the individual, we are all professionals, whether we are students, nurses, doctors, social workers, researchers, clinicians, educationalists, managers, service developers, religious ministers – and so on. However, the level of expertise may vary from one professional to another. We are also individuals. There is a need to distinguish between the person experiencing a mental health problem and the person interacting professionally (at whatever level) with that individual. To acknowledge and to differentiate between those who experience – in this context – and those who intervene, we have adopted the term *professional*.

It is indicative that we have had, or are receiving, education and training related specifically to help us meet the needs of the individual. We may or may not have experienced palliative care–mental health problems but we have some knowledge that may help the individual – an expertise to be shared. We have a specific knowledge that, hopefully, we wish to use to offer effective intervention and treatment to another human being. It is the need to make a clear differential, and for that purpose only, that forces the use of 'professional' over 'individual' to describe our role – our input into another person's life.

INTRA- INTER-DISCIPLINARY TEAMS

The term *intra- inter-disciplinary* has been chosen over *multidisciplinary* in that the latter is often hierarchical, usually with a consultant at the head. Intra- and inter-disciplinary teams function more democratically, with the person who has most interactions with the individual and family being chosen as the lead – indeed this need not be one person and the role will change as ill-health progresses. Intra- inter-disciplinary teams have a common purpose, and members have an understanding of one another's roles, the ability to pool resources, and the ability to step back and permit others to take over the lead in the interest of the individual and family.

Cautionary note

Wisdom and compassion should become the dominating influence that guide our thoughts, our words, and our actions.[1]

Never presume that what you say is understood. It is essential to check understanding, and what is expected of the individual and/or family, with each person. Each person needs to know what he or she can expect from you, and from other professionals involved in her or his care, at each meeting. Jargon is a professional language that excludes the individual and family. Never use it in conversation with the individual, unless requested to do so; it is easily misunderstood.

Remember, we all, as individuals, deal with life differently. It does not matter how many years we have spent studying human behaviour, listening and treating the individual and family. We may have spent many hours exploring with the individual his or her anxieties, fears, doubts, concerns and dilemmas, and the ill-health experience. Yet, we do not know what that person really feels, how she or he sees life, ill-health or death. We may have lived similar lives, experienced the same ill-health, but the individual will always be unique, each different from us, each independent of our thoughts, feelings, words, deeds and symptoms, each with an individual experience.

REFERENCE

1 Matthieu Ricard. As cited in: Föllmi D, Föllmi O. *Buddhist Offerings 365 Days*. London: Thames and Hudson; 2003.

Other books by the editors

Cooper DB. *Alcohol Home Detoxification and Assessment*. Oxford • New York: Radcliffe Medical Press; 1994 – reprinted 1996.

Cooper DB, editor. *Alcohol Use*. Oxford • New York: Radcliffe Medical Press; 2000 – reprinted 2008.

Cooper DB, editor. *Introduction to Mental Health–Substance Use*. Oxford • New York: Radcliffe Publishing Ltd; 2011.

Cooper DB, editor. *Developing Services in Mental Health–Substance Use*. Oxford • New York: Radcliffe Publishing Ltd; 2011.

Cooper DB, editor. *Responding in Mental Health–Substance Use*. Oxford • New York: Radcliffe Publishing Ltd; 2011.

Cooper DB, editor. *Intervention in Mental Health–Substance Use*. London • New York: Radcliffe Publishing Ltd; 2011.

Cooper DB, editor. *Care in Mental Health–Substance Use*. London • New York: Radcliffe Publishing Ltd; 2011.

Cooper DB, editor. *Practice in Mental Health–Substance Use*. London • New York: Radcliffe Publishing Ltd; 2011.

Cooper J, editor. *Stepping into Palliative Care 1: relationships and responses*. 2nd ed. Oxford • New York: Radcliffe Publishing Ltd; 2006.

Cooper J, editor. *Stepping into Palliative Care 2: care and practice*. 2nd ed. Oxford • New York: Radcliffe Publishing Ltd; 2006.

Acknowledgements

We are grateful to all the contributors for having the faith in us to produce a valued text and we thank them for their support and encouragement. We hope that faith proves correct. Thank you to those who have commented along the way, and whose patience has been outstanding.

Many people have helped us along our career paths and life – too many to name individually. Most do not even know what impact they have had on us. Most were individuals who touched our professional lives and who contributed most to our knowledge and understanding, leading us to appreciate the importance of compassion in care . . . and our effort to move towards this in our practice and life.

To Gillian Nineham of Radcliffe Publishing, our sincere thanks. Gillian had faith in this project from the outset and in our ability to deliver. Her patience is immeasurable and for that we are grateful. Thank you to Jessica Morofke, and Tanya Dean, for putting up with our too numerous questions and guiding us through the process of publication! Thank you to Jamie Etherington, Editorial Development Manager, and Alice French, of the book marketing department, both competent people who make our work look good. Thanks also to Camille Lowe, project manager and Dina Cloete, copy-editor and the production team at undercover, for bringing this book to publication, and to the many others who are nameless as we write but without whom this book would never come to print; each has placed his or her stamp on any successes of this book.

Our sincere thanks to our friends and colleagues along our career paths, to those who have touched our life in a positive way . . . and a minority, in a negative way (for we can learn from the negative to ensure we do better for others).

Last but not least, to our children (Phil, Marc and Caroline) who unfailingly take a valued interest in what the 'oldies' are doing . . . thank you.

A final heartfelt statement: any errors, omissions, inaccuracies, or deficiencies within these pages are our sole responsibility.

Dedication

This book is dedicated to those people whom we have been privileged to care for. They have been our true teachers and have shared with us so much about themselves, enabling us to learn the value of caring with respect, dignity and compassion, and showing us the importance of having courage to hope. They have been our natural teachers of humanity.

A dedication must also go to:

➤ Alfred (Alfie) John Ted Hall, born Friday, 6 July 2012 – absolutely beautiful – and a delightful addition to our five grandchildren (Ella Maisy, Megan Louise, Daisy Mae, Daniel John Charlie, Noah Jacob).

➤ 'Derry' – Audrey Keryk our sister – who is a mainstay and support in our extended family and the best child-minder ever!

➤ Our dear friend Brian Middleton who sadly died, aged 59, on New Year's day 2012. Throughout his life, Brian always had us in fits of uncontrolled laughter. But, more important, Brian was always there and is sadly missed.

CHAPTER 1

Embracing palliative care within mental health

Jo Cooper, David B Cooper

SETTING THE SCENE

> Perhaps our human purpose is no more or less than that of providing
> warmth, companionship and acceptance of our fellow women and men,
> rather than trying to fix them.[1]

INTRODUCTION

This book is about caring, applying the principles and philosophy of palliative
care within serious and enduring mental health practice. This includes:

➤ person-centred practice
➤ relationship-based connectedness
➤ a belief in compassionate care
➤ respect for autonomy and choice
➤ quality-of-life issues
➤ the family as the unit of care
➤ the need for democratic and intra- inter-disciplinary team work (*see*
  Terminology).

Palliative Care within Mental Health: principles and philosophy is *not* a treatment text per se. It is about the practice skills needed before we can be competent
to address intervention and treatment. Each chapter develops a theoretical
framework, and then broadens to include application in practice. Throughout,
we adopt a person-centred approach. It is anticipated that the reader will be able
to follow the reasons for palliative care, within her or his practice, from concept
through to application.

We look at the '*What, When, Where and Why*'. Overriding to the text is the '*How*' in practice. Consequently, each chapter moves from informing to implementation within practice – the '*how to*'. The aim is to improve, above all else, the relationships, responses, care and practice necessary to be effective in interventions and treatment with those experiencing serious and enduring mental health concerns and dilemmas. The emphasis is on the individual *and* the family, and the stigma of such problems for them as human beings.

For the individual and family experiencing serious and enduring mental health, life presents many concerns and dilemmas. The needs are complex and all-encompassing. For the professional, educator, researcher, manager and service providers/developers, this presents multifaceted challenges. To successfully and innovatively deliver interventions, treatment, care responses and comprehensive services, professionals need to continually explore and update knowledge and skills. *Palliative Care within Mental Health* provides a foundation for discussion and dissemination around the subject of palliative care within mental health. We do not address 'serious and enduring mental health' or 'palliative care' as individual subjects. Such concerns relate not only to the individual and family but also to the future direction of practice before we introduce interventions and treatment. While presenting a balanced view of what is best practice today, we aim to challenge concepts and stimulate debate, exploring all aspects of the development of palliative care principles and practices within serious and enduring mental health practice and care responses, and the adoption of research-led best practice.

WHAT IS PALLIATIVE CARE?

> You matter because you are you. You matter to the last moment of your life, and we will do all we can to help you not only to die peacefully, but also to live until you die.[2]

Palliative care is widely accepted as best-practice end-of-life care (*see* Chapter 13) and is concerned with promoting and maintaining the best possible quality of life. Connecting with the person is the central focus in both palliative care and mental health disciplines. The World Health Organization defines palliative care as:

> An approach that improves the quality of life of patients [people] and their families facing the problems associated with life threatening illness, through the *prevention and relief of suffering* by means of early identification and impeccable assessment and treatment of pain and other problems, physical, psychosocial and spiritual.[3] Affirms life and regards dying as a normal process that:
> - provides relief from pain and other symptoms [*see* Chapters 11 and 12]
> - intends neither to hasten nor to postpone death

- integrates psychological and spiritual aspects of care [*see* Chapters 5 and 8]
- offers a support system to help patients to live as actively as possible until death
- offers a support system to help the family cope during the patient's [person's] illness and in their own bereavement [*see* Chapter 14]
- uses a team approach to address the needs of patients and families, including bereavement counselling if indicated [*see* Chapter 16]
- enhances the quality of life, and may also positively influence the course of illness
- is applicable early in the course of the illness, in conjunction with other therapies that are intended to prolong life, such as chemotherapy or radiotherapy, and includes those investigations needed to better understand and manage distressing clinical complications.[3]

Every person has the right to receive high-quality palliative care whatever the ill-health, regardless of the course and nature of the ill-health (*see* Chapter 3). The principles of palliative care can be applied to any condition, irrespective of the clinical setting. The goal of palliative care is to meet individual need and to provide the best quality of life for the person and their family. This approach includes physical, psychological, social, and spiritual health, extending into bereavement, grief and loss, which can occur before, during and after death.

The philosophy and knowledge within the mental health and palliative care disciplines can be integrated, thus, providing the very highest standard of caring for individuals with serious and enduring health problems.

As in mental health, palliative care relies considerably on intra- inter-disciplinary team working, an integral part of the philosophy of both disciplines, providing a responsive and sustained approach to person-centred care (*see* Chapter 16).

RESPECTING LIFE

The mandate for palliative care offers a respect for life, and accepts the inevitability of death. Therefore, treatment is balanced against its inherent burdens. Supportive medical measures used in acute situations, such as the use of intravenous infusions, the taking of blood gases, recording of blood pressure, artificial feeding, etc. is responsible practice. However, when there is an acknowledgement that there is going to be no return to good health, and the person is diagnosed as dying, this becomes inappropriate practice, and all measures possible to ensure freedom from distressing symptoms, physical and psychological, are maintained.[4]

Good communication is a prime function and fundamental within mental health and palliative care. The essence of good communication is our ability to listen carefully to what we are being told, if the person is to feel fully heard and understood. It is not only about our interpretation of the information in order to manage complex needs and symptoms (*see* Chapter 4); it is about ensuring that we convey, with empathy, the validity of the person and their story.

Communication is imperative with and within the families, so that they are in no doubt about what we are doing (*see* Chapter 6). If we are to give the person free choices, then they must be properly informed about what those choices are, and the consequences of the choices they make. They are facing strong feelings and emotions as a direct consequence of their ill-health – such as anger, sadness, fear, anxiety – and are facing existential concerns, which demand exploration and sensitive approaches, in order to reduce and allay the many and varied emotions experienced (*see* Chapter 12). Improved awareness of palliative care is a first step towards reducing disparities in utilisation of important and useful services for persons with life-limiting ill-health. Lack of awareness may limit access to needed palliative care.[5]

HUMANITY IN CARING

> Humanity is the place where you will find someone who will enter into your suffering and never leave you there alone.[6]

The human condition encompasses the experiences of being human. Human nature refers to certain characteristics that humans have in common: as human beings, we have certain characteristics, such as empathy, compassion, aggression and fear.

Being human is about the acceptance of every human being for just being another human being, regardless of colour, religion, race or gender (*see* Chapters 2, 3 and 9). When caring for people who are ill, we are constantly challenged to provide support and care in a human and compassionate way. The person-centred philosophy of mental health and palliative care is based on humanness and compassion. The focus is not just on the ill-health or the complex symptoms it produces, but is actively involved in finding out the needs of the whole person. In order to carry out this level of holistic care, we must attend to the three indivisible facets of the human condition – the mind, body and spirit of humankind (*see* Chapter 8).[7]

THE ESSENCE OF CARING

Florence Nightingale[8] firmly believed that the essence of nursing rested on the nurse's capacity to provide humane, sensitive care to the sick, which she believed would allow healing. The therapeutic relationship (*see* Chapter 6) in mental health has its origins in the work of Peplau[9] who introduced her Theory of Interpersonal Relations, which focused on the human connection between the professional and individual. In today's healthcare environment, the human relationship is in danger of being overlooked in deference to computerised technology. We acknowledge the beneficial advantages of such technology – this registers the person's vital observations, but fails to provide information relevant to the person as a human being (*see* Chapter 10).[10]

When John was very ill, I would sit with him for hours on end. The nurses would come into the room, check the computers, which noted his pulse, breathing and blood pressure, check his drip, and take blood when needed. They were very efficient in this respect, but they never really talked to him, asked him '*how*' he was feeling, or really talked to me. I was desperate for someone to tell me what was happening – I thought he was dying – but no one said anything only that 'his obs [medical observations] are fine, he's just sleepy'. They concentrated on the technology, not on John as a person with feelings; they did not see his suffering.

WARMTH, COMPANIONSHIP AND ACCEPTANCE

Caring for someone should be a human activity . . . performed as humanly as possible . . . one person to another . . . an equal footing (*see* Chapter 2). We meet people at a time of emotional need. However, do we have the resources to meet that need? Do we, in fact, see that there is an emotional need to be met? The difficult situations that we meet may tempt us to run away from the emotional pain – it is easier to deal with physical pain. In 'doing', rather than 'being' we can easily fail to reach the 'meaning' of the situation, a meaning which will offer opportunity for us to discover how we can best help the person, in a compassionate way. We need to have a genuine desire to help, to acknowledge the pain of another – make a human response.

SUFFERING

Suffering is subjective, encompassing factors which diminish quality of life, a perception of distress, and ultimately an expression of a life not worth living (*see* Chapter 7).[11] Suffering can be physical, emotional, spiritual, mental, or all of these. Relief of suffering is an important goal for all members of the healthcare team and a mutual commitment exists to reduce and relieve suffering. However, no type of care can ever alleviate *all* suffering, and some issues will always defy explanation. It is not only the person themself that suffers, feeling isolated and desperate, but also the family and often the healthcare professional. Suffering is all-embracing; it affects us all. *It is part of life.*

A GENUINE DESIRE TO HELP

In order for us to try to help the person, we need to be fully present, to focus on the experience of that person – to listen fully to their story, for they will have one to tell, rather than be focused on ourselves, in order to protect us from the suffering of another. Watching someone suffer causes distress within ourselves and witnessing this suffering does not leave us untouched. As helpers we make human responses, showing compassion, empathy and understanding, and offering hope. We need the desire and competence to act, to acknowledge and share in the other's suffering and to make worthwhile and purposeful responses to the person's pain (*see* Chapters 16 and 10).

The family is important. Watching someone you love in pain and suffering causes distress that goes far beyond words.

> I sat with Carrie for days, feeling very alone, although I was not alone. The family, her husband and child were present and trying, as best as they could, to act as normally as possible, in a situation that was, to my mind, far from normal. Surgery had left her with complications. She was very ill, with fever and bad headaches as soon as she sat upright. Severe pain had been problematic for many months. We had had to watch her then, a young woman, in the throes of motherhood, struggling to walk, to sleep, to play with her child. It had been impossible for her to do normal daily things. Things that we would all take for granted, basic easy tasks like cooking or washing up. Pain prevented any quality of life. There was also the emotional pain for her; I watched her dawning realisation that she had lost so much already; her assumed world had crumbled. All that she had looked forward to in the future had been taken away . . . what was there left? This, for me, was the most painful of all her suffering. The surgery seemed so futile, so I sat, alone in my desperation, not knowing how best to help, and feeling unheard by the visiting professionals. I wanted to shout; I was helpless to relieve any of her distress. I could not make it better for her. I felt I knew what should be done to help her suffering and to alleviate some of her physical distress, but I sat alone, watching, waiting – until someone who recognised her pain, knew what needed to be done; listened to the family, managed the situation and changed the course of action. It only took one person to *see*, to *understand* and to *feel*.

The above is a brief extract of a mother's pain. Suffering affects the family, as much as it does the sufferer, and, as human beings, we try to find a way to help support the whole family. We also have to be realistic! We may not be able to fully relieve the person's suffering, but we are trying our best, motivated in the purest way possible. Whatever we do, even if it is not ultimately successful, it cannot be thought of as detrimental, or harmful to that person (*see* Chapters 7 and 14).

SELF-KNOWING

As adults, we have the capacity to *feel* and to *think*, as well as the capacity to think about feelings. Being able to imagine the feelings of others is the cognitive basis for empathy.[12] It is helpful to be self-aware and 'knowing' oneself is the fundamental axiom in both mental health and palliative care. Self-awareness enriches our own understanding of *who* we are.

Possessing self-awareness indicates that we have a philosophical belief about life, death and the human condition (*see* Chapter 2).[13] It is important to examine our own beliefs in order to influence the way we interpret and make use of the person's story about himself or herself. When we have been touched, as human beings, by the pain of others, we may try to find strategies to distance ourselves from that pain, in order for us to survive and move on to offer support to others within our care.

COMPASSION

Compassion becomes the dominant premise in provision and conservation of caring and the art of caring lies in the relationship with the person, the family and is inclusive of our colleagues within the intra- inter-disciplinary team. When offering a helping relationship, based on empathic understanding, it is important, as far as we can, to remain connected to that person. As we go through our own life, we learn to use our own experiences to help those we care for.[12] We all recognise and feel something about the benefits of compassion. In one way, we are all the same – we all want to avoid suffering. What, then, is compassion? It is not simply a sense of sympathy or caring for the person suffering. Rinpoche explains it as a sustained and practical determination to do whatever is possible and necessary to help alleviate the suffering of another.[14] Neither is it a sense of pity. Pity has its roots in fear; a sense of smugness, or arrogance. However, both sympathy and pity may be useful for a short period of time; both may bring some comfort to the sufferer during episodes of extreme suffering. At best, it is still an expression of sadness for the person who is suffering. It can also help to validate the person's suffering, as it can be so easy for a person's suffering to be minimised, for example, by being told to have a *positive attitude*!

> Nobody has much sympathy about my fear of taking so many tablets? This makes me feel undervalued and misunderstood. They say, it's this, or your life! I know that, and I don't need to be convinced. Of course I want my life, but they are just missing the point'.

Compassion provides some indication of acceptance of the person's dilemma, it is strength giving and affords comfort. This is not to say that feeling compassionate is easy. It is often challenging and difficult, and causes suffering for ourselves, as we share in the suffering of another.

> She (the nurse) sits quietly, nods as if she understands, holding my hand. It's so difficult and so complicated for you. We all feel for you and your children; it could be anyone of us . . . She stops; she gives full eye contact; it tells me, she knows; she understands . . .

Those we care for are our teachers. If we remain open, with a sense of allowingness, we can learn to develop our compassion for others. Each person we come into contact with who is ill, or who is dying, will teach us. *All we have to do is . . . listen.*

SUBSTANCE USE

The problems encountered by prolonged and excessive use of alcohol and other drugs (substance use) have an important consideration in the often long-term mental and physical health issues that accompany such use. Therefore, we need to be open to the types of problem encountered and our role in offering palliative care to these individuals and family. While Chapter 15 addresses some of these concerns and dilemmas, the reader is asked to be open-minded throughout this book to the problems that arise because of substance use and/or existing mental health problems among the people we care for.

CONCLUSION

Palliative care becomes important when we cannot offer a cure but can offer symptom management . . . but not total control. Therefore, it does apply to serious and enduring mental health . . . and substance-use problems. To some extent, mental health and substance-use professionals may offer such an approach; however, we have a lot to learn from specialist palliative care professionals.

When talking with mental health colleagues it was hard to convey that we were not talking about individuals experiencing mental health issues who also had a diagnosis of cancer – the concept was alien, and indeed, ridiculed by some. The employer of one potential author did not permit her to write for this book because 'it did not relate to mental health'. Clearly, a lot of work needs to be done before we can truly embrace the palliative care philosophy. This is despite a growing awareness that a palliative care approach – in the true sense of the term – can be meaningful to the individuals we have contact with on a daily basis. It offers hope – not of a cure – but that the professional is willing to work alongside the individual to manage symptoms that improve the quality of life for those individuals.

REFERENCES

1 Barker P, Buchanan-Barker P. Mental health in an age of celebrity: the courage to care. *Journal of Medical Ethics*. 2008; **34**: 110–14.
2 Saunders C. Care of the dying – the problem of euthanasia. *Nursing Times*. 1976; 1 July: 1003–5.
3 World Health Organization. *Definition of Palliative Care*. Geneva: WHO; 1990.
4 Twycross R. *Introducing Palliative Care*. 4th ed. Oxford: Radcliffe Publishing; 2002.
5 Matsuyama RK, Balliet W, Ingram K, *et al.* Will patients want hospice or palliative care if they do not know what it is? *Journal of Hospice and Palliative Nursing*. 2011; **13**: 41–6.
6 Roy DJ. Humanity: idea, image, reality. *Journal of Palliative Care*. 2004; **20**: 131–2.
7 Hopper A. Meeting the spiritual needs of patients through holistic practice. *European Journal of Palliative Care*. 2000; **7**: 60–3.
8 Nightingale F. *Notes on Nursing: what it is and what it is not*. Philadelphia JP: Lippincott; 1946.
9 Peplau, HE. The heart of nursing: Interpersonal Relations. *Canadian Nurse*. 1965; **61**: 273–5.
10 American Humanist Association. 2002. Available at: www.americanhumanist.org/humanism/Humanism_Unmodified (accessed 05 April 2012).

11 Cherny NI, Coyle C, Foley KM. Suffering in the advanced cancer patient: a definition and taxonomy. *Journal of Palliative Care.* 1994; **10**: 57–70.

12 Lendrum S, Syme G. *Gift of Tears: a practical approach to loss and bereavement in counselling and psychotherapy.* 2nd ed. East Sussex: Routledge; 2004.

13 Eckroth-Bucher M. Philosophical basis and practice of self-awareness in psychiatric nursing. *Journal of Psychosocial Nursing.* 2001; **39**: 32–9.

14 Rinpoche S. *The Tibetan Book of Living and Dying: a spiritual classic from one of the foremost interpreters of Tibetan Buddhism to the West.* Classic ed. London: Rider; 2008.

CHAPTER 2

The Tidal Model

Poppy Buchanan-Barker, Phil Barker

PALLIATIVE CARE RATHER THAN TREATMENT

It is now commonplace to claim that as many as one in four people might develop a 'mental illness'.[1] As a way of managing the potential panic over this rising tide, most Western nations now employ the concept of 'serious mental illness'[2] to distinguish states attributed to 'schizophrenia' or 'bipolar disorder', for example, from other less serious psychiatric conditions – the so-called common mental disorders such as depression or anxiety. If a parallel is drawn with physical illness, 'schizophrenia' and 'bipolar disorder' might be classed as highly malignant. Some people with a diagnosis of schizophrenia or bipolar disorder kill themselves or die as a consequence of self-neglect, their deaths often attributed to their 'illness'. Not surprisingly, many people – especially family members – believe that such risks, however remote, signal an urgent need for medical treatment, if necessary to be delivered by force.[3]

By contrast, 'common mental disorders' are often assumed to respond to some 'talking cure'. For example, for more than 40 years, 'depression' has been known as the 'common cold of psychiatry'.[4] The widespread assumption that 'mental illness is just like any other illness' encourages many people to assume that psychiatric drugs are necessary to 'treat' a discrete 'mental' condition. However, when someone appears, or complains of feeling 'mentally unwell', such a 'symptom' (self-report) is often considered sufficient to confer a psychiatric diagnosis. None of the bodily 'signs' shown in physical illness will be evident: the physical or physiological indications of the underlying disorder. No blood tests, biopsies, tissue samples or other forms of pathological examination confirm, or deny, that the person's 'symptoms' are, indeed, related to a discrete pathological process. Consequently, any psychiatric diagnosis is based on the person's self-report (symptoms) and a professional observation of some 'abnormal behaviour', or judgement that the reported 'symptoms' are abnormal (i.e. allegedly pathological). Psychiatric diagnoses are confirmed by circular logic: e.g. the person hears voices, *therefore*, he must be psychotic; the person is psychotic *because* he hears voices.[5]

We open with this honest observation since it has long been clear to us that the phenomena called 'mental illness' or 'psychiatric disorders' are *problems in human living*, which the person and/or the person's family, and/or society at large find difficult to understand. Consequently, people seek help with these problems, or someone else proposes that they need help, even if they do not request it.

In physical (actual) illness, the physician seeks to identify the pathological process, which underlies the 'symptom' (e.g. pain). This process becomes the target for treatment: e.g. infection by antibiotics or a malignant tumour by chemotherapy. Where such a process cannot be identified – as in a prescription of analgesics for a headache – most physicians acknowledge that they are not offering actual 'treatment' but merely providing 'symptomatic relief'.

> **KEY POINT 2.1**
>
> In the absence of evidence of any discrete pathological process underlying 'symptoms' such as 'low mood' or 'hearing voices' much, if not all, of the 'treatment' offered to people diagnosed with 'depression' or 'schizophrenia' is 'symptomatic relief'. In that sense, much – if not all – of the relief, which people try to provide in the name of mental health care or treatment, is 'palliative'.

THE TIDAL MODEL – FOCUS AND ASSUMPTIONS

The *Tidal Model* was developed originally in England in the mid- to late 1990s, as an alternative model for nursing practice in the care of people experiencing 'serious and enduring mental illnesses'. Over the past 15 years, the Tidal Model[6] has become recognised, internationally, as a key mid-range nursing theory[7] which is practised widely not just by nurses but by a range of disciplines in the mental health and social care field.

The Tidal Model adopts a dedicated person-centred focus, recognising that the problems or issues commonly diagnosed as 'mental illness' are, in effect, problems in human living. Tidal focuses on helping people, who have experienced some metaphorical 'breakdown', recover their lives as fully as possible. The key method employed is to help people reclaim the story of their distress or difficulty, couched in their own words. By helping people to explore, discuss or reflect upon their stories, we hope that they will be better placed to negotiate what might need to be done, to help them overcome, transcend or otherwise live more effectively with their problems in living.

Although 'recovery' models have become popular in contemporary mental health services, the Tidal Model has some distinguishing characteristics. It is:
➤ the *first* recovery-focused model developed *by* mental health nurses *for* mental health nursing practice
➤ the *first* mental health recovery model developed *conjointly* by mental health professionals *and* people in their care

> the *first* mental health recovery model developed for use in the most challenging situations; i.e. where people are 'at their lowest ebb'
> the *first* mental health recovery model to be *evaluated* rigorously in public-sector practice
> the *first* model to be used as the basis of recovery-focused care across the *hospital-community spectrum* – from child and adolescent services to older persons.[8,9]

The focus on caring

As noted, the Tidal Model assumes that many health and social problems are best viewed as 'problems in living'.[10] As such, practitioners aim to provide the person with 'the necessary conditions for the promotion of growth and development'.[11] The beginning point for this process involves helping people to describe and name their experiences in their *own language*, rather than in the language of medicine or psychology. This provides the basis for all the conversations leading to exploring how people might begin to deal better with, if not completely resolve, such problems in living.

The Tidal metaphor

Traditionally, people experiencing problems in living have been encouraged to think of themselves as being in some fixed state; e.g. 'I am an alcoholic' or 'I have schizophrenia'. The Tidal Model recognises that all human experience is ephemeral – ebbing and flowing like the tide. Sometimes a person is like 'this' and at other times is like 'that'. The experience of 'breakdown' and 'recovery' often seems to 'come and go'; 'two steps forward, one step back'. Most languages have nautical metaphors to describe such uncertain or dramatic states, e.g. drifting, washed up, wrecked, or drowning. Tidal practitioners try to discover and employ the person's own preferred metaphors, which best represent an experience, thus respecting the language the person uses to tell her or his own unique story.

REFLECTIVE PRACTICE EXERCISE 2.1

Time: 15 minutes
- Recall one of your recent 'problems in living'.
- Write down the different names you gave to it, or how you would have described the experience to a close friend.

The Tidal Theory of the person

The Tidal Model views the person as living in three *domains.*
1 The **Self-domain**: the place where people hold all their 'private' experiences, e.g. thoughts, feelings, and beliefs – about themselves, others and the world in general.
2 The **World Domain**: the place where people feel comfortable in *bringing out*

some 'private' experience into the world; sharing these experiences, selectively, with others through conversation.

3   The **Others Domain**: the place where people *act out* their life story with others; this results in them influencing – and being influenced by – others, through an infinite range of social encounters.

Tidal emphasises story telling since all any person ever can *be* is a story.

> **KEY POINT 2.2**
>
> We only 'know' who a person is by the stories she or he tells us. People grow and develop through story telling – they make themselves up as they talk.

The Tidal Model uses story telling as the key means of helping people to 'know themselves' and to 'know better' what is troubling them. This represents a vital step towards working out what might *need to be done* to begin to resolve these problems.

TIDAL PRACTICE

Tidal Model practice uses *individual* and *group* processes to help people address their problems in living. Each of these is linked to one of the three theoretical Tidal *domains*.

1 Self-domain

If the person believes that she or he is in any way at risk of harming her- or himself or others (or is believed by others to be so at risk), a person-centred *Personal Security Plan* is developed. This Plan focuses on identifying the *personal and interpersonal* resources which the person might use to address current 'risks or threats'.

> **KEY POINT 2.3**
>
> This is the opposite of the 'advice' that professionals often give to people, regarding how best to deal with a particular problem.

2 World Domain

Before people can begin to deal with their problems they need to 'tell the story' of how these problems emerged and developed to become part of their lives. The *Holistic Assessment* is a format aimed at developing an in-depth conversation, within which the person will feel comfortable in exploring the story of different problems, as a precursor for talking about what might 'need to be done', to begin to address them.

Further conversations take place within dedicated, confidential, *One-to-One Sessions*. These focus on working alongside the person to identify and discuss how problems are showing themselves, or being experienced *today* in the 'here and now'. This serves as a springboard for discussing what the person might do *and* what help might be received from others, as a way of addressing, or dealing with, such problems.

3 Others Domain

Tidal professionals use three forms of group work aiming to work alongside people to further reclaim their personal power and identify personal and inter-personal resources.

1   The **Discovery Group** helps people become more aware of aspects of life experience, which have shaped who and what they are, as persons.
2   The **Information Sharing Group** helps people learn more about services, issues or other topics, which the person has *chosen* to explore.
3   The **Solutions Group** helps people become more aware of the part other people might play in providing support and encouragement – people who are, metaphorically, 'in the same boat' as themselves.

All three groups help to build a sense of community, which, it is hoped, will help the person prepare to participate in more informal group activities in the natural community, where support and encouragement may prove mutually rewarding.

REFLECTIVE PRACTICE EXERCISE 2.2

Time: 15 minutes
- Recall the last time when you felt 'threatened'.
- Name *two* things, which you did *for yourself,* which appeared to reduce the sense of 'threat'.
- Name *two* things, which *other people did* – for you or with you – which appeared to lessen your sense of 'threat'.

Story telling *in situ*

Traditionally, professionals 'interview' people – either in an assessment or a ther-apy session. Usually, they then retire to an office to 'write up' the clinical notes of the encounter. This results in the person's natural story being 'translated' into a 'history', where much of the richness of the original story is lost and replaced with professional jargon. When a person is discharged from care, the service is likely to have amassed a large file of such 'notes', but the person may well go home with nothing more than an appointment card for a follow-up appointment. This may well be their only 'souvenir' of the experience of care.

The Tidal assumes that if a service is to be genuinely person-centred, then the person must have a realistic 'souvenir' of the caring relationship – something which he or she can re-read, reflect upon and use to recall the work that has been done. Consequently, in addition to any 'clinical records', which the professional needs to make, people must hold (and own) their own records of all the key interactions they have had with professionals, which they can use as a basis for developing their own, personalised, form of 'self-management'.

All the Tidal processes, briefly summarised earlier, involve *active conversations*, which are recorded *live – in situ* (as they occur). This also demonstrates the professional's commitment to the *collaborative* nature of the professional–person relationship. All the 'stories' which are told within the sessions are summarised, in the person's own voice – capturing the essential features as understood by the person her- or himself. The person receives a copy at the end of each session and the professional team members keep a copy for reference. This confirms that the person is the *agent* at the centre of the caring encounter, and the professional is merely making her- or himself available as a help or support.

REFLECTIVE PRACTICE EXERCISE 2.3

> **Time: 10 minutes**
> * Imagine that you tell someone – in your own words – about a deeply personal experience.
> * Imagine that the person says, 'So, what you really mean is . . .' and proceeds to 'translate' *your* words into *their* words.
> * How does this make you feel?

Self-management

One of the people 'experiencing mental health problems' who was involved in the original development of the Tidal Model described her experience of the various processes (described above) as the 'beginnings of *self-management*'.[12] Many recovery models also emphasise 'self-management' but often this takes the form of helping the person to 'stay well' or 'maintain progress', once the effects of the original crisis have passed. Tidal emphasises that 'self-management' should begin as soon as the person enters the service – *not* when the person is being prepared to return to 'normal life'. The various individual and group processes all help the person *rehearse* the kind of decision making and/or actions that might be needed as part of everyday living, when they have returned to ordinary life in the community.

The Tidal Model in practice

It is axiomatic that Tidal practice requires professionals to collaborate closely with the people in their care. Six guiding principles articulate the elements of this collaborative relationship.

1 Curiosity

The person's life story is a mystery, which requires careful exploration if needs are to be identified and met. Professionals try to understand what the person thinks, feels and knows about her- or himself, and the problems which have brought them into the healthcare setting.

2 Resourcefulness

People in care settings are often defined in terms of their problems, deficits, diagnosis, or illness. While recognising the existence of such 'problems', the Tidal Model is concerned mainly with how the person manages to *live* with these problems *now*. How might these personal and interpersonal resources be brought to bear to influence the person's recovery?

3 Respect

Care and treatment programmes are often based on what the care team believes is 'best' for the person. However, given that the person is the centre of the whole story of care and treatment, it is obvious that she or he should be the final judge as to what is, or is not, helpful.

4 Crisis as an opportunity

Traditionally, a crisis is something that needs to be 'managed' or 'contained'. The Tidal Model believes that crises are signs that something needs to change: natural indications that something 'needs to be done'. The crisis is an 'opportunity for change'.

5 Think small

Care and treatment programmes often emphasise the end-point of the care process: e.g. cure, resolution or discharge. The Tidal Model emphasises the small steps a person needs to take to move away from the circumstances that brought them into care in the first place. What simple, specific actions might help the person begin to move forward, or move away from the problem in living?

6 Think simple

Care and treatment programmes are often framed by professional jargon, and may involve multiple layers of action by different agencies. The Tidal Model stresses the need to identify the simplest action which might 'make a difference' for the person. Such a simple action can be understood and 'owned' by the person, thus representing the beginnings of 'self-help'.

The Tidal Model philosophy

The Tidal Model is primarily a way of thinking about the kind of help or support that people might need. In that sense, it is a *philosophy* and involves asking four basic questions.

1   **Why this, why now?** Why is the person experiencing this particular problem

in living *now*? The focus is on what the person is experiencing *at this moment* and what *needs to be done now* to begin to address the situation.

2 **What works?** Rather than offer advice or counsel, the Tidal practitioner seeks to establish what the person believes has worked in the past or what might work in the immediate future.

3 **What is the personal theory?** What does the person think is happening now; what is it all about; and what it might mean? What 'sense' does the person make of their problems? Rather than offering a 'professional' explanation of their difficulties – in the form of psychological theory or diagnosis – the professional tries to understand the experience from the person's perspective. 'What is the person's theory of what is going on?'

4 **How to limit restrictions?** To avoid fostering dependency, practitioners should aim to do as little as is necessary to help people begin to address their problems in living. The focus is on identifying what the *person* needs to do, which a negotiated form of support from the team supplements.

A personal story

Jay lost touch with his family years ago. He used to take various street drugs but now can afford to drink only cheap wine and cider. He is a 'sociable drunk', but suspicious of people when sober. He is in his early thirties and has a long-standing diagnosis of schizophrenia. He has been receiving depot injections of antipsychotics for over 10 years. Recently, he was sectioned under the Mental Health Act, following a violent outburst in a supermarket café, where he was refused service.

Escorted to hospital by police, Jay refuses to talk with the admitting doctor and nurse. Two days later Mike, a young staff nurse, tries to engage him, but receives the same mix of hostility and silence. Mike comes back six times over the next three days, to try to open a dialogue. Finally, Jay asks him angrily: 'What do you want from me?' Mike is uncertain.

> 'I'm not sure I want anything *from* you, but I feel that I should be doing something to help you. I don't know how I'm going to do that if I don't know you . . . don't know what's bothering you . . . don't know what *you want from me*.'

Over the next few days, Mike visits Jay and slowly opens up a conversation. From casual talk about weather, TV news and life on the ward, the conversation turns to Jay and the circumstances of his admission. With some difficulty, he begins to talk about the 'stuff going on in my head'.

Mike thinks of himself as a novice. However, honesty is important to Jay, who has never met a nurse or doctor who 'wasn't a smart-arse'. Mike talks about the team's approach and brings two copies of the *Holistic Assessment* to their next meeting, one for each of them. Mike explains: 'This is just a bunch of questions that might help me learn a bit about what's been happening for you, so we can talk about what *you* might find useful right now.'

When Mike offers him a pen to 'write down some of your answers as we talk', Jay becomes uncomfortable. Mike explains: 'I want to understand what is happening for you, and the best way to do that is to get the story "right from the horse's mouth", in your own words. When we are finished, I'll give you a copy, so you'll know what we've been talking about. It's your life after all. This is your stuff, not mine.'

Jay insists that Mike do the writing: 'It's your job anyway.' Slowly, he gets into his stride, and begins to talk.

Over the next few days Mike and his colleague Jenny spend dedicated time with Jay in *One-to-One Sessions*. They discuss what is on Jay's mind and explore practical ways that he might deal with these issues or problems. A record of these conversations also is made, in Jay's own words, and he keeps a copy as a reminder of what he needs to do to deal with his problems.

Jenny also helps Jay develop a *Personal Security Plan*. This addresses his feelings of fear and insecurity, which are associated with his violent outbursts. Jay is helped to identify how he managed these feeling in the past, or imagine what might help in the future. Again, he takes away a record of this conversation, in his own words, to use as an *aide memoire*.

With some encouragement, Jay agrees to go with Jenny to the *Discovery Group* she is facilitating. He enjoys listening to the other people talk about the things that are important in their lives, their hopes and dreams, and the obstacles they have overcome. Although he doesn't speak, he feels quite emotional afterwards. The mix of laughter and poignant stories was a new experience for him: nothing like his past experience of 'therapy groups'.

When discharged, Jay says two things made a difference for him.

1 He would never have started to talk about his voices, and the way people scared him, if 'Mike had not kept coming back, over and over again'. Jay could not understand why he wanted to know 'what was happening for me . . . usually, they only want to talk about my illness and stuff'.

2 Jay knew that doctors and nurses wrote things about him, but he had never seen what they had written. He was unnerved at first by Mike's willingness to share what he was writing with him, and to make copies for him to take away for reference. This took a lot of getting used to. Gradually, he came to realise that Mike was right: 'This is my life. This is all about me!'

REFLECTIVE PRACTICE EXERCISE 2.4

Time: 15 minutes
- How would you go about discovering the *person* who is Jay – his troubles, his strengths?
- How might you begin to help him to *palliate* his current difficulties?

CONCLUSION

The first step in the Tidal Model involves *reclaiming* the story of our lives. This does not apply especially to people with an 'illness' – whether 'mental' or physical – but applies to anyone who is overtaken or overcome by life events. This might involve a deeply private and personal sense of *shame* or *embarrassment* (e.g. feeling that you have made a fool of yourself in public). Or, the events might involve members of your family or local community – who, individually or collectively, have been 'knocked off balance'. In either case we must ask:

➤ What happened?

➤ How did it feel?

➤ How is it changing, over time?

➤ What made it so 'shameful', 'embarrassing', 'unbalancing' in the first place?

Owning the story of our lives is the first step in recovering our composure or 'balance'. Irrespective of the 'problem', we must own it, before we can begin to talk about what would need to be different for the problem to be resolved or at least rendered 'liveable'.

KEY POINT 2.4

In a very important sense, making a situation 'liveable' is one of the core meanings of the concept of *palliation*.

Helping a person feel sufficiently comfortable to begin to talk about some painful or disturbing experience can present a signficant challenge. The person needs to *trust* the professional. This very small word can shelter a wide range of emotions.

By making transparent the process of story telling and by continually negotiating the relationship – as Mike illustrated in his relationship with Jay – professionals can cast aside the trappings of power and authority, which hinder the active collaboration needed to help the person 'grow and develop'. The *process* could not be simpler – but its *practice* is often highly complex.

Palliation

As we noted at the outset, we believe that most of the work done in the name of mental health care could be described as 'palliative' – at least in the strict medical sense of the word. Only rarely does a person say that their original problem has 'disappeared' or been 'resolved completely', and has never returned. More commonly, people learn to 'manage', 'minimise' or otherwise 'deal with' their problems, in such a way that they are able to live their lives more effectively and purposefully. In our view this seems to be the most realistic attitude. Even when a problem does seem to have disappeared, who knows when it will 'rear its ugly head' again. We all learn to live with our 'demons'. However, few of us are able to do this alone. As GK Chesterton once remarked:

'we all are in the same boat and we owe each other a terrible loyalty'.[13]

Chesterton's philosophy is central to the Tidal Model. We do have a responsibility to help our fellow women and men, but to do this properly we first need to understand what 'ails' them. We can only do this by listening carefully to the story of their distress and difficulty, and, by working alongside, help the individual to tell us what we might need to do to help them manage better, if not overcome, their present difficulties. If we can do this we might help to reduce their distress – *which is one of the key objectives of palliative care.*

ACKNOWLEDGEMENT

We are grateful to the authors, editor, and publisher for permitting adaptation of a chapter first published in: Buchanan-Barker P, Barker P. The Tidal Model. In: Cooper DB, editor. *Intervention in Mental Health–Substance Use.* London: Radcliffe; 2011. pp. 22–8.

REFERENCES

1 National Alliance on Mental Illness (NAMI). Available at: www.nami.org/ (accessed 15 November 2011).

2 Barker P, Keady J, Croom S, *et al.* The concept of serious mental illness: modern myths and grim realities. *Journal of Psychiatric and Mental Health Nursing.* 1998; **5**: 247–54.

3 Patterson B. Restraint. In: Barker P, editor. *Mental Health Ethics: the human context.* London: Routledge; 2011. pp. 159–68.

4 Miller H. 'The Common Cold of Psychiatry'. Book Review. *British Medical Journal.* 1969; **2**: 563.

5 Barker P. The keystone of psychiatric ethics. In: Barker P, editor. *Mental Health Ethics: the human context.* London: Routledge; 2011. pp. 31–50.

6 Barker P, Buchanan-Barker P. *The Tidal Model: a guide for mental health professionals.* London: Brunner-Routledge; 2005.

7 Brookes N, Barker P. The Tidal Model of recovery and reclamation. In: Tomey AM, Alligood MR, editors. *Nursing Theorists and Their Work.* 6th ed. St Louis: Mosby; 2005. pp. 696–725.

8 Buchanan-Barker P, Barker P. The Tidal Commitments: extending the value base of recovery. *Journal of Psychiatric and Mental Health Nursing.* 2008; **15**: 93–100.

9 Barker P, Buchanan-Barker P. Reclaiming nursing: making it personal. *Mental Health Practice.* 2008; **11**: 12–16.

10 Barker P, Buchanan-Barker P. Mental health in an age of celebrity: the courage to care. *Medical Humanities.* 2008; **34**: 110–14.

11 Barker P. *The Philosophy and Practice of Psychiatric Nursing.* Edinburgh: Churchill Livingstone; 1999. p. 121.

12 Whitehill I. Foreword. In: Barker P, Buchanan-Barker P. *The Tidal Model: a guide for mental health professionals.* London: Brunner-Routledge; 2005. pp. v–ix.

13 Chesterton GK. Available at: www.worldofquotes.com/topic.Loyalty/1/index.html (accessed 20 April 2012).

TO LEARN MORE

- Barker P. The Tidal Model: the lived experience in person-centred mental health care. *Nursing Philosophy.* 2000; **2**: 213–23.
- Barker P. The Tidal Model: developing an empowering, person-centred approach to recovery within psychiatric and mental health nursing. *Journal of Psychiatric and Mental Health Nursing.* 2001; **8**: 233–40.
- Barker P. The Tidal Model: the healing potential of metaphor within the patient's narrative. *Journal of Psychosocial Nursing.* 2002: **40**: 42–50.
- Barker P, Buchanan-Barker P. Beyond empowerment: revering the storyteller. *Mental Health Practice.* 2003; **7**: 18–20.
- Barker P, Buchanan-Barker P. Bridging: talking meaningfully about the care of people at risk *Mental Health Practice.* 2004; **8**: 12–16.
- Barker P, Buchanan-Barker P. The Tidal Model of mental health recovery and reclamation: applications in acute care settings. *Issues in Mental Health Nursing.* 2010; **31**: 171–80.
- Buchanan-Barker P, Barker P. The Ten Commitments: a value base for mental health recovery. *Journal of Psychosocial Nursing and Mental Health Services.* 2006; **44**: 29–33.
- For an understanding of the Tidal Model. Available at: www.tidal-model.com (accessed 20 April 2012).
- For a *free copy* of the Tidal Model training manual, email: tidalmodel@btinternet.com

CHAPTER 3

Application of transcultural theory to practice: the Purnell Model

Larry D Purnell

Case study 3.1

Eun Kim, age 52 years, is of Korean heritage. She has experienced a serious bipolar disorder for over 20 years. Because of a decreased energy level, increased irritability, and lack of interest in her employment as an accountant, she has been unable to maintain steady employment. She has little interest in food and now weighs 40 kg. Three months ago, she decided to forego allopathic medical treatments and tried herbal therapies when she thought to take them. Eun states that life is no longer worth living and wants to move to Denmark because she has heard that euthanasia is legal there. Eun has never been married and currently lives with Angela, her life partner of 22 years. Eun refuses any more hospitalisations but is agreeable to have a home health nurse visit.

On the intake home assessment, the nurse asked who was the next of kin and was told that it was her partner, Angela. The nurse then asked what blood relative would make decisions about healthcare if she was unable to make decisions. Eun again gave Angela's name and explained their relationship. The nurse stated she was unsure if it was acceptable for Angela to make healthcare decisions and would ask her supervisor (*see* Chapter 4). Angela explained that Eun has not been on speaking terms with her family for many years because same-sex relationships carry a significant stigma in the Korean culture. In addition, her parents did not like the idea of Eun having an intimate relationship with anyone who is not of Korean ancestry. She is also estranged from her two older brothers and younger sister. At this point the nurse responded, 'I can understand why!'

CASE STUDY 3.1 – QUESTIONS (ANSWERS ON PP. 41–2)

Time: 45 minutes

1   What legally has to be done in your country for decision-making authority being delegated to Angela?

2   What do you know about euthanasia for serious mental health illnesses in Denmark?

3   Would you be supportive and assist Eun in obtaining more information about euthanasia in Denmark or other countries?

4   How do you feel about Eun discontinuing allopathic treatments and taking herbal therapies?

5   What family support systems does Eun have?

6   Would you ask Angela if her family is supportive of their relationship?

7   What resources besides family might be available for Eun and Angela?

8   How do you feel about Eun and Angela's same-sex intimate partnership?

9   If Eun and Angela were to seek support from the Catholic Church, how do you think church members would respond?

10 What is the Roman Catholic Church's view on same-sex intimate partner relationships?

INTRODUCTION

The professional literature on culturally competent palliative care for individuals experiencing serious and enduring mental health problems is exceedingly scarce and does not include stigma (*see* Chapter 5), making it difficult to provide high-quality intra- inter-disciplinary care. In addition, what denotes a stigma varies among and within cultures as does the role and expectations of family members who are frequently the ones who are the primary day-to-day caregivers for this population. The few empirical studies on hospice and palliative care report that minority individuals access and use palliative care at lower rates than the general population because they are either unaware the service exists or are unsure what palliative care really is.[1] The lack of literature on palliative care with culturally diverse peoples experiencing serious and enduring mental health issues has exaggerated the complexities of providing care.[2] These groups are among the most underrepresented populations in our society. Culture needs to become a focal point in the perspectives of palliative care and mental health professionals working alongside the individual experiencing serious and enduring mental health issues,[3] otherwise this population will be marginalised and will face further discrimination.

Culture is complex given that:

➤ the person has a culture

➤ each healthcare professional has a culture which may be different from that of the person needing care, intervention and treatment

➤ each profession – nursing, medicine, physical therapy, occupational therapy, social services, etc. – has a culture

➤ each specialty – oncology, paediatrics, rehabilitation, psychiatry, palliative care, etc. – has its own culture
➤ each healthcare facility has a culture which can vary between service units.

When all these competing cultures and subcultures are combined, a significant mismatch may occur, resulting in an increased complexity for providing culturally competent palliative care to people experiencing serious and enduring mental health problems. Thus, providers must become competent in culture, mental health and palliative care as well as possess the ability to work with intra- inter-disciplinary teams that include the family – which is defined by the individual – and who can be blood relatives, staff in in-patient facilities, and the community.

This chapter uses the Purnell Model for Cultural Competence as a guide to providing palliative care to individuals experiencing serious and enduring mental health. Because the professional literature related to terminology has not been standardised on a global basis, essential terminology is reviewed. The literature on cultural and ethnic-specific palliative care within serious and enduring mental health is non-existent. Because space does not permit an extensive review on the beliefs and values of multiple cultures, aggregate data on collectivistic cultures and on individualistic cultures are presented using the Purnell Model.[4]

ESSENTIAL TERMINOLOGY

The literature reports many definitions for the terms *culture*, *cultural awareness*, *cultural sensitivity*, and *cultural competence*. Sometimes these definitions are used interchangeably.

Culture is defined as the totality of socially transmitted behavioural patterns, arts, beliefs, values, customs, lifeways, and all other products of human work and thought characteristics of a population of people that guide their worldview and decision making. Health and healthcare beliefs and values are assumed in this definition. These patterns may be explicit or implicit, are primarily learned and transmitted within the family, are shared by most (but not all) members of the culture, and are emergent phenomena that change in response to global phenomena.[4]

Culture, a combined anthropological and social construct, can be seen as having three levels:
1 a tertiary level that is visible to outsiders, such as things that can be seen, worn, or otherwise observed
2 a secondary level, in which only members know the rules of behaviour and can articulate them
3 a primary level that represents the deepest level in which rules are known by all, observed by all, implicit, and taken for granted.[5]

Cultural beliefs, values and practices are largely unconscious and have powerful influences on health and illness. They are learned from birth: first at home, then in the church and other places where people congregate, and then in educational settings.

➤ Cultural awareness has more to do with an appreciation of the external or material signs of diversity, such as the arts, music, dress, or physical characteristics.[6,7]

➤ Cultural sensitivity has more to do with personal attitudes and not saying things that might be seen as offensive to someone from a cultural or ethnic background different from that of the professional.[6,7]

➤ Cultural competence, as used in this chapter, means having the knowledge, abilities and skills to deliver care congruent with the person's cultural beliefs and practices. Engaging in cultural competence is a conscious process and not necessarily a linear one.[4,7]

➤ Cultural relativism is the belief that the behaviours and practices of people should be judged only from the context of their cultural system. Cultural relativism, relating one's own cultural experiences to those from another setting, requires knowledge about other cultures complemented by cultural values, biases and subjectivity. Proponents of cultural relativism argue that issues such as abortion, euthanasia, female circumcision and physical punishment in child rearing should be accepted as cultural values without judgement from the outside world. Opponents argue that cultural relativism may undermine condemnation of human rights violations, and family violence cannot be justified or excused on a cultural basis.[4,7]

➤ Cultural imposition is the intrusive application of the majority groups' cultural view upon individuals and families.[4,8] The practice of prescribing special diets without regard to individuals' cultural food choices borders on cultural imposition. Professionals must continually recognise that their beliefs and values may differ from those of the individual and family.

➤ Cultural imperialism is the practice of extending policies and procedure of one organisation (usually the dominant one) to disenfranchised and minority groups. Proponents appeal to universal human rights values and standards. Opponents posit that universal standards are a disguise for the dominant culture to destroy or eradicate traditional cultures through worldwide public policy.[4,7]

REFLECTIVE PRACTICE EXERCISE 3.1

Time: 10 minutes
- What practices have you seen in mental health services and/or palliative care that might be considered a cultural imposition?
- What practices have you seen in mental health services and/or palliative care that might be considered cultural imperialism?
- What practices have you seen in mental health services and/or palliative care that might be considered cultural relativism?
- What have you done to address them when you have seen them occurring?

Ethnocentrism and stereotyping

➤ Ethnocentrism is a universal tendency to believe that one's own worldview is superior to another's.[9] It is often experienced in the healthcare arena, in particular when the professional's own culture or ethnic group is considered superior to another.

➤ Stereotyping is having a simplified and standardised conception, opinion, or belief about a person or group. The professional who fails to recognise individuality within a group is jumping to conclusions about the individual or family. If one concentrates on the variant characteristics of culture when assessing the individual, the tendency can be ameliorated.[9] A generalisation begins with assumptions about the individual or family within an ethnocultural group but leads to further information seeking about the individual or family.[10]

REFLECTIVE PRACTICE EXERCISE 3.2

Time: 5 minutes

- Ethnocentrism and stereotyping are universal tendencies. Can you think of times when you were ethnocentric and/or stereotyped?
- What have you done to address your personal ethnocentrism and stereotyping in palliative care alongside people experiencing serious and enduring mental health problems?

CULTURAL SELF-AWARENESS

The process of professional development and diversity competence begins with self-awareness, sometimes referred to as self-exploration or critical reflection. Before addressing the multicultural backgrounds and unique perspectives of the individual, family and communities, professionals must first address their own personal and professional views regarding culture and palliative mental healthcare.

The way professionals perceive themselves as competent providers is often reflected in the way they communicate with the individual. They should also examine the impact their beliefs have on those who are culturally diverse.

Self-knowledge and understanding promote strong professional perceptions that free professionals from prejudice and allow them to interact with others in a manner that preserves personal integrity and respects uniqueness and differences among individual patients.[6,11,12]

REFLECTIVE PRACTICE EXERCISE 3.3

Time: 5 minutes
- In your opinion, why is there conflict about working alongside people who are culturally diverse?
- What attitudes are necessary to deliver palliative care to people experiencing serious and enduring mental health problems and whose culture is different from yours?

Critically analysing our own values and beliefs in terms of how we see differences enables us to be less fearful of others whose values and beliefs are different from our own.[11] The ability to understand oneself sets the stage for integrating new knowledge into the professional's knowledge base, perceptions of health, interventions, and the impact these factors have on the various roles of professionals when providing palliative care to multicultural individuals experiencing serious and enduring mental health problems.

REFLECTIVE PRACTICE EXERCISE 3.4

Time: 5 minutes
- What have you done in the last 5 to 10 years to increase your cultural self-awareness?
- Has increasing your self-awareness resulted in an increased appreciation for cultural diversity?
- How might you increase your knowledge about the diversity in your community? In your school/workplace?

VARIANT CULTURAL CHARACTERISTICS
Major influences that shape people's worldview and the extent to which people identify with their cultural group of origin are called variant cultural characteristic. Some variants are attributes that either cannot be changed or, if they are changed, a significant stigma may occur for the individual or family.

The variant cultural characteristics are listed below.
➤ **Nationality** – cannot be changed but people have changed their surname because of a stigma attached to it.
➤ **Race** – cannot be changed but it can carry a stigma in some communities.
➤ **Colour** – cannot be changed but it can carry a stigma in some communities.
➤ **Gender** – can be altered with reassignment surgery but can cause a significant sigma for some people and/or their families
➤ **Age** – cannot be changed but as a result of ageism, age can carry a stigma for a few in some cultures.

➤ **Religious affiliation** – can be changed but may cause a stigma for some; e.g. changing from Baptist to Islam or vice versa.
➤ **Educational status** – can change, resulting in a change in worldview.
➤ **Socio-economic status** – can change even on short notice, resulting in loss of insurance benefits in some countries, resulting in a stigma for the individual.
➤ **Occupation** – can change and cause a stigma; e.g. if the person decides to practise prostitution.
➤ **Military experience** – changes worldview.
➤ **Political beliefs** – can change and may cause a stigma for some; e.g. changing political affiliation to communism for some in a Western culture.
➤ **Urban versus rural residence** – can change.
➤ **Enclave identity** – can change, but people who live and work in an enclave – e.g. China Town, Little Italy – may be marginalised.
➤ **Marital status** – can change but divorce can carry a stigma in some cultures.
➤ **Parental status** – it can change but may cause a stigma in some cultures; e.g. having children out of wedlock.
➤ **Physical characteristics** – can change with hair colour and style, facial hair, etc. For those with a physical disability, a stigma may occur.
➤ **Sexual orientation/preference** – can change (prisoners) and if it does, a stigma may occur for the individual or family (*see* Chapter 9).
➤ **Gender issues** – change over time but the issue itself does not cause the problem but rather the person supporting or not supporting the issue may create a stigma; e.g. extreme feminist views.
➤ **Reason for migration** (sojourner, immigrant, or undocumented status) – immigration status can cause a stigma for some, resulting in marginalisation.[4,9]

REFLECTIVE PRACTICE EXERCISE 3.5

Time: 10 minutes
- What are your primary and secondary characteristics of culture?
- What effect have they had on your mental health practice?
- What effect have they had on your palliative care practice?
- How have they changed over time?
- Has any of them resulted in your being stigmatised or marginalised?

THE PURNELL MODEL FOR CULTURAL COMPETENCE

The Purnell Model for Cultural Competence and its organising framework can be used in all practice settings and by all professionals. The model is a circle, with an outlying rim representing global society, a second rim representing community, a third rim representing family, and an inner rim representing the

The Purnell Model for Cultural Competence

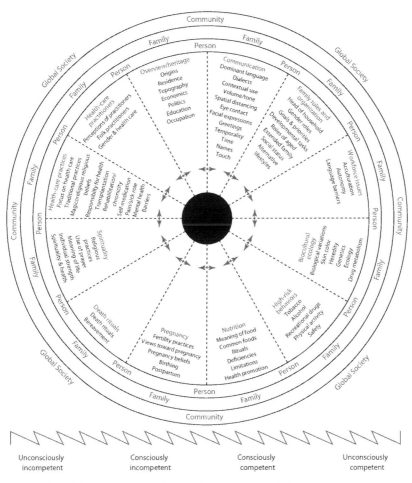

Figure 3.1 The Purnell Model of Cultural Competence
© **Reproduced with the kind permission of Professor Larry Purnell**

person (*see* Figure 3.1). The interior of the circle is divided into 12 pie-shaped wedges depicting cultural domains (constructs) and their associated concepts. The dark centre of the circle represents unknown phenomena. Along the bottom of the model is a jagged line representing the non-linear concept of cultural consciousness. The 12 cultural domains and their concepts provide the organising framework. Each domain includes concepts that need to be addressed when assessing the individual in various settings. Moreover, professionals can use these same concepts to understand their own cultural beliefs, attitudes, values, practices and behaviours. An important concept to understand is that no single domain stands alone; they are all interconnected.[4,9] The 12 domains are:

1 Overview/heritage
2 Communications
3 Family roles and organisation
4 Workforce issues
5 Biocultural ecology
6 High-risk health behaviours
7 Nutrition
8 Pregnancy and the childbearing family
9 Death rituals
10 Spirituality
11 Healthcare practices
12 Healthcare professionals

COLLECTIVIST VERSUS INDIVIDUALISTIC CULTURES

All cultures vary along the individualism and collectivism scale and are subsets of broad worldviews. Individualistic cultures are also seen as being low contexted while collectivist cultures are seen as being highly contexted. In individualistic low-contexted cultures, ties between groups are loose; in collectivistic high-contexted cultures, people from birth onwards are integrated into strong cohesive in-groups and often extended families.[13] A continuum of values for individualistic and collectivistic cultures includes:

➤ orientation to self or group, including family
➤ decision making
➤ autonomy
➤ knowledge transmission
➤ individual choice and personal responsibility
➤ concepts of progress
➤ competitiveness
➤ shame and guilt
➤ stigma
➤ gender roles
➤ views of after-life
➤ beneficence
➤ help-seeking
➤ expression of identity
➤ interaction/communication style.[14–17]

Elements of individualism and collectivism exist in every culture. People from an individualist culture will more strongly identify with the values at the individualistic end of the scale. People from a collectivist culture will adhere more closely to the values at the collectivist end of the scale. Moreover, individualism and collectivism fall along a continuum, and some people from an individualistic culture will, to some degree, align themselves towards the collectivistic end of the scale. Some people from a collectivist culture will, to some degree, hold values along the individualistic end of the scale. Acculturation is a key component of adapting individualistic and collectivistic values. Those who live in ethnic enclaves *usually but not always* adhere more strongly to their dominant cultural values. Acculturation and the variant cultural characteristics determine the degree of adherence to traditional individualistic and collectivist cultural values, beliefs and practices.

Counselling a person from an individualistic culture where the most important person in society is the individual may require different techniques than for a person in a collectivist culture where the group is seen as more important than the individual.[9] The professional must not confuse individualism with individuality, the degree that varies by culture and is usually more prevalent in individualistic countries. Individuality is the sense that each person has a separate and equal place in the community and where individuals who are considered 'eccentrics or local characters' are tolerated.[14]

Some examples of highly individualistic cultures are:
➤ *Traditional* American (USA)
➤ British
➤ Canadian
➤ German
➤ Norwegian
➤ Swedish.

Examples of collectivist cultures are:
➤ *Traditional* Arab
➤ Chinese
➤ Filipino
➤ Korean
➤ Japanese
➤ Latin American
➤ Mexican
➤ Native American Indians (and most other indigenous Indian groups)
➤ Taiwanese
➤ Thai
➤ Turkish
➤ Vietnamese.

Far more world cultures are collectivistic than are individualistic.[15,16,18,19,20]

CULTURAL DOMAINS WITH INDIVIDUALISTIC AND COLLECTIVIST CULTURES

Dominant aggregate values for individualistic cultures include individualism, free choice, independence, self-reliance, confidence, doing rather than being, egalitarian relationships, non-hierarchical status, achievement over ascribed status, truth telling, friendliness, openness, futuristic temporality and the ability to control the environment. Dominant aggregate values for collectivistic cultures include the importance of family, the group over the individual, men over women, age over youth, education, formality, harmony, co-operation, smooth interpersonal indirect communication, and not displaying emotions to outsiders. Remember that aggregate cultural characteristics are true for the group but not necessarily for the individual (Table 3.1).

TABLE 3.1 Cultural domains with individualistic and collectivist cultures

Domain from the Purnell Model	'Typical' individualistic low-context aggregate cultural characteristics	'Typical' collectivistic high-context aggregate cultural characteristics
Communication Includes concepts related to the dominant language, dialects, and contextual use of the language.	Low-contexted, explicit communication is valued over implicit communication that is clearly stated or further explanation is expected. Communication is direct, linear, and precise.	High-contexted implicit communication may be valued over explicit communication: meaning is usually embedded in the information and the listener must 'read between the lines'.
Paralanguage variations include voice volume and tone, intonations, inflections, and willingness to share thoughts and feelings.	Although interrupting someone who is talking is considered rude, it is common practice and forgiven.	To interrupt another in a conversation is considered extremely rude.
	Sharing personal feelings is encouraged, even for sensitive issues because the stigma does not necessarily extend to the family.	Do not reveal sensitive issues that may cause a stigma to family or others unless agreed upon by the individual.
Non-verbal communication includes the use of eye contact, gesturing and facial expressions, use of touch, body language, spatial distancing practices, and acceptable greetings.	Direct explicit communication is expected with serious and enduring mental health so plans for the future can be made.	Direct communication with serious and enduring mental health and discussing palliative care may mean giving up hope: approach these issues subtly (*see* Chapter 7).
Temporality in terms of past, present, and future orientation of worldview and clock versus social time.	If a question is asked that can be answered with 'yes' or 'no', the expectation is to tell the truth.	Many have difficulty with saying 'no' because it is seen as disrespectful: do not ask questions that have a 'yes' or 'no' answer.

Domain from the Purnell Model	'Typical' individualistic low-context aggregate cultural characteristics	'Typical' collectivistic high-context aggregate cultural characteristics
	Minimal touching unless very close family and friends and is reinforced by sexual harassment policies. One is expected to ask permission before touching another person.	Touching is common among same-gender friends and new acquaintances but a high degree of modesty necessitates explaining the necessity of touching: ask permission before doing so.
	Conversants are expected to maintain eye contact regardless of class or social standing: lack of eye contact is usually interpreted as not listening, not caring, or not telling the truth.	Eye contact may vary according to age and status of conversants. Those of lower status or of opposite gender might not maintain eye contact with those of higher status as a sign of respect.
	Unless close family and friends, conversants stand 18 to 24 inches (45–60 cm) apart.	Most are comfortable with conversants standing less than 18 inches (45 cm) apart.
	Punctuality is valued in both business and social settings.	Time is more relaxed; punctuality is valued only in business and situations where it is essential such as in making transportation connections.
	Futuristic temporality dominates; want to know the possible ramifications of an ill-health in the future.	Many are past oriented; to engage individuals experiencing serious and enduring mental health, seek topics from the past before addressing the present or future.
	Value on informality commonly using first names in most situations.	Most value formality: always greet the individual and family members formally until told to do otherwise.
Family roles and organisation	High value is placed on egalitarian spousal relationships with shared responsibilities and decision making.	In most traditional cultures, but not all, men have decision-making authority. May be reluctant to appoint a family member for decision making for fear of isolating other family members and increasing family conflict. Ask the person who has decision-making authority without the presence of family.

(continued)

Domain from the Purnell Model	'Typical' individualistic low-context aggregate cultural characteristics	'Typical' collectivistic high-context aggregate cultural characteristics
Includes concepts related to the head of the household, gender roles (a product of biology and culture), family goals and priorities, developmental tasks of children and young adults, roles of the aged and extended family, individual and family social status in the community, acceptance of alternative lifestyles, such as single parenting, non-traditional sexual orientations, childless marriages, and divorce.	Ask the individual (if not cognitively impaired) directly who has decision-making authority.	Even though an adult may be able to give consent, a son or other family member may be the spokesperson. For legal documents, have the person or legal next of kin as well as their designated spokesperson sign the document.
	Autonomy is encouraged in children and adolescents; children and young adults are encouraged to speak up on issues and wishes and make their own choices. Young adults are encouraged to have a job to learn responsibility.	Children and young adults are not encouraged to speak up on issues. Parenting is usually authoritarian.
	Children and teenagers have friends of both genders with fluid gender roles.	Gender roles are less fluid; expectations upon immigration may cause significant family discord.
	Intimate sexual behaviour before marriage is not encouraged, is tolerated when it does occur, but may still carry a stigma for some.	Sexually intimate relationship outside marriage is stigmatised, especially for women. Pregnancy outside marriage is highly stigmatised.
	Adult children are expected to leave parental home at age 18 or upon completion of education.	Adult children are encouraged and expected to live with their parents until marriage.
	Social attitudes towards gay and lesbian relationships vary widely but may still cause a stigma for some.	Lesbian and gay relationships are frowned upon and personal disclosure to family and friends jeopardises the family name and may lead to ostracism.
	Substance use (smoking, alcohol, recreational drugs) is tolerated but still carries a minor stigma.	Substance use can carry a significant stigma and may not be revealed to outsiders. May be very reluctant to participate in group therapy.

Domain from the Purnell Model	'Typical' individualistic low-context aggregate cultural characteristics	'Typical' collectivistic high-context aggregate cultural characteristics
	Nuclear family is the norm but divorce is accepted as an unfortunate circumstance without a significant stigma.	Women who divorce may be stigmatised.
	Long-term care for those for whom self-care is a concern is common so as to not disrupt family life.	Placing a family member in a long-term care facility is frowned upon and may cause a stigma for the family.
Death rituals and bereavement Includes how the individual and the society view death and euthanasia, palliative care, rituals to prepare for death, burial practices, and bereavement behaviours.	Most value mastery over the environment: terminal physical illnesses and serious and enduring mental health problems may be seen as a personal failure.	Most do not favour truth telling with serious physical or mental ill-health, believing that the individual should not be told so that they do not give up hope. Direct communication about the severity of a mental illness may be seen as self-fulfilling.
	Most are accepting of and prefer palliative care if made aware of the services.	Palliative care is well accepted by most when the concept is explained.
	Bereavement, whether for an actual death or for serious chronic illness, varies significantly but women are usually more verbal than are men.	Family may bereave histrionically to denote their love for a family member.
Spirituality Includes formal religious beliefs related to faith and affiliation and the use of prayer, behaviour practices that give meaning to life, and individual sources of strength.	Religion is not a usual topic of conversation in countries that have separation of church and state. A visit by a chaplain may be welcome either at home or in-patient facilities.	The church is a strong social support for many in collectivistic cultures. A visit by a chaplain either at home or in an in-patient facility is expected.
	Prayer is commonly used in times of serious physical and mental illness as well as other times.	Some believe the spirit starts a new life as another person or as an animal.
	May ask the religious congregation to say prayers to improve the health of a member experiencing serious physical and/or mental health problems.	Suffering may be seen as a spiritual/religious event. Ask: 'What do I need to know about your religious/spiritual beliefs in providing care to you?'
	Primary source of strength may not be family or religion but work and even material possessions.	Primary sources of strength are frequently religion and the nuclear and extended family.

(*continued*)

Domain from the Purnell Model	'Typical' individualistic low-context aggregate cultural characteristics	'Typical' collectivistic high-context aggregate cultural characteristics
Healthcare practices Include the focus of healthcare (acute versus preventive); traditional, magicoreligious, and biomedical beliefs and practices, individual responsibility for health; self-medicating practices; views on mental illness; chronicity; rehabilitation; acceptance of blood and blood products; and organ donation and transplantation.	The person is responsible for his or her good or bad health and is expected to be fully engaged in decision making for his or her care.	The primary treatment unit is the family.
	Autonomy in healthcare decision making is an enlightened perspective. Advance Directives are an important part of medical care (see Chapter 4).	Autonomy in decision making for healthcare may be seen as isolating rather than empowering.
	Aggressiveness of treatment and palliative care services are addressed directly to the person unless he or she is cognitively impaired.	'Do no harm' means protecting individuals from decision making and by not disclosing the severity of physical and mental ill-health.
	Illness is primarily an individual event.	Illness is a family event.
	Common practice is to incorporate complementary and alternative practices with allopathic medicine.	Herbal medicines are a mainstay and combined with allopathic treatments.
	Even though mental healthcare is a mainstay in healthcare and is supposed to be accepted, it can still cause a stigma for the individual or family.	Mental illness is highly stigmatised in most collectivistic cultures.
	Mental or physical disabilities are seen as an unfortunate circumstance.	Families who have children with mental or physical disabilities often question what they have done wrong to make their ancestors angry. Children with physical disabilities and those with a mental handicap may be hidden from society.
	Most favour organ donation which is seen as a humanitarian endeavour.	Asking about organ donation may be seen as an excuse to prematurely terminate treatment.
		Organ donation and transplantation are rare, reflecting traditional attitudes towards integrity and purity.

Domain from the Purnell Model	'Typical' individualistic low-context aggregate cultural characteristics	'Typical' collectivistic high-context aggregate cultural characteristics
	'Do Not Resuscitate' orders are accepted and seen as humanitarian to prevent pain and suffering.	'Do Not Resuscitate' orders may be seen as cost saving instead of relieving pain and suffering.

Case study 3.2

Paul Williams, age 32 years, was born in Scotland of naturalised parents formerly from the United States. By the time he was 16, he weighed 150 kg and was marginalised by some of his peers at a private school with a strong Church of Scotland (The Kirk) orientation. Shortly before graduation at the age of 18, he decided to go on a strict weight-reduction diet and changed his religious affiliation to Islam. Although his parents were displeased with his religious change, they accepted it but did not talk about it in the community or with relatives, even though he still lived at home with his parents.

Over the next several years, Paul would lose significant weight and then regain it. Eventually, he became a vegan and consistently lost weight. As an incentive to continue losing weight, he had pictures of very thin men and women on the walls of his room. Four years ago he was unable to lose more weight and began purging after each meal and taking laxatives. When he collapsed at home, his parents took him to the local Accident and Emergency room where he was diagnosed with congestive heart failure resulting from anorexia nervosa. He was referred to a general Islamic practitioner whom he saw for a year. Eventually, the practitioner suggested he see the local Imam for counselling but his parents refused to take him for his appointments. The parents did agree to an allopathic specialist who diagnosed the anorexia nervosa as serious and life threatening.

CASE STUDY 3.2 – QUESTIONS (ANSWERS ON P. 42)

Time: 15 minutes
1 Identify several stigmas that Paul has.
2 Would these same stigmas for Paul cause a stigma in your culture?
3 How supportive is his family?
4 Do you think that interventions at age 18 might have prevented Paul becoming anorexic?
5 Is Paul a candidate for palliative care?
6 What team of professionals is needed to adequately address Paul's health problems?

Case study 3.3

Jon is a 14-year-old male of mixed race (African-American and Hispanic) who has had numerous psychiatric in-patient admissions due to aggressive behaviour, extreme mood lability, and accompanying poor adherence to medication regime. His behaviour problems are of long standing and began soon after his placement in this family. This most recent stay, in the state hospital, was for aggressive behaviour directed towards his father. Jon has received a diagnosis of bipolar disorder. Adopted by a childless couple of Irish/Catholic descent when he was around three years of age, he is their only child. His early history was problematic and characterised by foetal alcohol syndrome, placement in foster care before the age of six months, developmental delays, and multiple care providers. The current hospitalisation is one of 10 previous in-patient stays.

Jon's parents, a couple now in their early fifties, are saying they cannot have him return home. They are fearful that he will physically hurt them. Jon is unable to give reassurance about this and is resistant to many milieu treatment interventions. He has had two physical restraints even with a complex medication regime involving neuroleptics and mood stabilisers.

CASE STUDY 3.3 QUESTIONS (ANSWERS ON PP. 42–4)

Time: 25 minutes

1 What is the most complex treatment issue currently facing this young man and his parents?
2 How will you ascertain the eventual discharge plan that needs to be in place for Jon?
3 How do you understand the cultural issues of being a mixed-race adolescent living in a Caucasian family?
4 How do you mobilise treatment resources for Jon's parents?
5 What needs to occur in the milieu environment before Jon's parents could consider taking him home?
6 Is it possible for parents of adopted or birth children to decide they 'can't take them home' and what is involved in this process?
7 What are the possible stigmas that Jon's parents experience as they have been adoptive parents to a severely disturbed child?

CONCLUSION

Palliative care for individuals experiencing serious and enduring mental health problems requires an intra- inter-disciplinary team that includes the family and the community. Individuals who come from a culture different from the intra-inter-discipline, multicultural team require special attention because:

➤ all mental health issues have a cultural component

➤ cultural conflicts are intensified when there is a mismatch between and among providers, the individual and organisation

➤ ethical issues are always involved with palliative care, mental health and cultural diversity.

Health professionals can use the Purnell Model for Cultural Competence and characteristics of individualism, collectivism and individuality as guides for assessment. The more one knows about the culture of the individual and family, the better the assessment. Becoming culturally self-aware and knowledgeable about diverse cultures is a life-long process, which can decrease ethnocentrism, stereotyping, cultural imposition and cultural imperialism.

REFERENCES

1 Matsuyama RK, Balliet W, Ingram K, *et al.* Will patients want hospice or palliative care if they do not know what it is? *Journal of Hospice and Palliative Nursing.* 2011; **13**: 41–6.

2 Ellison N. *Mental Health and Palliative Care Literature Review.* London Mental Health Foundation; 2008. Available at: www.mentalhealth.org.uk/content/assets/PDF/publications/mental_health_palliative_care.pdf (accessed 21 April 2012).

3 Owens A, Randhawa G. 'It's different from my culture; they're very different': providing community based culturally competent palliative care for South Asian people in the UK. *Health & Social Care in the Community.* 2004; **12**: 414–21.

4 Purnell L. *Guide to Culturally Competent Health Care.* Philadelphia: F.A. Davis; 2009.

5 Koffman J. Transcultural and ethical issues at the end of life. In: Cooper J, editor. *Stepping into Palliative Care.* Oxon: Radcliffe. 2006. pp. 171–86.

6 Giger J, Davidhizar R, Purnell L, *et al.* American Academy of Nursing Expert Panel Report: developing cultural competence to eliminate health disparities in ethnic minorities and other vulnerable populations. *Journal of Transcultural Nursing.* 2007; **18**: 95–102.

7 Purnell L. Cultural competence in a changing healthcare environment. In: Chaska N. *The Nursing Profession: tomorrow's vision.* Thousand Oaks, CA: Sage; 2001. pp. 451–61.

8 United Nationals. *The Universal Declaration of Human Rights.* 2001. Available at: www.un.org/Overview/rights.html (accessed 21 April 2012).

9 Purnell L, Paulanka, B. *Transcultural Health Care: a culturally competent approach.* Philadelphia: F.A. Davis; 2008.

10 Lipson J, Dibble S. *Culture and Clinical Care.* San Francisco: University of California Nursing Press; 2005.

11 Calvillo E, Clark L, Purnell L, *et al.* Cultural competencies in health care: emerging changes in baccalaureate nursing education. *Journal of Transcultural Nursing.* 2007; **20**: 137–45.

12 Teekman B. Exploring reflective thinking in nursing practice. *Journal of Advanced Nursing.* 2000; **31**: 1125–35.

13 Hofstede G, Hofstede J. *Cultures and Organizations: comparing values, behaviours, institutions, and organizations across nations.* 2nd ed. Thousand Oaks, CA: Sage; 2005.

14 Triandis H, Bontempo R, Villareal M, *et al.* Individualism and collectivism: cross cultural perspectives on self-group relationships. *Journal of Personality and Social Psychiatry.* 1998; **54**: 323–38.

15 Gudykunst WB, Ting-Toomey S, Nishida T. *Communication in Personal Relationships Across Cultures.* Thousand Oaks, CA: Sage; 1996.

16 Hall ET. *Beyond Culture.* NY: Anchor; 1989.

17 Hofstede, G. *Cultures and Organizations*. Berkshire, England: McGraw Hill; 1991.

18 Hofstede G. Cultural dimensions. (2009). Available at: www.geert-hofstede.com/ (accessed 21 April 2012).

19 Nishimura S, Nevgi A, Tella S. *Communication Style and Cultural Features in High/Low Context Communication Cultures: a case study of Finland, Japan and India*. Teoksessa A. Kallioniemi (toim.), *Uudistuva ja kehittyvä ainedidaktiikka. Ainedidaktinen symposiumi 8.2.2008 Helsingissä. Osa 2* (ss. 783–796). [In: Kallioniemi A, editor. *Renovating and developing subject didactics. Proceedings of a subject-didactic symposium in Helsinki on Feb. 2, 2008. Part 2* (pp. 783–796). University of Helsinki. Department of Applied Sciences of Education. Research Report 299]; 2008. Available at: www.helsinki.fi/~tella/nishimuranevgitella299.pdf (accessed 21 April 2012).

20 Kim D, Pan Y, Park HS. High- versus low-context culture: a comparison of Chinese, Korean, and American Cultures. *Psychology of Marketing*. 1998; **15**: 507–21.

21 Zolta E. *Stanford Encyclopaedia: voluntary euthanasia*. 2010. Available at: http://plato.stanford.edu/entries/euthanasia-voluntary/ (accessed 21 April 2012).

22 Dignity USA. (2011). Available at: www.dignityusa.org/ (accessed 21 April 2012).

TO LEARN MORE

- Purnell L, Paulanka B. *Transcultural Healthcare: a culturally competent approach*. 3rd ed. Philadelphia: FA Davis; 2008. Accompanying this textbook is an extensive guide for web resources and it includes documents on health disparities/inequalities and cultural information from several countries in Europe as well as from Australia, Canada, New Zealand, the United States and the World Health Organization. Additional chapters, case studies, a test bank, and instructor resources are also included. Available at: http://davisplus.fadavis.com/landing_page.cfm?publication_id=2417 (accessed 21 April 2012).

- U.S. Department of Health and Human Services Office of Minority Health. Think Cultural Health: bridging the healthcare gap through cultural competency continuing education programs. Available at: www.thinkculturalhealth.hhs.gov (accessed 21 April 2012). The content of this site was developed by a multicultural, multidiscipline team of 18 people, and has content for all health professionals. The web site now features a section dedicated to the National Standards for Culturally and Linguistically Appropriate Services (CLAS Standards) and discusses how states are legislating cultural and linguistic competency. The information can be used as a guide for other counties.

- Owens A, Randhawa G. 'It's different from my culture; they're very different': providing community based culturally competent palliative care for South Asian people in the UK. *Health & Social Care in the Community*. 2004; **12**: 414–21.

- Ellison N. Mental health and palliative care literature review. London Mental Health Foundation; 2008. Available at: www.mentalhealth.org.uk/content/assets/PDF/publications/mental_health_palliative_care.pdf (accessed 21 April 2012).

- Lynch M, Dahlin C, Hultman T, *et al.* Palliative care nursing: defining the discipline? *Journal of Hospice and Palliative Care Nursing*. 2011; **13**: 106–11.

- Yearwood EL, Pearson GS, Newland JA. *Child and Adolescent Behavioral Health: a resource for advanced practice psychiatric and primary care practitioners*. West Sussex: Wiley-Blackwell; 2012.

ANSWERS TO CASE STUDY 3.1 – P. 23

1 Regardless of a person's ethnicity or culture, professionals must first follow the legal mandates of the country. In most Western cultures when a person is cognitively impaired and unable to make a healthcare decision, the next of kin is a spouse or, in the absence of a spouse, then the oldest child. If there are no children or a spouse, the next of kin is an older brother or sister. In some collectivist cultures, the oldest son or daughter is the next of kin for decision-making authority. In this case, the spouse may agree to sign consent for treatment if the oldest child also signs. Thus, cultural and legal requirements are met. Legal documents such as Durable Power of Attorney or fully notarised Living Wills are accepted by most countries (*see* Chapter 4).

2 Some countries have legalised voluntary euthanasia. The person must be a legal citizen of that country; the length of time varies among countries. For most countries, five quite restrictive conditions have to be met. The person:
   i. is suffering from a terminal illness
   ii. is unlikely to benefit from a cure for that illness
   iii. is, as a direct result of the illness, either suffering intolerable pain, or only has available a life that is unacceptably burdensome
   iv. has an enduring, voluntary, and competent wish to die (or has, prior to losing the competence to do so, expressed a wish to die in the event that conditions i to iii are satisfied
   v. is unable without assistance to commit suicide.[21]

3 There is not a correct answer to this ethical dilemma and it relies heavily on the philosophy of the healthcare professional.

4 Complementary and alternative therapies in conjunction with and as stand-alone therapies have been beneficial for some, regardless of ethnicity or cultural background.

5 Eun does have support from her life partner, Angela, who is considered family. It is unknown to what extent Eun's family and Angela's family might be supportive with the assistance of a healthcare professional who should concentrate on the importance of family in a collectivist culture.

6 In an individualistic low-context culture, this question would be stated directly and explicitly. In a collectivist high-context culture, the question would need to be approached subtly and indirectly.

7 Depending on the country, community resources should be garnered to assist Eun and Angela, whether such resources be emotional, social, or financial.

8 There is not a correct answer to this ethical dilemma and it relies heavily on the philosophy of the healthcare professional. Regardless of the professional's philosophy, care should be delivered in a non-judgemental, caring, accepting and respectful manner.

9 Church members' responses will be highly varied from complete acceptance to rejection.

10 The views of the Catholic Church on gay and lesbian issues vary among and within

countries and are continuously changing. The views vary from highly stigmatised to accepting same-gender marriage as in Spain and parts of Mexico. Dignity USA is a support organisation for gay and lesbian Catholics and has expanded its mission worldwide.[22]

ANSWERS TO CASE STUDY 3.2 – P. 37

1 Paul has a number of potential major or minor stigmas for him and his family and these include:
    i. having naturalised parents
    ii. having strong affiliation with the Church of Scotland
    iii. attending a private school
    iv. being severely overweight
    v. becoming a vegan
    vi. becoming anorexic
    vii. converting to Islam.
In different contexts and settings, many of these may not be stigmatised.
2 The answer to this question depends on the cultural and individual views of the professional.
3 Paul's parents seem to be less than supportive at this time in his life, especially since he converted to Islam. Family care and support from healthcare professionals is extremely important at this time.
4 This hypothetical question cannot be answered with any certainty. However, as a rule, the earlier the intervention with emotional and mental health concerns the better is the outcome.
5 With a 16-year history of some mental health concerns and the diagnosis of serious and life-threatening anorexia nervosa, Paul is, as most health professionals would agree, a candidate for palliative care.
6 Paul needs a culturally competent team of professionals:
    i. a physician mental health specialist
    ii. a professional mental health nurse
    iii. a religious leader of his choice
    iv. a family counsellor
    v. a nutritionist.

ANSWERS TO CASE STUDY 3.3 – P. 38

1 There are actually two complex treatment issues that need to be dealt with in the care of Jon. The first involves his parents' hesitancy to take him home and continue to be a living resource and parental support source for him. This needs to be explored thoroughly by the professional assigned to his care on the unit. The second treatment issue involves the complexity of his serious psychiatric illness.

Bipolar disorder, diagnosed in a young teen, has devastating effects on the young-ster's ability to master the developmental tasks necessary to grow up and become an independent adult. Jon needs a comprehensive treatment plan that combines medication management strategies with psychosocial interventions, including fam-ily treatment, vocational training and interpersonal support. Teaching for Jon and his family should focus on helping them understand his illness, the chronic nature of its presentation and the supports he will need to function.

2   This will depend on what his parents eventually decide to do about his return home and how much behaviour stabilisation can be achieved in the in-patient setting. Regardless, a return to the community must include an array of supports for Jon, including:
   i. therapy
   ii. medication management services
   iii. educational services
   iv. comprehensive case management
   v. a possible mentor.

3   In this family, the issue of race was rarely acknowledged or discussed; this tended to cause Jon anxiety and anger. He had many questions about his birth origins and neither of his adoptive parents wanted to discuss this with him. In reality, as he became an adolescent, his racial differences from his parents became more of an issue for him and their inability to address this contributed to his behaviour problems and rage.

4   In many communities there are intensive case management services available for severely disturbed individuals. Jon's school should be approached about his educational needs. Ideally, his clinical care would be centred in one agency that could co-ordinate services for him and his family. If parents absolutely refuse to have him return home, an alternative placement will be needed. This would usu-ally be arranged with the child welfare department and could be group home or therapeutic foster care.

5   Jon needs to behaviourally stabilise and show some change in his acuity. The clinician needs to explore the roots of his parents' reluctance to take him home and then try to address this.
   i. Have they made use of community services?
   ii. Do they think these issues can be mediated by psychotherapy?
   iii. What would they need to consider for a return home?
   iv. Would a partial hospital programme ease this transition?

6   Once a child is adopted, they legally belong to the adoptive parents. Like any family choosing to relinquish their child, this process becomes legal, in which in the extreme case, custody is given back to the state and the welfare department becomes involved. It is not a simple or easy process. Given Jon's clinical complexity and age, it would be difficult to plan for his placement in another environment.

7   The stigma involves mental health issues and the reluctance of society to acknowl-edge and understand what this means to a family. These parents are conservative, Irish Catholic, Caucasian and at the time they pursued adoption, only older

children of colour were available for placement. It was unclear whether or not they were told of his history and his complex potential mental health problems. While they stated that his race did not matter to them, the level of their self-reflection about this was unclear. It has to be noted that parents of any child with chronic, serious mental health problems must go through the same grieving process experienced by parents of mentally challenged children: loss of the idealised, healthy, and perfect child.

ACKNOWLEDGEMENTS

1 We would like to thank Dr Geraldine S Pearson, PhD, RN, FAAN for her contribution to Case Study 3.3. Dr Pearson is the Director of the HomeCare Program and Associate Professor, Child and Adolescent Division at the University of Connecticut Health Center School of Medicine. She is also the Editor of *Perspectives in Psychiatric Care.*
2 The editors and publisher would like to thank Professor Larry Purnell for granting permission to reproduce the Purnell Model for Cultural Competence.
3 The author, editors and publisher are grateful to the following for permitting the adaptation of this chapter from:
   i. The Purnell Model for Cultural Competence. In: Cooper DB. *Intervention in Mental Health–Substance Use.* London and New York: Radcliffe; 2011. pp. 29–50.
   ii. Purnell LD. Application of transcultural theory to mental health–substance use in an international context. In: Cooper DB. *Intervention in Mental Health–Substance Use.* London and New York: Radcliffe; 2011. pp. 51–68.

Ethics

Cynthia MA Geppert, Philip J Candilis

Time: 45 minutes

One of the most difficult situations facing both palliative and mental health profession-als is the lack of healthcare facilities and staff able to meet both the psychiatric and palliative care needs of individuals experiencing serious and enduring mental health (SEMH) and medical ill-health.

Read the **case scenario** carefully:

- identify the ethical issues involved
- present some possible approaches to the dilemmas.

Consider the clinical, psychological, emotional and spiritual features of the case for the individual, the family and the professionals responsible for the person's short- and long-term care and for you as a fellow professional.

Case scenario

John is a 48-year-old man diagnosed with chronic paranoid schizophrenia who has lived most of his life in a residential unit attached to a government mental hospital. Recently he was diagnosed with advanced stomach cancer that presented as a gastric outlet obstruction. Unable to eat or take oral medications, including his antipsychotic, and suffering from severe abdominal pain and dehydration, John was transferred to the medical ward of an acute-care community hospital.

In the hospital, he has become paranoid, believing the staff are trying to poison him: this is the reason he cannot eat and that his stomach hurts. He refuses pain medications because these also are contaminated. When professionals try to place an intravenous infusion (IV) or draw blood samples, he becomes agitated and strikes out, requiring restraints. These only worsen his delusions of being harmed. Over the past decades, John's family has only seen him on weekend and holidays. In view of his relatively young age, they would like everything done that can possibly prolong his life. John's mother, a nurse, asks about possible chemotherapy for his cancer. John does not have an advance directive, but keeps asking to return home so he can 'get better'. Members of the treatment team from the residential unit believe that hospice would be the most compassionate option for John.

Comment

This case scenario poignantly illustrates many of the major themes of this chapter, most notably the need for cross-training of palliative and mental health professionals so they can provide appropriate care for John's physical and psychic pain. The fact that few persons experiencing serious and enduring mental health have completed advance directives and are estranged from their families of origin complicates already difficult end-of-life decision making. This lacuna in *advance care planning* (ACP) is amplified when the person's capacity to make medical decisions is in question. The professionals in the residential programme, the acute-care hospital and John's family all have different interpretations of John's wishes and best interests.

INTRODUCTION

There are no other areas of healthcare ethics as contextually rich and diverse, legally and morally complex, as mental health and palliative care. When the two domains intersect, an individual confronts the existential dilemmas of life and death, meaning and hopelessness, alienation and relationship – themes that characterise both serious and enduring mental health and physical illness. The related ethical dilemmas faced by persons experiencing SEMH and the professionals that treat them become even more profound and complicated.

BOX 4.1 Ethics issues common to mental health and palliative care

- Centrality of suffering
- Stigma and discrimination
- Multiple and overlapping vulnerabilities:
  - medical
  - cultural
  - economic
  - social
  - spiritual
- Potentially diminished decisional capacity and voluntarism
- Family conflicts
- Interdisciplinary conflicts

Historically, the communities of mental health and palliative care have been strangers to each other's philosophies and practices. This separation has made the provision of comprehensive and empathic care ethically problematic. Ethical considerations are nonetheless remarkably similar in the two disciplines and their mutual commitment to relieve suffering provides a common ground on which the two professions can stand[1] (*see* Box 4.1).

SELF-ASSESSMENT EXERCISE 4.1

Time: 15 minutes

Reflect on the core ethical concerns you have encountered in your specialty area, e.g. mental health, and identify whether and in what way these concerns would be relevant for palliative care. For example, persons who are experiencing mental health problems or at the end-of-life (EOL) are often stigmatised and marginalised by contemporary society's emphasis on youth and productivity.

ETHICAL PRINCIPLES AND THEORIES

Principles are the general norms or rules that help guide ethical decision making. Beauchamp and Childress, two leaders of the school of principle-based ethics, have called them 'action guides or maxims' that help clinicians justify, specify and balance ethical arguments and issues.[2] Moreover, there are a number of ethical theories or models that enrich principles for professionals identifying and analysing ethical concerns.[3]

KEY POINT 4.1

Two of the most salient theories for the palliative care of persons experiencing SEMH are:

- virtue ethics
- the ethics of care.

Virtues are qualities of character or habits of behaviour that help persons to do good even when it is difficult or against their own self-interest. Ethical decisions are those that virtuous persons would make in similar situations and that express this habitual character of moral excellence.[4] Care ethics, in its overarching focus on fostering relationships of commitment and caring, incorporates many of the cardinal virtues such as trust and altruism. Rights and duty-based theories may exclude emotions and relational values by overemphasising rationality and justice – principles that ignore the more subjective, personal influences frequently found in person-centred care. In order to reinforce the importance of virtues and relationships, we offer (*see* Table 4.1) definitions of core ethics principles and mini-case examples of their significance.

TABLE 4.1 Core ethics principles

Principle	Definition	Case-example
Autonomy	Literally 'self-rule'; the right of an individual to self-determination.	A 45 year old experiencing chronic schizophrenia and metastatic breast cancer refuses aggressive treatment or hospice in favour of returning to the hotel where she has lived her life.
Beneficence	The holistic good or benefit to a person; to act to promote one's well-being and interests above all other priorities.	Palliative care and mental health professionals collaborate to provide integrated care on the in-patient psychiatric unit for an individual experiencing psychotic depression and lung cancer. The individual is fearful of the general hospital and has been treated on the in-patient psychiatric service many times.
Fidelity	Holding faithfully to duty; perseverance in service.	The professionals of an intensive case management programme visit a person experiencing a psychotic disorder and chronic obstructive pulmonary disorder daily in the in-patient hospice unit of a university hospital.
Justice	Aristotle defined justice as treating 'equals equally and unequals unequally'.[5] More generally in healthcare, this term often refers to the fair allocation of resources.	In some settings, individuals experiencing schizophrenia and cancer receive the same standard of care and have comparable outcomes to persons with cancer alone.[6-8]
Non-maleficence	A classic foundational duty of clinicians: *primum non nocere*, 'first, do no harm'.	Mental health and palliative care professionals support the decision of a 35-year-old individual experiencing melanoma and bipolar disorder not to undergo the aggressive treatment his oncologist recommends.
Respect for persons	Unqualified respect for the intrinsic dignity, individuality and values of a human being regardless of: • diagnosis • ethnicity • religion • sexuality • economic status • social status.	A 45-year-old homeless person with serious borderline personality disorder, methamphetamine dependence and acquired immune deficiency syndrome (AIDS) receives hospice and psychiatric care in a specialised shelter.
Veracity	The professional obligation to disclose health information accurately and compassionately.	Professionals caring for an individual experiencing chronic schizophrenia refuse the family's request that he not be told he has advanced heart failure for fear it will upset him.

SELF-ASSESSMENT EXERCISE 4.2

> **Time: 30 minutes**
> Do you think individuals experiencing serious and enduring mental health are capable of making decisions about palliative care such as whether to be resuscitated? Propose an argument using the virtues and/or principles in Table 4.1, and then offer a counter-argument to your initial position.

DECISIONAL CAPACITY

The concept of decisional capacity is an essential consideration in ethical dilemmas commonly encountered in end-of-life and SEMH care. For the essential elements of decisional capacity illustrated with case examples, *see* Table 4.2. Persons experiencing SEMH may suffer not only from impairments of thought, reasoning, insight and judgement, but also from affective, volitional and appraisal dysfunction that undermines contributions to the more demanding requirements of decision making. Components of decision making like reasoning and appreciation are particularly vulnerable to mental and pain syndromes.[9,10] Enhanced consent procedures such as repeating information, offering feedback and applying computerised teaching materials have improved decisional capacity in numerous studies of SEMH individuals.[11–13]

TABLE 4.2 Elements of decisional capacity[14]

Elements	Definition	Case example
Communication	The capacity to express a choice by any means.	A 32-year-old person experiencing serious post-traumatic stress disorder is intubated for two years after rehabilitation for a motorcycle accident. He consistently signals with eye-blinks that he wants the ventilator disconnected.
Comprehension	The capacity to understand (retain and order) information presented at an appropriate level.	A 64-year-old person experiencing chronic psychosis has radiation treatment explained to him through a demonstration in the radiation suite and is able to answer all post-test questions correctly.
Reasoning	The capacity to manipulate facts rationally to arrive at a logical conclusion.	A 57-year-old individual experiencing melancholic depression and cardiac disease watches a video on electroconvulsive therapy (ECT) and is then able to weigh the risks and benefits of the therapy for his refractory depression.
Appreciation	The capacity to appreciate the implications of a choice at a more emotional level.	A 70-year-old person experiencing schizoaffective disorder who spends most of his time in day-treatment studying nature and taking long walks is diagnosed with end-stage renal disease. He refuses dialysis so he can be free to enjoy his life in the time he has left.

(continued)

Elements	Definition	Case example
Voluntarism	The capacity to make a decision free from excessive internal or external coercion.	A devout 35-year-old Hindu experiencing bipolar disorder and non-Hodgkin's lymphoma resists the wishes of his family and doctors for palliative chemotherapy in favour of a final pilgrimage to India.

ADVANCE CARE PLANNING

Intact decisional capacity is crucial to mental ill-health and palliative care because it allows individuals experiencing SEMH to engage in advance care planning, an under-utilised component of EOL care. A broad definition of ACP is:

> A *process of communication* between the patient, the family/healthcare proxy, and staff for the purpose of prospectively identifying a surrogate, clarifying treatment preferences, and developing individualized goals of care near the end of life.[15]

Several important aspects of ACP (*see* Box 4.2) are critical for mental health professionals who work alongside the individual experiencing this critical piece of healthcare communication.

BOX 4.2 Aspects of advance care planning (ACP)

- The goal of ACP is for persons who possess decisional capacity to express their wishes for healthcare at a future time when they have lost decision-making capacity.
- ACP does not have to be performed in a healthcare setting. Mental health and other professionals can engage in ACP in shelters, day-treatment programmes, or group homes.
- Although written documents may carry more legal weight, ACP need not require extensive written documentation. It can be accomplished through a brief conversation or in pieces over the lifetime of the individual.
- ACP does not require the participation of a healthcare professional or the authorisation of a legal professional to be valid.
- ACP does not go into effect until the individual loses decision-making capacity.
- The individual can rescind or modify ACP at any time, so long as they retain capacity.
- ACP does not and should not be delayed until a person is diagnosed with a life-limiting illness. Optimal ACP occurs when an individual is healthy. Goals of care can then be revised as medical conditions evolve.
- ACP for SEMH should be completed when the individual is psychiatrically stable because the process may not be possible when a person is in a physical or psychological crisis.
- The professional who has the strongest therapeutic alliance with the person experiencing SEMH may be in the best position to conduct ACP discussions.

Advance directives

Advance directives are legal, usually written documents that codify an individual's treatment preferences. *See* Table 4.3 for a description of the types of advance directive. Because the nature, scope and limitations of these documents vary in different jurisdictions, professionals should have access to up-to-date legal counsel.

TABLE 4.3 Types of advance directives

Directive	Purpose
Living Will or Advance Healthcare Directive or Statement	• Contains written or verbal instructions regarding end-of-life beliefs, values and desires. • May include declining a feeding tube or requesting a time-limited course of life-sustaining therapy.
Durable Powers of Attorney for Healthcare, Medical Powers of Attorney, or Healthcare Proxy	• Designate a person who makes treatment decisions on behalf of the individual once capacity is lost. • Decision-making surrogate is termed a 'healthcare proxy' or 'healthcare agent'.
Guardianship orders	• The court appointment of an individual to make decisions on behalf of a decisionally incapable person. • Does not always grant the power to make healthcare decisions.
Psychiatric Advance Directives	• A legal document executed when a person is decisionally capable. • Specific instructions for future mental health care. • Designates an agent to make mental healthcare decisions when the person loses capacity secondary to acute psychiatric illness.

There are several elements of uncertainty and contradiction restricting – and in some instances annulling – the autonomy of individuals experiencing SEMH making EOL decisions. For instance, psychiatric advance directives that allow individuals to express their preferences for psychiatric care and appoint a proxy to assist in making decisions[16] generally do not cover non-psychiatric treatment. Similarly, traditional advance directives usually only apply to 'medical' care, leading to considerable confusion, lack of co-ordination and failure to respect the autonomy of the individual experiencing SEMH. A detailed examination of the diverse legal aspects of ACP in various countries is beyond the scope of this chapter, but a few clinically relevant issues under debate worldwide are outlined below. Many of these are unique to the individual experiencing SEMH, and underscore the role of stigma in ACP. Moreover, they underscore the need for both palliative and mental health care professionals to advocate for the right of individuals experiencing SEMH to exercise self-determination.

Surrogates

For decades, legislation has been in place in North America, the United Kingdom and Australia that establishes the right of citizens to execute advance directives.

Yet despite education efforts, it is estimated that only around 30% of Americans and fewer than 50% of seriously ill individuals have completed an advance directive.[17] Members of disadvantaged populations, including those experiencing SEMH, are even less likely to complete the documents.[18] One group of American researchers conducted an innovative study that persuasively addressed these difficulties. One-hundred-and-forty-two persons experiencing SEMH completed a structured interview called the Health Care Preferences Questionnaire. The survey examined preferences regarding the experiences, beliefs, values and concerns of individuals considering healthcare surrogates and end-of-life issues in general.

In this study, 27% of respondents experiencing SEMH had thought about EOL preferences, but only 2% of respondents had documented their healthcare preferences; and only 5% had discussed them with their doctor.[19] This means that only a small percentage of this group with higher morbidity and mortality[20] have provided healthcare professionals with their treatment preferences or named anyone to assist in interpreting their values and wishes. To address this widespread ethical and clinical problem, most governments and healthcare systems establish an order of surrogacy through law or policy. This is a hierarchy of individuals authorised to make healthcare decisions on behalf of incapacitated persons. Generally, the surrogates are family members in a particular order:

➤ spouses
➤ adult children
➤ parents
➤ other relatives.

This order is based on the social acceptance of the moral authority of family members to know their loved ones' values, care about their well-being and respect their wishes.[21]

The primacy of family, however, is problematic for persons experiencing SEMH. The social isolation of many individuals experiencing SEMH, who are frequently estranged from their family of origin, never married and without children, makes the obligatory choice of family members an ethically dubious proposition. Indeed, it may be psychologically harmful and constitute a form of social discrimination.[22] The American researchers found that, compared with the 85%–90% of non-SEMH individuals who would name a family member as proxy, only 63% of SEMH persons would do so.[19,23]

Most often, the 'family' of the person experiencing SEMH are those who care for their health. It is mental health professionals who are familiar with the lives and beliefs of the person experiencing SEMH, and who are frequently in the best position to know what they would choose if they were able. In fact, in the study described above, 23% of respondents would name a professional as their proxy if allowed to do so.[19] Ironically, legislation or facility policies[24] may bar these persons from serving as surrogate decision makers because it is considered a conflict of interest that could place the priorities of the professional above those of the individual.

From a humanistic perspective, if a healthcare professional is the only one that the person trusts with her or his deepest hopes and fears, that professional has moral licence to serve as a surrogate. Appropriate institutional oversight, such as the involvement of an ethics consultant or committee, may help legitimise this option.[22] This problem becomes even more poignant when the legal and ethical standards of surrogate or proxy decision making are considered. Legal and ethical consensus establishes that when the explicit (or often implicit) wishes of a person are known, then these must guide decision making. This is the 'substituted judgement standard' that makes decisions as the individual would if able. When, as is common, those values and wishes are not known, surrogates use a best-interest standard. This standard uses the individual's best interests as the touchstone for medical decisions, applying truisms like 'health is better than illness', 'life is better than death' to guide decision making.[2] Moreover, it is the criterion employed when an individual has no surrogate, and a professional or a court-appointed guardian must be assigned the decision-making role.[25]

Treatment preferences

The EOL treatment preferences of persons experiencing a SEMH diagnosis warrant further research. A related study to the one described above presented 150 individuals experiencing SEMH in the community with hypothetical EOL scenarios to elicit their treatment preferences for an imaginary 'other' and for themselves. Respondents demonstrated a strong practical ability to express their wishes.[26] Their choices were most similar to those of other minority groups and were more conservative than those of the general population – especially in wishing to continue life-sustaining treatments even when they are low-yield. It is likely that this similarity reflects a shared experience of disparity in healthcare and a lack of trust for the system that delivers it.[27,28] *See* Box 4.3 for a summary of the findings.

BOX 4.3 Summary of treatment preferences from Foti *et al.*[26]

- 66% of respondents experiencing SEMH desired aggressive pain management if they had incurable cancer, even if it affected thinking.
- 34% believed a professional should provide the individual with enough medication to end their life.
- Given a scenario of irreversible coma, 29% would terminate life support immediately and 45% would end it after a set period.[26]

Three misunderstandings or myths[29] regarding people experiencing serious and enduring mental health and physical ill-health frequently contribute to ethical and legal conflicts. One common misunderstanding is the difference between decisional incapacity and incompetence. The first is a clinical judgement; the second is a legal determination. Certainly, clinical judgement informs the legal determination, but competence is ultimately the purview of the courts. Any physician, and in some jurisdictions, other practitioners, can assess decisional capacity, but only the legal system can formally adjudicate an individual incompetent. This preserves individual rights by providing a public forum for disputes over the autonomy of the individual.

The second misunderstanding is that decisional capacity is a once-and-for-all or all-or-none assessment. In fact, clinical decision-making capacity is task-specific and may change over time. For instance, an individual with disorganised schizophrenia may not be able to make financial decisions, yet be quite able to express a treatment preference for his lung cancer. The capacity to make medical decisions is also very sensitive to changes in medical and psychosocial status. An individual with a mood disorder and respiratory distress secondary to chronic obstructive pulmonary disease may be delirious and unable to provide consent for cardiopulmonary resuscitation (CPR). Yet once he or she is stabilised in intensive care, she or he may well be able to communicate her or his wishes.

Two further detrimental and prevalent myths are that persons experiencing SEMH *de facto* lack decision-making capacity, and that even people who are capable find the subject of dying too distressing to discuss.[30] The research group above persuasively dispelled these myths. Fifty-eight per cent of individuals completing their interviews were comfortable discussing EOL issues, and only 4% reported a great amount of stress from the process. In addition, the results suggest that persons experiencing SEMH are cognitively and emotionally able to engage in ACP discussions, and are interested in having their preferences for treatment and surrogacy known and respected. Seventy per cent were comfortable with the EOL interview and 71% understood the content without additional explanation. Indeed 69% wanted to receive more information about appointing a healthcare proxy.[19,31]

FORCE, FUTILITY AND THE FUTURE OF END-OF-LIFE IN SERIOUS AND ENDURING MENTAL HEALTH

One of the most controversial concepts in end-of-life ethics is that of futility. Futility, even outside mental health, is a troubled and troubling concept that is of special relevance to vulnerable and disadvantaged individuals considering palliative and EOL care.[32] Futility is technically defined as:

> an effort to provide a benefit to a patient which reason and experience suggest is highly likely to fail and whose rare exceptions cannot be systematically produced.[33]

How the definition is applied to vulnerable populations is the crux of the ethical problem.

Critiques of the concept of futility argue that it masks quality-of-life judgements that should be the prerogative of the ill person, not the treating professional – judgements which are often strikingly discordant.[34] Indeed, empirical research suggests that interventions for disadvantaged individuals are more likely to be deemed futile, leading to concerns that these are reflections of social bias rather than objective clinical judgements.[35]

Futility arises in two specific areas. The first is whether SEMH itself is ever so burdensome and so refractory to treatment that its treatment can legitimately be considered futile. Is SEMH itself more appropriate for palliative care than continued aggressive treatment? Some authors fit chronic eating disorders into this category because of the poor prognosis and frequent forced feeding.[36] Some prominent commentators have opined that aggressive psychiatric treatment for depression may ultimately prove burdensome.[37]

The second area of futility is that of forced treatment for those who refuse life-saving treatment. The traditional presumption of Hippocratic ethics, reinforced through rulings in Anglo-American law, is that the preservation of life takes precedence in uncertain prognoses. Similarly, a proxy, family member or professional can submit individuals who are not thought to be decisionally capable to involuntary medical treatment. Consider the 2009 case report of a woman with terminal breast cancer and psychosis who refused treatment and asked to be allowed to go into the mountains to die.[38] There is always the danger of erring on the side of paternalism and overruling the authentic voice of a competent person on the mistaken assumption it is the illness speaking.[22] Conversely, professionals may be so concerned with violating a person's autonomy that they allow her to choose death when the choice is not truly autonomous but the manifestation of depression or paranoia.[38]

However, even when individuals experiencing SEMH possess decisional capacity to refuse treatment, their wishes have not always been respected. This is especially true if the person resides in a state hospital or community residential programme where deaths from medical causes can be the subject of criminal investigation.[39] Risk managers and hospital attorneys may order treatment, rightly concerned that professionals and facility are more liable to charges of medical negligence than battery.[30]

One of the greatest barriers to providing competent and compassionate EOL care to people experiencing SEMH is the lack of facilities, and professionals, able and willing to serve both the medical and psychiatric needs of individuals with overlapping conditions.[6] Indeed, some hospice programmes have admission criteria which exclude persons experiencing SEMH, especially those with acute psychotic symptoms and threatening behaviour.[38]

CONCLUSION

> **KEY POINT 4.2**
>
> Education related to these ethical problems is crucial.

If the vision of collaboration between palliative and mental health professionals in the EOL care of people experiencing SEMH is to be realised, education on these ethical problems will be crucial. For example, better training in the assessment of functional capacity might enhance the likelihood that people will have their wishes documented and honoured. Research has shown that professionals, especially those who provide hands-on care, desire and benefit from this kind of training.[7] Legal reforms such as more flexible proxy statutes that allow professionals to serve as surrogates must join educational efforts if individuals experiencing SEMH are to have their wishes honoured. It is the ethical obligation of all professionals in palliative and mental healthcare to advocate these changes so that persons who have endured lives of suffering and stigma may end their lives with an experience of comfort and compassion.

REFERENCES

1 Billings JA, Block SD. Integrating psychiatry and palliative medicine: the challenges and opportunites. In: Chochinov HM, Breitbart W, editors. *Handbook of Psychiatry in Palliative Medicine.* 2nd ed. New York: Oxford University Press; 2009. pp. 13–19.

2 Beauchamp TL, Childress JF. *Principles of Biomedical Ethics.* 6th ed. New York: Oxford University Press; 2009.

3 Rachels J. Ethical theory and bioethics. In: Kuhse H, Singer P, editors. *A Companion to Bioethics.* Malden, MA: Blackwell; 2001. pp. 15–24.

4 Pellegrino ED, Thomasma DC. *The Virtues in Medical Practice.* New York: Oxford University Press; 1993.

5 Aristotle. *The Ethics of Aristotle: the Nicomachean Ethics.* New York: Penguin; 1976. p. 244.

6 Kelly BD, Shanley D. Terminal illness and schizophrenia. *Journal of Palliative Care.* 2000 Summer; **16**: 55–7.

7 Foti ME. 'Do it your way': a demonstration project on end-of-life care for persons with serious mental illness. *Journal of Palliative Medicine.* [Review]. 2003 Aug; **6**: 661–9.

8 Ganzini L, Socherman R, Duckart J, *et al.* End-of-life care for veterans with schizophrenia and cancer. [Comparative Study Research Support, U.S. Gov't, Non-P.H.S.]. *Psychiatric Services.* 2010 July; **61**: 725–8.

9 Bursztajn HJ, Harding HP, Jr., Gutheil TG, *et al.* Beyond cognition: the role of disordered affective states in impairing competence to consent to treatment. [Case Reports]. *The Bulletin of the American Academy of Psychiatry and the Law.* 1991; **19**: 383–8.

10 Geppert CM, Abbott C. Voluntarism in consultation psychiatry: the forgotten capacity. *American Journal of Psychiatry.* 2007; **164**: 409–13.

11 Dunn LB, Lindamer LA, Palmer BW, *et al.* Enhancing comprehension of consent for research in older patients with psychosis: a randomized study of a novel consent procedure. *American Journal of Psychiatry.* 2001; **158**: 1911–3.

12 Stiles PG, Poythress NG, Hall A, *et al.* Improving understanding of research consent disclosures among persons with mental illness. *Psychiatric Services.* 2001; **52**: 780–5.

13 Palmer BW, Dunn LB, Depp CA, *et al.* Decisional capacity to consent to research among patients with bipolar disorder: comparison with schizophrenia patients and healthy subjects. *Journal of Clinical Psychiatry.* 2007; **68**: 689–96.

14 Appelbaum PS. Clinical practice. Assessment of patients' competence to consent to treatment. *New England Journal of Medicine.* 2007; **357**: 1834–40.

15 Davison SN. Advance care planning in chronic illness. Fast Facts and Concepts [serial on the Internet]. 2006. Available at: www.eperc.mcw.edu/fastfact/ff_162.htm (accessed 13 October 2011).

16 Srebnik DS, Rutherford LT, Peto T, *et al.* The content and clinical utility of psychiatric advance directives. *Psychiatric Services.* 2005; **56**: 592–8.

17 Riker RR, Fraser GL. Altering intensive care sedation paradigms to improve patient outcomes. *Critical Care Clinics.* 2009; **25**: 527–38, viii–ix.

18 Perkins HS, Geppert CM, Gonzales A, *et al.* Cross-cultural similarities and differences in attitudes about advance care planning. *Journal of General Internal Medicine.* 2002; **17**: 48–57.

19 Foti ME, Bartels SJ, Merriman MP, *et al.* Medical advance care planning for persons with serious mental illness. [Comparative Study Research Support, Non-U.S. Gov't]. *Psychiatric Services.* 2005; **56**: 576–84.

20 Dembling BP, Chen DT, Vachon L. Life expectancy and causes of death in a population treated for serious mental illness. [Research Support, U.S. Gov't, P.H.S.]. *Psychiatric Services.* 1999; **50**: 1036–42.

21 Swisher KN. Implementing the PSDA for psychiatric patients: a common-sense approach. *The Journal of Clinical Ethics.* 1991; **2**: 199–205.

22 Lee MA, Ganzini L, Heintz R. The PSDA and treatment refusal by a depressed older patient committed to the state mental hospital. *HEC Forum.* 1993; **5**: 289–301.

23 Emanuel LL, Barry MJ, Stoeckle JD, *et al.* Advance directives for medical care: a case for greater use. [Research Support, Non-U.S. Gov't Research Support, U.S. Gov't, P.H.S.]. *The New England Journal of Medicine.* 1991; **324**: 889–95.

24 Beth Israel Deaconess Medical Center. Advance Directive Planning – Massachusetts Health Care Proxy. 2010. Available at: www.bidmc.org/CentersandDepartments/Departments/SocialWork/AdvanceDirectivePlanningMassachusettsHealthCareProxy.aspx (accessed 13 October 2011).

25 Buchanan AE, Brock DW. *Deciding for Others: the ethics of surrogate decision making.* New York: Cambridge University Press; 1990.

26 Foti ME, Bartels SJ, Van Citters AD, *et al.* End-of-life treatment preferences of persons with serious mental illness. [Research Support, Non-U.S. Gov't]. *Psychiatric Services.* 2005; **56**: 585–91.

27 Blackhall LJ, Frank G, Murphy ST, *et al.* Ethnicity and attitudes towards life sustaining technology. [Research Support, U.S. Gov't, P.H.S.]. *Social Science & Medicine.* 1999; **48**: 1779–89.

28 Cort MA. Cultural mistrust and use of hospice care: challenges and remedies. *Journal of Palliative Medicine.* [Review]. 2004; **7**: 63–71.

29 Ganzini L, Volicer L, Nelson WA, *et al.* Ten myths about decision-making capacity. *Journal of the American Medical Directors Association.* 2005; **6**(Suppl): S100–4.

30 Candilis PJ, Foti ME, Holzer JC. End-of-life care and mental illness: a model for community psychiatry and beyond. [Research Support, Non-U.S. Gov't]. *Community Mental Health Journal.* 2004; **40**: 3–16.

31 Geller JL. The use of advance directives by persons with serious mental illness for psychiatric treatment. *The Psychiatric Quarterly*. 2000; **71**: 1–13.

32 Brody BA, Halevy A. Is futility a futile concept? *Journal of Medicine and Philosophy*. 1995; **20**: 123–44.

33 Jonsen AR, Seigler M, Winslade WJ. *Clinical Ethics: a practical approach to ethical decisions in clinical medicine*. 7th ed. New York: McGraw-Hill; 2010.

34 Pearlman RA, Uhlmann RF. Quality of life in chronic diseases: perceptions of elderly patients. [Research Support, U.S. Gov't, Non-P.H.S. Research Support, U.S. Govt, P.H.S.]. *Journal of Gerontology*. 1988; **43**: M25–30.

35 Truog RD, Brett AS, Frader J. The problem with futility. *The New England Journal of Medicine*. 1992; **326**: 1560–4.

36 Lopez A, Yager J, Feinstein RE. Medical futility and psychiatry: palliative care and hospice care as a last resort in the treatment of refractory anorexia nervosa. *The International Journal of Eating Disorders*. [Case Reports]. 2010; **43**: 372–7.

37 Sullivan MD, Youngner SJ. Depression, competence, and the right to refuse lifesaving medical treatment. *American Journal of Psychiatry*. 1994; **151**: 971–8.

38 Levin SM, Feldman MB. Terminal illness in a psychiatric patient – issues and ethics. *South African Medical Journal*. 1983; **63**: 492–4.

39 McGrath PD, Forrester K. Ethico-legal issues in relation to end-of-life care and institutional mental health. *Australian Health Review*. 2006; **30**: 286–97.

TO LEARN MORE

- Craun MJ, Watkins M, Hefty A. Hospice care of the psychotic patients. *American Journal of Hospice & Palliative Care*. 1997; **14**: 205–8.
- Woods A, Willison K, Kington C, Gavin A. Palliative care for people with serious persistent mental illness: a review of the literature. *The Canadian Journal of Psychiatry*. 2008; **53**: 725–36.
- McCasland LA. Providing hospice and palliative care to the seriously and persistently mentally ill. *Journal of Hospice and Palliative Nursing*. 2007; **9**: 305–13.
- Massachusetts Department of Health. 'Do it your way': end of life care for persons with serious mental illness. Available at www.promotingexcellence.org/mentalillness/index.html (accessed 18 April 2012).
- Promoting excellence in end-of-life care. *Innovative Models and Approaches for End-of-Life Care*. Available at www.promotingexcellence.org/ (accessed 18 April 2012).
- McGrath P, Holewa H. Mental health and palliative care: exploring the ideological interface. *The International Journal of Psychosocial Rehabilitation*. Available at www.psychosocial.com/ IJPR_9/Palliative_Care_McGraph.html (accessed 18 April 2012).

CHAPTER 5

Psychological impact of serious and enduring mental health

Alyna Turner, Brian Kelly, Amanda L Baker

INTRODUCTION

Mental health problems can take a variety of forms, ranging from mild symptoms of depression or anxiety to serious and enduring conditions, such as schizophrenia, bipolar affective disorder, and chronic depression. For some, the symptoms of mental health problems might be transient, while for others the condition might be life changing, taking a chronic and persistent course.

SELF-ASSESSMENT EXERCISE 5.1

Time: 20 minutes

Consider the ethos of palliative care. If you are unsure of the philosophy of this discipline, take 15 minutes to find out about the main principles.

On an individual level, how a person reacts to and expresses their distress, whether or not they choose to inform others, and the response of others to that person, will vary. Social, cultural, religious and generational influences play a role in the person's experience of mental health problems and the experience of stigma. These influences will also influence the individual's, and family's, beliefs around whether the condition is considered problematic and whether or not assistance should be sought.[1]

REFLECTIVE PRACTICE EXERCISE 5.1

Time: 15 minutes

Reflect on how you might manage a person experiencing serious and enduring mental health, using a palliative care approach to maximise and improve quality of life.

The course of SEMH may be defined by ongoing impairments in functioning, and the goals of treatment will vary over time and across individuals. Treatment goals span acute recovery through to stabilisation, focusing on increasing or maintaining functioning with recognition of limited capacity for complete resolution of disorder. In this respect, these goals are not dissimilar from those that may occur with chronic physical illness, although the affected functions may differ.

While end-of-life care of individuals experiencing SEMH has been reviewed elsewhere[2] (*see* Chapter 13), the following discussion will draw on the principles fundamental to palliative care that can be applied to diverse populations and relevant to the needs of people experiencing SEMH, their families and those caring for them. Common themes in palliative care include:
➤ the process of coping with persistent symptoms and disability
➤ the impact of illness on future hopes and expectations (*see* Chapter 7)
➤ attention to spiritual and existential dimension of illness (*see* Chapter 8)
➤ the task of redefining goals of care
➤ the focus on maximising psychosocial and physical function rather than complete resolution of disease.

Furthermore, focus is given to the impact of persistent ill-health on the treating practitioner.

SELF-ASSESSMENT EXERCISE 5.2

Time: 10 minutes
How might a person experiencing serious and enduring mental health impact on:
● you directly?
● other people within your care?
● the family?

LIVING WITH ILLNESS AND FINDING WELLNESS: THE PSYCHOLOGICAL IMPACT OF SEMH ON THE INDIVIDUAL

An individual's journey experiencing SEMH begins with first onset of symptoms, which may vary in intensity and form. Often there is a 'prodromal' period, and some may experience a serious decline in functioning, without acute symptoms in the beginning. Whatever the picture, the change can be a confusing and frightening experience, filled with uncertainty around the cause of the problem. Many people will not seek assistance and may never receive any treatment, particularly in less-developed countries.[3] Fewer still will receive adequate treatment and follow-up care.[3] For those who do receive treatment, the process of assessment, diagnosis, and finding and maintaining adequate treatment strategies, brings additional challenges for the individual, their family and the professional.

From time of onset, uncertainty about the course of the condition, and the degree of expected recovery, if any, is the norm regardless of whether adequate treatment is received.[4] Stereotypes of people experiencing SEMH often paint the condition as chronic, deteriorating and associated with poor outcomes.

KEY POINT 5.1

While for some this trajectory of ill-health will fit, research indicates that many individuals will show significant improvements in both their illness and their lives.[4]

In schizophrenia, 'complete recovery' (loss of psychotic symptoms and return to the pre-illness level of functioning) is seen in 20% of people experiencing the condition, while 'social recovery' (economic and residential independence and low social disruption) is seen in 40%.[5] A challenge for the individual, family and healthcare provider is balancing the need and impact of ongoing, possibly lifetime care, while fostering hope.

The potential erosion of future personal expectations, self-esteem and sense of competence are important elements of the psychological impact of SEMH.

KEY POINT 5.2

Personal accounts[6] of individuals experiencing SEMH consistently describe the experience of loss of the sense of self and previous identity, either in totality or specific parts (for example, work, or parental role).

Previous identity can become replaced by a focus on deficit and dysfunction. Individuals describe the sense of dual 'ill' and 'well' selves, and the struggle to reconcile the 'ill' self with the other identities or roles so it is seen as a part of a larger whole rather than a defining characteristic. In this respect the experience of SEMH links closely with the work undertaken relating to the impact of advanced physical illness on sense of personal dignity.[7]

While previous roles are lost, decisions to take on new potential roles, for example, becoming a parent, become more challenging. Striving to 'act normal', lead a 'normal' life and reach 'normal' developmental milestones might coexist with an underlying recognition of the changes induced by the ill-health. The age, and therefore the developmental stage, of the person when the illness is at its peak will determine which developmental milestones are affected. Schizophrenia emerging in late adolescence, for example, will have a profound impact on ability to negotiate almost all 'adult' milestones and tasks.

Ongoing personal and public stigma and discrimination[8] can have a pervasive and detrimental impact on all facets of the person's life and underlie much of the negative psychological impact of SEMH. Coping strategies have been identified that enhance psychological adjustment over time in a range of health conditions (for example, problem-focused coping, active engagement of social support, and strategies that enhance meaning and purpose).

KEY POINT 5.3

Maintenance of hope can be a vital element of coping and an important target for these therapeutic interventions (*see* Chapters 4 and 5).[9]

Stigma

> The stigma attached to mental illness is the main obstacle to the provision of care for people with this disorder. Stigma does not stop at illness: it marks those who are ill, their families across generations, institutions that provide treatment, psychotropic drugs, and mental health workers.[10]

REFLECTIVE PRACTICE EXERCISE 5.2

Time: 5 minutes
Think carefully about how we, as the professional, may add to the feelings of stigma in the provision of care we offer to the individual.

KEY POINT 5.4

The process of marginalisation and ostracism, rejection or disapproval due to being perceived as different, or 'not normal', in some way compared with others[1] is potentially worse for the person and their loved ones than the illness itself.

People experiencing SEMH are often seen as inherently different and they therefore engender misunderstanding, prejudice, confusion and fear in the general public,[1] and at times among health professionals. For example, people experiencing psychotic conditions are often viewed with fear and as potentially violent or dangerous, incompetent and unpredictable, while people experiencing depression may be seen as negative, morose and weak willed.[1]

REFLECTIVE PRACTICE EXERCISE 5.3

Time: 10 minutes
Reflect on your own personal view about the above statement.
- Does it resonate with the above?
- If yes, why?
- Were you aware of this?
- Are your own views different now?

The process of stigmatisation has been well described.[11] Identifiable character-istics, or 'markers' such as a visible abnormality or a label, become loaded with negative attitudes or emotions as a result of previous knowledge, information or memories (for example, through movies, the press or personal contact). In this way, the marker becomes a 'stigma'. Once stigmatisation occurs it may lead to differential treatment of the individual. This negative discrimination due to 'public stigma' can result in loss of opportunities, coercion due to perceived lack of competence, and segregation[12] through to abuse and 'social death'.[13] This may lead to numerous experiences that impact negatively on the person's self-esteem and result in other negative psychological outcomes such as increased stress. The individual may internalise the stereotypes and experience 'self-stigma', resulting in further loss of self-esteem and self-efficacy.[14] The consequences of stigma from the public and self may result in a worsening of the condition, amplifying the 'marker' and making identification easier.

Public stigma resulting in marginalisation can bring about social isolation should the person be rejected from employment, friendship groups, activities and even family, depriving individuals of important sources of social support. Differential treatment might be received from services, including core services such as health, housing and legal. Awareness of these public attitudes may result in individuals avoiding care and concealing their condition, which may lead to a worsening of symptoms or even death. Should the condition be revealed, however, the consequences of public stigma and resulting fear and stress on the individual may also lead to a worsening of symptoms and suffering. Despite often being the primary support, family may compound the situation by either assisting to hide their relative or the condition or rejecting the individual.[15]

While public stigma might result in marginalisation and inequities in care, self-stigma can:
➤ increase self-imposed isolation
➤ decrease behaviours directed towards life goals
➤ impact on involvement in and response to care.[14]

For self-stigma to occur, the individual must first be aware of the pervasive stereotypes, agree with them, and then apply them to one's self. If stereotypes are internalised, the individual may see himself or herself as unworthy of help, respect and social inclusion, and consequently they may isolate themselves further and exacerbate the existing mental health problems. Demoralisation and devaluation resulting from the self-stigma lead to reduced self-esteem and self-efficacy, which may compromise the likelihood of the individual engaging in behaviours to achieve specific life goals.[14]

While insight into the condition is often perceived as a positive sign by the professional and a goal of treatment, high levels of internalised stigma appear to undermine the possibility that insight will lead to positive outcomes.[16]

KEY POINT 5.5

Insight, or acceptance of the diagnosis, combined with high levels of internalised stigma, is associated with lower levels of hope and self-esteem which results in avoidant coping, social avoidance and depression and decreased quality of life.[4]

Studies among people experiencing mental health–substance use problems (*see* Chapter 15) suggest the impact of stigma persists despite successful treatment of the condition/s, particularly with regard to contribution to the person's remaining symptoms of depression.[17] The impact of this remaining stigma can be as strong as the impact of stress and social factors such as:

➤ social support
➤ mastery
➤ stressful life events
➤ chronic stressors.[1]

In treatment studies (for example, integrated treatment for mental health–substance use problems[18,19]) depression often does not return to a non-clinical level, potentially due to losses experienced (family, friends, jobs, roles) and/or the impact of stigma in regaining esteem and functioning in their own and others' eyes.[1]

The profound impact of stigma on the individual's health, well-being and treatment outcome highlight the importance of considering and counteracting these stigma effects. This can be done on an individual level by working to avoid perpetuating public stigma, and helping the individual decrease self-stigma and its negative effects through strategies that work to increase personal empowerment. At an international level, the World Health Organization (WHO) has implemented multilevel approaches to combat stigma.[20] These include interventions to combat self-stigma as well as promoting social support and networks among individuals and families to combat isolation, including methods to enhance understanding of illness, its causes and treatment. System-wide interventions have also been utilised, to improve quality and breadth of services and addressing attitudinal tone of care for people experiencing mental ill-health, to ensure services are delivered in a way that does not compound stigma.

SELF-ASSESSMENT EXERCISE 5.3

Time: 20 minutes
- What do you know about the WHO's approaches to combating stigma?
- Review these interventions.
- Would these be helpful in your own practice?
- How would you implement these changes in your practice?

Diagnosis and treatment

Coping strategies to protect the person against public and self-stigma, such as secrecy, denial and withdrawal, are essentially undermined by the process of seeking treatment. Being assessed and diagnosed by a health professional, while being beneficial for the purpose of treatment, can lead to negative stigma effects.[17] A label once given never really goes away, and the person can never return to the point at which the SEMH was undefined and, therefore, potentially non-existent.

SELF-ASSESSMENT EXERCISE 5.4

> **Time: 5 minutes**
> Whilst denial can be a useful coping strategy initially, what could be the longer-term negative effects on the individual and the family?

For some people, seeking treatment may be akin to admitting failure or weakness. The person may have believed that the problem would get better on its own; to recover from depression they just needed to 'put their chin up' and 'get over it'.[1] Others may not have acknowledged or recognised the problem, or the symptoms of the condition may have impacted on treatment-seeking behaviour. For example, depression might impact on motivation; fear and anxiety may result in avoidance;[1] and psychosis may be associated with a lack of awareness of the need for treatment.

However, as mentioned above, many people experiencing SEMH experience clinical and personal recovery, and appropriate treatment can play a vital role. In addition, while seeking assistance risks stigma effects, effective treatment may reduce the appearance of the illness marker/s (for example, adequate management of positive symptoms, and side effects such as extra-pyramidal symptoms). However, shadowing these benefits are the losses associated with effective treatment, or attempts to find effective treatments, such as:

➤ restrictions in day-to-day life resulting from treatment regimes
➤ loss of symptoms perceived as pleasant
➤ living with side effects of medications
➤ loss of resources (such as time and money) due to cost of the treatment
➤ change to relationships precipitated through changes resulting from treatment.

Medication: friend or foe?

KEY POINT 5.6

For many, medication is presented as the dominant treatment tool, with a focus on symptom management and reduction of side effects.

For individuals experiencing SEMH, while medication is only part of the equation, one study found that 72% of respondents considered it important[21] and it has been described as a safety net to protect from relapse and re-hospitalisation.[22] When 60 individuals experiencing SEMH were asked about the things that they needed to help their recovery, 70% mentioned medication.[23] For some, medication was seen to aid recovery, in particular finding a medication that works and complying with medication. For others, medication was important as part of a larger plan; that is, taking medication in combination with services and supports, and having a say about medication. For a third of respondents, recovery would mean no longer being on medication either because it meant they were recovered from the condition, or because they no longer had to deal with the negative side effects.

In some cases, individuals experiencing SEMH describe the treatment as worse than the illness, with the potential for significant side effects, for example weight gain and lethargy. Medication can sometimes be perceived as hindering recovery. In addition, many individuals have experienced coercive treatment at some point, or pressure is placed on them to comply by well-meaning professionals, family or friends.

SELF-ASSESSMENT EXERCISE 5.5

Time: 5 minutes

Whether or not to withdraw medication due to intolerable side effects is an ethical dilemma (*see* Chapters 4 and 11).

- How might you begin to resolve such dilemmas for the individual within your care?

Dealing with co-occurring conditions

People experiencing SEMH are at higher risk of a range of other conditions, including additional mental health problems, substance use problems and physical health conditions. Post-traumatic stress disorder is common in people experiencing SEMH, but commonly overlooked.[24] Co-occurring mental health and substance use problems are very common, especially in those people attending treatment services.[25,26] Once two conditions co-exist, this can worsen the course of both conditions and can compromise the treatment response compared to either disorder alone.[27] Substance use problems are still often regarded by professionals as self-inflicted and so stigma is often greater among people experiencing this comorbidity. Treatment may be denied until substance use has ceased, which for many people is very difficult to accomplish in the absence of professional help.

SELF-ASSESSMENT EXERCISE 5.6

> **Time: 10 minutes**
> - Carefully consider the judgement values of the above statement.
> - Think how difficult it might be to have an open, non-judgemental approach.
> - How could you help yourself over this potential barrier (*see* Chapters 5 and 6)?

Self-esteem is often eroded among people experiencing SEMH by the physical health problems that often accompany SEMH. For example, weight gain associated with antipsychotic medication is common.[28] This can be particularly demoralising in young people and is associated with treatment non-compliance. Until recently, smoking was allowed in mental health treatment settings and many people experiencing SEMH have taken up smoking. Smoking is stigmatised in the wider community and therefore acts to isolate those experiencing SEMH.

Of particular concern are the poorer medical outcomes of people experiencing SEMH. Cardiovascular disease in particular is higher among people experiencing SEMH, with increased risk of death from coronary heart disease events or stroke even after controlling for smoking, antipsychotic medication and social deprivation.[29]

KEY POINT 5.7

Despite poorer mortality outcomes overall and from physical comorbidities, people experiencing SEMH are less likely to receive appropriate screening and care for physical ill-health and are often treated differently within the medical system.

Physical health care provided to people experiencing mental ill-health and/or substance use disorders has been found to be inferior to that provided to those with no comparable mental disorder.[30] Depression is increasingly recognised as a risk factor for coronary heart disease; however, people with a charted history of depression attending emergency for an acute myocardial infarction have been found to be more likely to receive a low-priority triage score and miss benchmark time for key screening and treatment procedures than people with other comorbidities.[31]

Medical problems may be misdiagnosed as being due to the psychiatric illness or drug and alcohol issues; treatment may be refused or adjusted; and stigma may be encountered. The impairments in communication (for example, thought disorder) that can accompany conditions such as chronic schizophrenia may interfere with ability to relate problems or concerns to professionals in a manner that is clearly understood. Consequently, individuals and families may avoid presenting to clinical services with problematic symptoms, or the person and/or their family may need to resort to less socially appropriate behaviours to get the person medical attention, with 'the squeaky wheel getting the oil,' which may serve to increase existing tension between the individual and the professional.[1] All of these factors can make an already stressful and challenging situation – being medically unwell – more difficult.[1] The person may feel unworthy of treatment; they or their family may experience anger at the system; or their medical situation may be more confusing and difficult for the professions to determine[1] because of the psychiatric symptoms, adding to the person's uncertainty.

Work and money

Any illness comes at high financial cost. Costs include medication and other interventions for the mental health problem. Additionally, people experiencing SEMH are at greater risk of many physical health problems, which bring additional financial burden. People experiencing SEMH may also have compromised earning ability, potentially having greater difficulty gaining and keeping employment. World Health Organization data from 19 countries found that people experiencing SEMH earned a third less than median earnings, with no significant between-country differences.[32] Employment barriers may be due to disability resulting from the condition or treatment, but can also be a consequence of public stigma such as prejudicial attitudes from employers and workmates, indirect discrimination from historical patterns of disadvantage, structural disincentive against competitive employment and generalised policy neglect.[33]

For some, loss of income or potential to earn, combined with increased costs and insufficient functional support, can lead to poverty. Poverty has a greater impact on the individual and society than simply compromising day-to-day life.[1] Poverty may be the factor that links mental disorder with social problems, such as crime, unemployment and homelessness.[34]

Conversely, employment is associated with positive outcomes for people experiencing SEMH. Working has been found to be related to increased quality of life, improved self-esteem, enhanced functioning and expanded social network, while at times of economic downturns, worse outcomes are seen for individuals experiencing schizophrenia and increases are seen in psychiatric admissions.[4] Qualitative studies with individuals experiencing SEMH support the notion that work facilitates the process of recovery by fostering pride and self-esteem, providing coping strategies for psychiatric symptoms as well as offering financial benefits.[35] Steady work has also been found to be associated with a greater decline in use of outpatient services and lower service costs.[36]

Striving for wellness while living with ill-health: hope, meaning and empowerment

Diagnosis, treatment and progression of a person experiencing SEMH can result in countless real and symbolic losses for the individual and family.[37] As mentioned previously, these losses can include:

➤ threats to identity

➤ loss of role
➤ loss of future dreams
➤ barriers to achieving 'normal' psychosocial developmental milestones of peers (e.g. individuation from family).

Individuals might lose jobs, relationships with partners, relatives and friends, and custody of children.

The mounting losses, public and self-stigma, adverse experiences of involuntary treatment (however necessary these may be), social disadvantages including isolation and loneliness, and the impact of ill-health on self-esteem that can all accompany persistent mental ill-health might lead individuals to be demoralised. Demoralisation is commonly observed in people with physical and psychiatric ill-health and is experienced as existential despair, hopelessness, helplessness and a loss of meaning and purpose in life (*see* Chapter 7).[38] Hopelessness, the hallmark symptom of demoralisation, is associated with poor outcomes in physical and psychiatric illness, and suicidal ideation and the wish to die.

KEY POINT 5.8

Loss of hope, loss of meaning and disempowerment can stand in the way of individuals living well despite having ill-health.

Becoming well, or recovery, from SEMH can refer to improvement in the condition itself as well as having a better life despite having the condition, as opposed to the notion of a 'cure' or complete recovery as might be the case for acute medical conditions. Clinical recovery might occur when professional rated improvements are seen in traditional clinical outcomes, such as diagnosis and objective measures of symptom management, remission from symptoms and improvements in psychosocial functioning. Personal recovery is the more subjective process of living a hopeful, satisfying and contributing life despite the presence of symptoms or disability.[39] Key elements identified in reaching this goal have included hope, personal responsibility, self-advocacy, wellness, empowerment, self-determination and acceptance.[40] Professionals are increasingly being encouraged to consider broader goals than symptom removal in treatment; with social, vocational and other functioning and quality of life being given greater recognition. This runs parallel with the palliative care approach.

THE PSYCHOLOGICAL IMPACT OF SEMH ON THE FAMILY

Serious and enduring mental health (SEMH) can have a profound impact on the family and close network of the individual. In addition to factors relating to the time of onset, chronicity, severity and symptom presentation of the ill-health, the impact will also vary depending on the structure and dynamics of these social networks and the role of the individual within that structure.

> **KEY POINT 5.9**
>
> Ill-health is stressful for a family and can significantly affect family relationships and roles.[1]

Existing tensions may be exacerbated and new ones arise. Old patterns of behaviour may be disrupted and over time new ones will emerge which may serve to either bring the family closer as a unit or move them further apart.[1]

When diagnosis first occurs, an initial reaction of family members might be relief that the problem is named and hope that it is not as serious as feared and will be successfully treated.[41] These temporary feelings might then be replaced by sadness and grief as awareness of the seriousness (*see* Chapter 14) of the condition increases and losses mount, including loss of the person as they knew them, loss of future hopes and dreams for the relative and the family, and changes to the family's life and relationships.[37] The increasing focus on genetic and heritable factors in mental ill-health may inadvertently accentuate guilt among family members, feeling responsible for the transmission of ill-health, and become a powerful influence on subsequent reactions to the person and their symptoms. This may be especially important among families with a transgenerational history of mental ill-health.

Family and friends are also not immune to the experience of – or the use of – stigma. They may marginalise the person within their own family or friendship network by focusing on their differences, their problems and the difficulties they cause for the family.[1] Family may experience judgement or even ostracism from their own peer group, or receive 'helpful advice' on how they 'should' handle the situation with their relative.[1] If greatly involved in the person's care, they may have to deal with health and legal systems, as well as expressed or unexpressed judgements that they are partly responsible for causing or maintaining the situation.[1] Should they choose to remove themselves from a close or carer relationship, they may then face stigma regarding their 'abandonment' of the person.[1]

People experiencing SEMH are up to 11 times more likely to be victims of violent crime[42] with the risk increasing with co-existing substance use,[43] rendering them an extremely vulnerable group. For the family, the experience of seeing their loved one become a victim of violence can be very distressing.[1]

If the individual experiencing SEMH is a parent of young children additional issues emerge.[44] Facing stigma, they may feel they have to prove themselves, and be uncertain whether the child's difficult behaviour is normal or a result of the impact of the condition on their parenting. Role strain issues, accompanied by stress and guilt, are felt by many parents – but can become exaggerated. Similarly, there can be uncertainty around whether stress experienced is normal stress experienced by parents or symptoms of the illness. They may experience conflict between the need to manage their condition versus meeting their child's needs, with the child possibly contributing to stress or even serving as a motivation to recover.

Families of people experiencing SEMH are often their primary and only support. Even when the relative lives in supported accommodation, families are identified as those who most believe in the person and their recovery.[40] Support may include provision of affection and a sense of belonging, staying actively involved, and providing emotional support, instrumental support such as assisting with activities of daily living, and financial support. Financial support may prevent the person from suffering the negative consequences of poverty. Clark[45] found that family and informal caregiver support was related to a greater reduction in substance use during treatment in people experiencing schizophrenia, and that financial support had a greater impact on reducing their substance use than did the amount of informal care given.

Particular family members may become long-term carers for their relative. Carers of people with ill-health are at increased risk of stress, burnout, physical problems and their own mental health problems, particularly depression symptoms.[1] Risk factors for caregiving burden among the family of people experiencing SEMH include:

➤ strain
➤ stigma
➤ dependence of the individual
➤ disruption to the family.[46]

Parent carers of a child experiencing SEMH reported less subjective burden and more gains if they received more assistance from their relatives.[47] Moreover, a positive relationship with the individual can be a protective factor.[48]

KEY POINT 5.10

Hope has also been a strategy identified as important for coping by relatives as well as the individual.[49]

SERIOUS AND ENDURING MENTAL HEALTH AND THE PROFESSIONAL

Dealing with any serious illness, including SEMH, can render a person vulnerable and dependent on the system of care they find themselves in. This care system has the potential to undermine an individual's identity or sense of self, particularly if the person feels that they are not being treated with dignity and respect.[6]

KEY POINT 5.11

A person is more likely to feel this way if they perceive themselves to be seen for the illness they have rather than for who they are or were as a whole person; i.e. when the whole person is not recognised, acknowledged, or affirmed.

Individuals who are not treated with dignity and respect find their sense of value undermined, feel that life no longer has worth meaning or purpose, and are more likely to feel a burden to others.[6] They may then start to question the point of continued existence.

Chochinov[50,51] writes about the notion of 'dignity conserving care', emerging from the palliative care literature but applicable across medicine in general. The A, B, C, D's of this approach:

➤ Attitude
➤ Behaviour
➤ Compassion
➤ Dialogue

. . . guide the professional to examine their internal stereotypes or assumptions towards groups of people and actions that impact on the care of the individual; they ensure their behaviours towards the person are based on:

➤ kindness and respect
➤ experiencing a deep awareness of the suffering of the person and the wish to relieve it
➤ person-centred communication strategies that aim to get to know the whole person and their story, rather than just details of the illness and symptomology.

The attitudes and beliefs of the professional shape the care received by the individual. Professionals can be vulnerable to perpetuating the stigma of mental illness. This can negatively influence their behaviour towards the individual to whom they are providing care[52] and may be a significant barrier to the provision of appropriate or best treatment. Even attitudes that are based on caution rather than negativity towards the individual can greatly influence the care of the individual and psychological well-being. If the condition is perceived as being chronic, deteriorating and associated with poor outcomes and incompetency, the professional may not offer additional interventions that may support personal and clinical recovery and increase individual empowerment, such as:

➤ encouraging the individual to be actively involved in decisions around treatment options
➤ offering talking and alternative therapies as well as medication
➤ discussing future occupational and educational opportunities.

The professional may also interpret and respond to the behaviour of the individual in varying ways depending on their beliefs and attitudes. For example, refusal by the individual to take medication or follow other treatment recommendations may lead to labelling the individual as 'difficult' or 'non-compliant'. Worsening of the condition might be blamed on the individual without consideration of the reasons behind the individual's choice to not engage in the treatment. In addition, the professional may experience feelings of anger, helplessness, or frustration, resulting in increased distance between themselves and the individual to whom they are providing care.

SELF-ASSESSMENT EXERCISE 5.7

Time: 10 minutes

With this in mind, the purpose of clinical supervision is paramount in helping explore our own negative feelings (*see* Chapter 16).

- What support is available to you in your team?
- Do you make effective use of the time allowed?

A study of veterans experiencing SEMH looking at barriers to care found that personal barriers were more often cited than were practical barriers (structural, financial, transport and distance).[53] The authors suggest this may have to do with a belief that formal treatment is ineffective or unnecessary. This suggests that individuals have internalised the stereotypes of the treatability of the condition and/or their experiences have not provided evidence that treatment does improve their overall life. These results may have also been due to perceptions of the quality of communication and their relationship with the professional.

Communication between the professional, the individual and their family is a vital tool in the therapeutic relationship from point of first contact. Better communication between the professional and individual is associated with:

➤ improved treatment adherence[54]
➤ improved individual symptom profiles[55]
➤ greater satisfaction with care.[56]

One of the major milestones in the relationship between the individual and the professional occurs at the time of communication of diagnosis. This is a challenging time not only for the individual but also for the treating professional, in whom there may be a struggle as to:

➤ the best approach balancing uncertainties about factors including accuracy of diagnosis and treatment efficacy
➤ concerns about stigma
➤ ability of the individual to process the information.

Such struggles may also intensify if experience is lacking.[57] In the case of schizophrenia, only 30%–46% of psychiatrists worldwide explicitly state the diagnosis of schizophrenia to the individual, instead using terms such as 'psychosis' or 'breakdown'.[58] However, studies suggest individuals experiencing SEMH want to be accurately informed, and improved communication can lead to greater shared decision making.[54]

SELF-ASSESSMENT EXERCISE 5.8

Time: 10 minutes

Think of your own area of work.

● How active are you in encouraging the individual to share in the decision-making process?

● How could you improve the decision-making process in your own work?

● How might you improve the decision-making process in your fellow professionals?

The importance of good communication goes beyond the time of diagnosis. A focus group with professionals and individuals experiencing SEMH revealed that professionals often referred to the notion of chronic disease management, using analogies to physical health conditions such as heart disease and diabetes.[52] Conversely, none of the individuals experiencing SEMH use the term 'chronic' to describe their ill-health. One participant commented that the focus on chronic disease management (including analogies to physical illness) without reference to the possibility of improvement or recovery made them feel like there was no hope, and therefore life was not worth living. Individuals experiencing SEMH were keen to talk about the elements of care that promoted recovery and the need for health professionals to understand the importance of the concept in structured reviews and other consultations.

The challenge of how to best balance the maintenance of hope without encouraging unrealistic expectations has been investigated in the area of terminal ill-health. A systematic review[58] revealed that although a minority of individuals, family and professionals avoided detailed information as a way to promote hope, other individuals have identified that the avoidance of negative outcomes can raise false hopes. Furthermore, if people are aware that their professional is avoiding delivering difficult information, it may be even more frightening.

KEY POINT 5.12

The majority of individuals and their family preferred the professional to be honest when providing information, and identified that honesty, when combined with sensitivity and empathy, can give hope.

Moreover, individuals and the family identified that 'being there' with the person, and treating the person as a whole, helped to maintain hope. In contrast, the family reported that difficulties communicating with professionals, feeling depersonalised, and receiving too many negative messages lead to an erosion of hope. Other ways to nurture hope included:

➤ emphasising what can be done – such as the control of physical symptoms

➤ practical support
➤ emotional support, care and dignity
➤ exploring realistic goals
➤ discussing day-to-day living.

Thus, the ethos of the palliative care approach can be applied here.

CONCLUSIONS

Mental health problems take a variety of forms, from transient and/or mild symptoms through to serious and enduring mental health problems. Serious and enduring mental health can have a profound impact on the individual and their family; however, many people experiencing SEMH do not seek or receive treatment due to perceived and actual barriers to care. Public stigma can lead to marginalisation and inequities in care, while self-stigma can:
➤ increase self-imposed isolation
➤ decrease behaviours directed towards life goals
➤ impact on involvement in and response to care.

Individuals experiencing SEMH and their families experience countless losses, including the loss of previous roles, identity and future plans, as well as the erosion of self-esteem and self-efficacy, processes that may increase the negative impact of the conditions on the person. As in the case of chronic and/or serious physical ill-health, goals of treatment will vary over time and across individuals, often with a focus on not only acute recovery, but also maintaining functioning in the face of low likelihood of complete clinical recovery. The professional can help facilitate recovery by working to address the stigma in themselves, and the system of care, as well as assisting the individual to reduce self-stigma. Dignity and hope can be fostered and maintained by using person-centred communication, knowing and treating the individual as a whole person – offering person-centred and person-led care – rather than focusing on deficit or dysfunction, and focusing on what can be done.

The approach in treating and working alongside the individual experiencing SEMH, and the approaches of humanistic care found in the palliative care approach, have been identified in this chapter. It is important to acknowledge and understand that palliative care crosses all boundaries – it is not solely for the person experiencing cancer – and can be effectively applied to any given situation within healthcare. That is, where human-to-human encounters and interventions aid well-being and potential therapeutic recovery.

REFLECTIVE PRACTICE EXERCISE 5.4

Time: 20 minutes
Take time to reflect on the following. Write down: your thoughts – how you feel – your beliefs.

- What are the main themes relating to the psychological impact of serious and enduring mental health?
- What is the impact on family and other caregivers?
- How do common forms of SEMH affect a person's functioning?
- What is stigma?
- How might stigma affect a person experiencing mental health problems in their day-to-day life? Consider family, social network, work/school, medical and mental health services.
- How can professionals reduce stigma in their interaction with the individual and family?
- How can professionals assist the individual and the family in coping with stigma?
- When working with a person experiencing SEMH, what situations might bring up feelings of frustration, anger and helplessness in a professional?
- What might be the underlying beliefs leading to these feelings?
- What might be the impact of these beliefs and feelings on the behaviour of the health professional, the individual and the family?
- What is meant by recovery-focused care and how can this be promoted?
- What strategies can promote realistic hope among people experiencing mental illness?

REFERENCES

1 Turner A, Baker AL. The psychological impact of serious illness. In: Cooper DB, editor. *Introduction to Mental Health–Substance Use.* Oxon: Radcliffe; 2011. pp. 94–106.
2 Woods A, Willison K, Kington C, *et al.* Palliative care for people with severe persistent mental illness: a review of the literature. *The Canadian Journal of Psychiatry.* 2008; **53**: 725–36.
3 Wang PS, Aguilar-Gaxiola S, Alonso J, *et al.* Use of mental health services for anxiety, mood, and substance disorders in 17 countries in the WHO world mental health surveys. *Lancet.* 2007; **370**: 841–50.
4 Warner R. Does the scientific evidence support the recovery model? *The Psychiatrist.* 2010; **34**: 3–5.
5 Warner R. *Recovery from Schizophrenia: psychiatry and political economy.* 3rd ed. East Sussex: Brunner-Routledge; 2004.
6 Wisdom JP, Bruce K, Saedi GA, Weis T, Green CA. 'Stealing me from myself': identity and recovery in personal accounts of mental illness. *Australian and New Zealand Journal of Psychiatry.* 2008; **42**: 489–95.
7 Chochinov HM, Krisjanson LJ, Hack TF, *et al.* Dignity in the terminally ill: revisited. *Journal of Palliative Medicine.* 2006; **9**: 666–72.
8 Thornicroft G, Brohan E, Rose D, *et al.* Global pattern of experienced and anticipated discrimination against people with schizophrenia: a cross-sectional survey. *Lancet.* 2009; **373**: 408–15.
9 Folkman S. Stress, coping, and hope. *Psycho-Oncology.* 2010; **19**: 901–8.
10 Sartorius N. Stigma and mental health. *Lancet.* 2007; **370**: 810–1.
11 Sartorius N, Schulze H. *Reducing the Stigma of Mental Illness: a report from a global programme of the World Psychiatric Association.* Cambridge: Cambridge University Press; 2005.
12 Corrigan PW. *On the Stigma of Mental Illness: practical strategies for research and social change.* Washington: American Psychological Association; 2005.

13 Kleinman A. Global mental health: a failure of humanity. *Lancet.* 2009; **374**: 603–4.

14 Corrigan PW, Larson JE, Rusch N. Self-stigma and the 'why try' effect: impact on life goals and evidence-based practices. *World Psychiatry.* 2009; **8**: 75–81.

15 Keusch GT, Wilentz J, Kleinman A. Stigma and global health: developing a research agenda. *Lancet.* 2006; **367**: 525–7.

16 Warner R, Taylor D, Powers M, *et al.* Acceptance of the mental illness label by psychotic patients: effects on functioning. *American Journal of Orthopsychiatry.* 1989; **59**: 398–409.

17 Link BG, Struening EL, Rahav M, *et al.* On stigma and its consequences: evidence from a longitudinal study on men with dual diagnoses of mental illness and substance abuse. *Journal of Health and Social Behavior.* 1997; **38**: 177–90.

18 Baker A, Bucci S, Lewin TJ, *et al.* Cognitive-behavioural therapy for substance use disorders in people with psychotic disorders: randomised controlled trial. *British Journal of Psychiatry.* 2006; **188**: 439–48.

19 Kay-Lambkin FJ, Baker AL, Lewin TJ, *et al.* Computer-based psychological treatment for comorbid depression and problematic alcohol and/or cannabis use: a randomized controlled trial of clinical efficacy. *Addiction.* 2009; **104**: 378–88.

20 Sartorius N. Lessons from a 10-year global programme against stigma and discrimination because of an illness. *Psychology, Health and Medicine.* 2006; **11**: 383–8.

21 Sullivan WP. A long and winding road. The process of recovery from severe mental illness. *Innovations and Research in Clinical Services, Community Support and Rehabilitation.* 1994; **3**: 19–27.

22 Svedberg B, Backenroth-Ohsako G, Lutzen K. On the path to recovery: patients' experiences of treatment with long-acting injections of antipsychotic medication. *International Journal of Mental Health Nursing.* 2003; **12**: 110–8.

23 Piat M, Sabetti J, Bloom D. The importance of medication in consumer definitions of recovery from serious mental illness: a qualitative study. *Issues in Mental Health Nursing.* 2009; **30**: 482–90.

24 Mueser KT, Goodman LB, Trumbetta SL, *et al.* Trauma and posttraumatic stress disorder in severe mental illness. *Journal of Consulting and Clinical Psychology.* 1998; **66**: 493–9.

25 Havassy BE, Alvidrez J, Owen KK. Comparisons of patients with comorbid psychiatric and substance use disorders: implications for treatment and service delivery. *American Journal of Psychiatry.* 2004; **161**: 139–45.

26 Kessler RC, Chiu WT, Demler O, *et al.* Prevalence, severity, and comorbidity of 12-month DSM-IV disorders in the National Comorbidity Survey Replication. *Archives of General Psychiatry.* 2005; **62**: 617–27.

27 Johnson J. Cost-effectiveness of mental health services for persons with a dual diagnosis: a literature review and the CCMHCP. The Cost-Effectiveness of Community Mental Health Care for Single and Dually Diagnosed Project. *Journal of Substance Abuse Treatment.* 2000; **18**: 119–27.

28 Tarricone I, Ferrari Gozzi B, Serretti A, *et al.* Weight gain in antipsychotic-naive patients: a review and meta-analysis. *Psychological Medicine.* 2010; **40**: 187–200.

29 Osborn DP, Nazareth I, King MB. Risk for coronary heart disease in people with severe mental illness: cross-sectional comparative study in primary care. *British Journal of Psychiatry.* 2006; **188**: 271–7.

30 Mitchell AJ, Malone D, Doebbeling CC. Quality of medical care for people with and without comorbid mental illness and substance misuse: systematic review of comparative studies. *British Journal of Psychiatry.* 2009; **194**: 491–9.

31 Atzema CL, Schull MJ, Tu JV. The effect of a charted history of depression on emergency

department triage and outcomes in patients with acute myocardial infarction. *Canadian Medical Association Journal.* 2011; **183**: 663–9.

32 Levinson D, Lakoma MD, Petukhova M, *et al.* Associations of serious mental illness with earnings: results from the WHO World Mental Health surveys. *British Journal of Psychiatry.* 2010; **197**: 114–21.

33 Stuart H. Mental illness and employment discrimination. *Current Opinion in Psychiatry.* 2006; **19**: 522–6.

34 Draine J, Salzer MS, Culhane DP, *et al.* Role of social disadvantage in crime, joblessness, and homelessness among persons with serious mental illness. *Psychiatric Services.* 2002; **53**: 565–73.

35 Dunn EC, Wewiorski NJ, Rogers ES. The meaning and importance of employment to people in recovery from serious mental illness: results of a qualitative study. *Psychiatric Rehabilitation Journal.* 2008; **32**: 59–62.

36 Bush PW, Drake RE, Xie H, *et al.* The long-term impact of employment on mental health service use and costs for persons with severe mental illness. *Psychiatric Services.* 2009; **60**: 1024–31.

37 Willick MS. Schizophrenia: a parent's perspective: mourning without end. In: Andreasen NC, editor. *Schizophrenia: from mind to molecule.* Washington, DC: Americal Psychiatric Press; 1994. pp. 5–19.

38 Clarke DM, Kissane DW. Demoralization: its phenomenology and importance. *Australia and New Zealand Journal of Psychiatry.* 2002; **36**: 733–42.

39 Davidson L, Roe D. Recovery from versus recovery in serious mental illness: one strategy for lessening confusion plaguing recovery. *Journal of Mental Health.* 2007; **16**: 459–70.

40 Piat M, Sabetti J, Fleury MJ, *et al.* 'Who believes most in me and in my recovery': the importance of families for persons with serious mental illness living in structured community housing. *Journal of Social Work in Disability and Rehabilitation.* 2011; **10**: 49–65.

41 Ozgul S. Parental grief and serious mental illness: a narrative. *Australia and New Zealand Journal of Family Therapy.* 2004; **25**: 183–7.

42 Teplin LA, McClelland GM, Abram KM, *et al.* Crime victimization in adults with severe mental illness: comparison with the National Crime Victimization Survey. *Archives of General Psychiatry.* 2005; **62**: 911–21.

43 Hiday VA, Swartz MS, Swanson JW, *et al.* Criminal victimization of persons with severe mental illness. *Psychiatric Services.* 1999; **50**: 62–8.

44 Nicholson J, Sweeney EM, Geller JL. Mothers with mental illness: I. The competing demands of parenting and living with mental illness. *Psychiatric Services.* 1998; **49**: 635–42.

45 Clark RE. Family support and substance use outcomes for persons with mental illness and substance use disorders. *Schizophrenia Bulletin.* 2001; **27**: 93–101.

46 Zauszniewski JA, Bekhet AK, Suresky MJ. Effects on resilience of women family caregivers of adults with serious mental illness: the role of positive cognitions. *Archives of Psychiatric Nursing.* 2009; **23**: 412–22.

47 Aschbrenner KA, Greenberg JS, Allen SM, *et al.* Subjective burden and personal gains among older parents of adults with serious mental illness. *Psychiatric Services.* 2010; **61**: 605–11.

48 Pickett SA, Cook JA, Cohler BJ, *et al.* Positive parent/adult child relationships: impact of severe mental illness and caregiver burden. *American Journal of Orthopsychiatry.* 1997; **67**: 220–30.

49 Nordby K, Kjonsberg K, Hummelvoll JK. Relatives of persons with recently discovered serious mental illness: in need of support to become resource persons in treatment and recovery. *Journal of Psychiatric and Mental Health Nursing.* 2010; **17**: 304–11.

50 Chochinov HM. Dignity-conserving care – a new model for palliative care: helping the patient feel valued. *Journal of the American Medical Association.* 2002; **287**: 2253–60.

51 Chochinov HM. Dignity and the essence of medicine: the A, B, C, and D of dignity-conserving care. *British Medical Journal.* 2007; **335**: 184–7.

52 Lester H, Tritter JQ, Sorohan H. Patients' and health professionals' views on primary care for people with serious mental illness: focus group study. *British Medical Journal.* 2005; **330**: 1122.

53 Drapalski AL, Milford J, Goldberg RW, *et al.* Perceived barriers to medical care and mental health care among veterans with serious mental illness. *Psychiatric Services.* 2008; **59**: 921–4.

54 Deegan PE, Drake RE. Shared decision making and medication management in the recovery process. *Psychiatric Services.* 2006; **57**: 1636–9.

55 Little P, Everitt H, Williamson I, *et al.* Observational study of effect of patient centredness and positive approach on outcomes of general practice consultations. *British Medical Journal.* 2001; **323**: 908–11.

56 Brody DS, Miller SM, Lerman CE, *et al.* The relationship between patients' satisfaction with their physicians and perceptions about interventions they desired and received. *Medical Care.* 1989; **27**: 1027–35.

57 Levin TT, Kelly BJ, Cohen M, *et al.* Case studies in public-sector leadership: using a psychiatry e-list to develop a model for discussing a schizophrenia diagnosis. *Psychiatric Services.* 2011; **62**: 244–6.

58 Clayton JM, Hancock K, Parker S, *et al.* Sustaining hope when communicating with terminally ill patients and their families: a systematic review. *Psycho-Oncology.* 2008; **17**: 641–59.

TO LEARN MORE

- Andreasen NC, editor. *Schizophrenia: from mind to molecule.* Washington, DC: American Psychiatric Press; 1994.
- Kleinman, A. *The Illness Narratives: suffering, healing, and the human condition.* New York: Basic Books; 1988.
- Corrigan P. *On Stigma and Mental Illness: practical strategies for research and social change.* American Psychological Association; 2004.
- The Lancet Global Mental Health Series, 2007, September 3. Available at: www.thelancet.com/series/global-mental-health# (accessed 19 April 2012).
- Stigma-related sites and resources. Available at: www.stopstigma.samhsa.gov/ (accessed 19 April 2012).
- www.rcpsych.ac.uk/campaigns/changingminds/whatisstigma/mentaldisorderschallenging.aspx (accessed 19 April 2012).
- Mind, for better mental health (UK). Available at: www.mind.org.uk/ (accessed 19 April 2012).
- National Institute of Mental Health (US). Available at: www.nimh.nih.gov/index.shtml (accessed 19 April 2012).
- National Institute for Health and Clinical Excellence (UK), Mental health and behavioural conditions guidelines. Available at: http://guidance.nice.org.uk/Topic/MentalHealthBehavioural (accessed 19 April 2012).
- beyondblue, the national depression initiative, Australia. Available at: www.beyondblue.org.au (accessed 19 April 2012).
- SANE Australia. Available at: www.sane.org/ (accessed 19 April 2012).

CHAPTER 6

Caring relationships

Jo Cooper

COMMENT

The case representations are in the first person to emphasise the human interactions between two people and the caring relationship that has evolved.

KEY POINT 6.1

- The terms 'caring' and 'therapeutic' are interchangeable. Whilst therapeutic is the acknowledged professional term, caring relates to the premise of a human relationship.

LEARNING OUTCOMES

➤ Understand the elements of a caring (therapeutic) relationship.
➤ Define the terms 'therapeutic' and 'relationship'.
➤ Recognise the importance of being human.
➤ Understand how caring with dignity and respect underpins the relationship.

INTRODUCTION

This chapter will focus on:
➤ the meaning of the caring (therapeutic) relationship
➤ our understanding of this relationship.

The work we do is primarily concerned with the essence and quality of the relationships we make, whether this is with the individual, the family, carers or professionals. It is not something that we *do* to people. It is a way of *being*, and should be part of our everyday life with each other: a human-to-human experience.

The essence of the relationship is the engagement ... the desire to follow an understanding of where the person *is* in his or her situation and how she or he *perceives* this situation.[1] Such relationships have been described as being rewarding for both parties, and the reciprocal nature of the relationship should reduce rather than increase risk of burnout in the professional. When working in the palliative care-mental health field, where we meet the distress and suffering of those we care for on a daily basis, the risk of emotional burnout is high (*see* Chapter 16).

There are two aspects to consider in the theory and practice of caring. For the individual, we are both professionals and fellow human beings. In the context of caring, we must use both aesthetic and empirical knowledge to understand and manage ill-health, together with an understanding of the person as a unique individual.

KEY POINT 6.2

- A fundamental premise of 'caring' is that professionals use themselves as the therapeutic instrument.[2]

The reason for this strong emphasis on the therapeutic relationship is the fact that when people are ill, they often have problems in communicating and forming relationships.[3]

By definition, the relationship needs both professional and personal closeness in order for a meaningful connection to be made. However, there must be a balance between human closeness and professional distance.[4]

REFLECTIVE PRACTICE EXERCISE 6.1

Time: 15 minutes
- What does the term 'caring (therapeutic) relationship' mean to you?
- Think about a person in your care whom you have worked with recently and with whom you had a good relationship. Consider:
  — what made it 'good'?
  — why was it different from other relationships?

What does the term 'therapeutic relationship' mean?

The word 'therapy' comes from the Greek word *therapeia*, meaning to care. The word 'relationship' comes from the Latin *relatus*, which denotes a 'connection'. Therefore, to work effectively with the individual and their family, we need to make a caring connection.[5] There is potential for the professional to act as the 'therapeutic tool'. The therapeutic nature of the relations is not so much *what* we say, but *how* we say it. It is a set of behaviours around a way of 'being', which should be practised in our everyday life. The relationship is dependent on the effectiveness of our interpersonal communication, both verbal and non-verbal. *How* we say something is often more important than the words we use.

In her seminal work on relationships, Muetzel[6] provides us with a simple framework which clarifies the elements within the relationship:

➤ reciprocity
➤ intimacy
➤ partnership.

These elements make up the caring process. Communication and interpersonal skills link the elements forming dynamic fluidity. In addition, it has been proposed that the *condition* of . . .

➤ genuineness
➤ empathy
➤ unconditional positive regard[7]

. . . are central to the therapeutic relationship.

REFLECTIVE PRACTICE EXERCISE 6.2

Time: 5 minutes
- Is there anything that you would like to add?
- Consider the possibility of adding compassion, dignity and respect.

RECIPROCITY

REFLECTIVE PRACTICE EXERCISE 6.3

Time: 10 minutes
- In reviewing the elements of Muetzel's[6] framework, consider the meaning of 'reciprocity'.
- How does this fit with your idea of the *caring relationship*?

The people for whom we care are constantly negotiating with us. They want to know a little about us as people. *Can I relate to this person? Can I trust them? How can they help me?* It is about making the connection; investing in the relationship, being 'in touch' and entering their world.[8] Exploring their situation, being available and making a quick response are central to connecting. We could say that reciprocity is about sharing together. It needs us to remain functional and not fall 'into the pit', while acknowledging and understanding the pain and distress of another.

REFLECTIVE PRACTICE EXERCISE 6.4

Time: 5 minutes
- What might you share with this person?
- Consider what is and what is not appropriate to share.

Often all we have is ourselves, and simply saying . . . *Thank you, I can see how hard that was for you* . . . is sufficient. It is more important to genuinely care than to get the right words.

In examining the concept of reciprocity, one author suggests its therapeutic properties lie in its mutual exchange, an action or relation given in return. In assuming therapeutic value, reciprocity becomes positive in its effect for both the professional and the individual in terms of sharing.[9]

We can share everyday events, something simple and ordinary. The acknowledgement of another's feelings and difficulties shows that we are *present* . . . that we have heard. This helps the individual to feel understood and legitimises their feelings. Being present to, and in contact with, the other person is at the heart of the caring relationship.[10] *Presencing* highlights the need to think of communication as more than just speaking. We all communicate differently: sometimes by just being 'present' and saying nothing. Silence is useful and of great value. It allows the gathering of thoughts, giving both sides the time to reflect and consider. It is a *mindful* silence. It is tempting to fill every silence with words. However, we need to step back [*silence*], allowing the person space to hear themself.

REFLECTIVE PRACTICE EXERCISE 6.5

Time: 5 minutes
- Reflect on the word 'present'.
- Think about absence of presence.
- How could you show someone you are present?

Sometimes, being present just involves sitting with someone, saying very little, being silent. This is not an empty silence but, rather, contains acceptance and understanding. It lets the person know that you value them and what they are telling you about their experience. It also tells the person, without words, that you know they must struggle to find their own words.[11] As you listen and give attention they will begin to trust you not to rush in with thoughtless words.

KEY POINT 6.3

People take a risk when they share their feelings with us.

REFLECTIVE PRACTICE EXERCISE 6.6

Time: 15 minutes
- With a colleague, discuss how your silence with an individual you are 'caring' for is different from the silence of people just sitting in a waiting area.
- Try to think of the *quality* of your silence and how this could be helpful.

The reciprocity of sharing

Case study 6.1

Bob was dying. He had metastatic prostate carcinoma. He was referred for management of intractable pain. He had been a keen gardener and every year had grown runner beans in his small garden. On one visit, Bob was showing his wife Gill how to plant the beans as he was no longer able to do this. I shared with him how much I had always wanted to grow them, but did not know where to start. Bob carefully explained to me exactly what I needed to know, sharing his knowledge generously with me. Later I planted my beans, not really expecting great results. On each of my visits to Bob, he would ask, with great interest, how they were doing and always wanted to know if they were as good as his! I was able to share my stories about how the beans were coming along, what I should have done to them; how I forgot last night to water them; how my granddaughters had loved to pick them for dinner, etc. Bob and I shared a mutual interest unrelated to his medical diagnosis. It provided an opportunity for our relationship to grow; he learned to trust me and found out a little about what sort of a person I was, without my disclosing any 'personal' information. In a big way, this made it a little easier for Bob to disclose some of his own distress and fears around dying. I was not just the professional; I was also a human being. I had knowledge (about Bob's condition and treatment needed); Bob had knowledge that I did not have (about growing vegetables!). I told Bob that I would never forget him – for many reasons. Mostly because of his inordinate faith and courage and also for sharing his knowledge with me about growing runner beans. In turn, he thanked me for taking an interest and being a good 'student'. Long after his death, the story of the beans remains with Gill, his wife, and will always remain with me.

Reciprocity does not mean that we share everything about ourselves. This would not be helpful to the relationship. Some basic essentials for caring encounters lie within the nature of being human. Human qualities are ordinary in that they are commonplace. The foundations of genuine helping lie in being ordinary, 'nothing special'.[12] The relationship requires us to think about ourselves: who we are, and what we are. It gives us the opportunity of self-reflection, a chance to be honest with what and whom we see. If we have a guest in our house, we remember to act with courtesy and respect for our guest. The same principles can be applied to those we care for.

Ordinariness has been offered as having the potential to describe everyday human qualities and activities. When professionals and individuals were 'just themselves' in clinical settings, they were happier with each other. Ordinariness is therapeutic, through the effects of genuine human relationships.[12] There is reciprocity in *allowingness*. Allowing individuals to disclose or not to disclose if they so wish. We have an opportunity of opening up possibilities for connectedness, because the everyday dramas of caring for ill and unhappy people encourage us to put aside our own feelings of importance and superiority. The foundation for this related connection lies in the authenticity of the helping relationship. It starts and ends with being open and honest not only with our own self but with other professionals with whom we work.

DIGNITY

Caring with dignity ensures that we not only value our own self-worth but that we acknowledge and value those for whom we give care, and for colleagues within the intra- and inter-professional team.

REFLECTIVE PRACTICE EXERCISE 6.7

> **Time: 20 minutes**
> - How do you interpret dignity?
> - What does it mean to you?
> - How can we *care* with dignity?
> - What changes do you need to make?
> - Think about how you would like to be treated and cared for.
> - If you were receiving care and were treated with lack of respect, how might this leave you feeling?

Dignity means we care about that person – she or he matters – and about what happens to him or her. We value that person's abilities, feelings and ideas and treat her or him in a way which shows that that person has worth.

Treating people with respect allows them to make their own choices – or at least to be helped to do so – giving them privacy, and treating older people like adults and not like children. We have to try to understand how traumatic some people's lives are and not sit in judgement of them.

> **KEY POINT 6.4**
>
> Every person has the right to be treated as a human being – with compassion, dignity and respect.

PARTNERSHIP

REFLECTIVE PRACTICE EXERCISE 6.8

Time: 20 minutes
- What do you think partnership involves?
- Think about your association within the caring relationship.
- How were you a partner in the care you gave?
- What made this a partnership?
- How might you gain from the partnership?
- Is the partnership an equal one?
- What happens to the balance of power?
- Is there a difference in caring for the individual in their home, as opposed to caring for them on the hospital ward?
- Consider the individual's need for privacy.
- How might we invade this?

Muetzel[6] considers partnership as a working association between two parties, implying a gain for both sides. There is so much gain for us when working with individuals and their families. If we remain open, we can learn so much; people have much to teach us. In the case of 'Bob', knowledge was gained, not only on a practical level, but insightful knowledge on how a person copes when their world is threatened. In turn, this helps when working with others, and when you can say . . . *Yes, your feelings are a normal reaction – other people often feel like this too* . . . you can reduce emotional isolation, normalising and validating their own perceptions and feelings.

Often the little things count. Benner[13] describes these as the 'hallmark of [professional] expertise':
➤ **making someone comfortable** – takes time and is a skill in itself
➤ **helping the person to eat or drink** – a fundamental, rather than a basic skill, often dismissed as basic and often an underused skill
➤ **admiring a family photo** – part of making the connection
➤ **accepting the offer of a cup of tea** – says I am not rushing off; I am here to listen
➤ **attention to detail** – psychological, emotional, physical, spiritual and financial
➤ **sitting quietly with someone** – words are not always necessary
➤ **giving our full attention** – eye-to-eye contact, listening and responding
➤ **being respectful** – about cultures different from our own (*see* Chapter 3).

All these help to build a relationship of trust, of emotionally engaging with another.

KEY POINT 6.5

The provision of comfort may be a part, and an expression, of caring and within the relationship it is a key function.[5]

These functions are therapeutic beyond their physical effect. They provide psychological and emotional comfort and are an expression of 'caring'. Development of these skills is essential if we are to work therapeutically and effectively with those in our care. It has been suggested that individuals put a high value on physical comfort and information sharing.[14] Information sharing, with the focus not only on what is shared but on how and when, is perceived as being an important enabler in the development of both optimal therapeutic relationships and care outcomes.[15] Being honest and genuine when sharing information was also perceived as important.

We cannot claim to know what is 'best' for people. We are human ourselves, and have many failings. We can only be alongside and help the person to choose what he or she feels is best. We can show respect in acknowledging that each individual has the right to choose what is best for them and their family. Each person travels their own unique journey, and has a story to tell, if they choose.

Whenever possible we encourage the person to work alongside us in planning their care; after all, it affects them. Their road to recovery may encounter many difficult setbacks. Hope is an important enabler in fostering a sense of optimism and achievement (*see* Chapter 7). This is very difficult when a person feels at their most hopeless, and it lies with us to maintain a sense of hope, even when things seem hopeless.

INTIMACY

REFLECTIVE PRACTICE EXERCISE 6.9

Time: 5 minutes
- What do you think intimacy involves?
- Is this an area that you have given thought to?

Intimacy implies closeness, a friendship – both professional and compassionate. It is about having the opportunity to have meaningful communication, the central focus to the relationship. Acting as an authentic person with competence as a professional and as a person does not mean that the relationship is a friendship.[20] A true friendship is characterised by mutuality. Each party has equal rights and obligations for the needs of the other. In contrast, the needs of the individual are the primary concern. Emotional closeness is based on trust, not exclusiveness. There is no ownership. Sometimes, as professionals, we behave as if we own the person for whom we are caring. This approach is unhelpful and not therapeutic, even though it is probably based on our innate need to provide loving care for that individual. Working together within the professional team, attending supervision and self-reflection, helps us to maintain emotional equilibrium, so that we share more openly, and address together, the needs of the individual.

Intimacy is about being human, about treating the other with respect, dignity and compassion; much how we would like to be treated ourselves. We do not have to have all the answers or have to be something that we are not. It is about getting close to the world of the individual, formed often by the caring and intimate physical care, which often provides opportunities and a level of trust that supports emotional closeness.

REFLECTIVE PRACTICE EXERCISE 6.10

> **Time: 5 minutes**
> Reflect on what being 'human' means to you.

Perhaps our human purpose is to provide warmth, companionship and acceptance of our fellow women and men, rather than trying to control, contain or 'fix' them.[17]

Insight into our own vulnerabilities and limitations will teach us that we cannot 'fix' the other person's problems. We cannot make their world, their life, their ill-health or their death different. We can only be 'alongside'. It is their journey, their story, and they are taking big courageous steps in sharing it with us. It is in this sharing and within our listening that takes place that we can make a difference. Some people feel that they have never been truly heard.

Can we make people 'feel' better, rather than 'get' better?

We can be 'ourselves', giving something of ourselves, working alongside that person, listening with compassion, and understanding from within. In order to practise an act of compassion, we need to be compassionate to ourselves. It is easy to forget our own needs when we are dealing with the grief and distress of others, but it is by looking after ourselves that we maintain emotional stamina needed to care for others. Acknowledge and accept our own weaknesses and vulnerabilities, learning from our fears and our own personal distress.

REFLECTIVE PRACTICE EXERCISE 6.11

> **Time: 10 minutes**
> - Think deeply about compassion, dignity and respect.
> - What do these things mean to you?
> - How can we practise compassion, dignity and respect – for ourselves and for others?
> - What is the difference between pity and compassion?

It is not simply warmth of heart, or a sharp clarity of recognition of the individual's needs and pain, it is also a sustained and practical determination to do whatever is necessary and possible to help alleviate suffering.[18] Suffering has been described as a state of severe distress caused by events that threaten the integrity of a person.[19] Suffering is an inevitable and inescapable part of life, for the individual, for their family and for ourselves. Although pain is often associated with physical hurt, the perception of the discomfort is always modified by the person's cognitive and emotional reaction.[20] Therefore, what we think must be a major cause of suffering for the individual may not be so. It is important not to assume. It can be helpful to ask . . . *What causes you the most suffering at the moment?*

> **KEY POINT 6.6**
>
> Suffering, distress, grief – all human experiences – sometimes offer an opportunity for learning and change.

When an individual is deeply distressed, their ability to see or to think clearly is often impaired. With a confused and often tormented mind, they are often unable to express verbally their troubled thoughts. Sometimes, it can be helpful to ask . . . *What do you feel in your heart?* We know what is in our heart, even if our mind is chaotic and confused.

Case study 6.2

Harry lived in a mobile home. He had few possessions, and his home was his pride and joy. He was elderly, frail, ill and intermittently confused. He had no family and had been a loner throughout his life. It was clear that he could not remain in his home and needed full-time care. It was such a tremendously difficult decision for Harry to make. He had no one to guide or help him make the decision and it was difficult for him to see a future outside of his home.

He was bewildered and at a loss as to how to express his obvious grief and sadness. His mind was in turmoil. One day as we sat together, I asked, 'What do you feel in your heart Harry?' He sat for several moments as if he had not really heard me, then looked directly at me and, with a degree of resignation, acknowledged that the time had come for him to be cared for.

This does not work every time. It was helpful for Harry. It is about *knowing* something about the person you are working with, and taking a risk, in order to help reduce emotional distress. It is also about truthfulness. As professionals, we were honest with Harry about his social and medical situation; we did not want to destroy his hope or make him feel that he had 'no choice'. Truth is one of the most powerful therapeutic agents available to us, but we need to develop a proper understanding of its clinical pharmacology, and to recognise optimum timing and dosage in its use.[21] Sometimes, it is wiser to be kind, rather than give the stark and painful truth. This is not about lying to the person but encouraging reflection, enabling the answer to be delivered in a more thoughtful way.

In palliative care-mental health, often on a daily basis, we work alongside despairing and distressed individuals. In order to work closely with them, we need to repair and maintain our own mental and physical well-being. We try to avoid thoughts of having serious ill-health for ourselves, of body or mind. Ill-health, such as those affecting mental or physical health, disrupts life, destroying our hopes and dreams for our future . . . taking away our meaning of life as we understand it. In our own mind, we each hold a picture of our assumed future, as we would like it to be. We have hopes and dreams for our future, which become the foundation for a 'certain' way of living. However, nothing in life is certain – only the finality of it. We live only with the illusion of certainty. It is important that we focus on the *person* and not on the ill-health.

Being able to think about our own feelings and being able to imagine the feeling of others is the cognitive basis for empathy and understanding.[11]

REFLECTIVE PRACTICE EXERCISE 6.12

Time: 15 minutes
- Think about a time in your life that was painful. Try to recall the event.
- Think about how other people responded.
- What was helpful? What was not helpful?
- Consider both the practical and emotional elements.
- Notice what feelings arise in you.
- Think about how using your own experience could help you to work alongside others, using the components of compassion and empathy.

FINDING MEANING

REFLECTIVE PRACTICE EXERCISE 6.13

Time: 5 minutes
Consider how you find meaning and purpose in your own life

Ill-health often provides strength and opportunities for change. People work hard to make sense of their situation. In working alongside, we try to help this process by exploring difficulties and dilemmas. In providing a space for the person to talk, they will often find their own answers. Speaking openly about a problem is often liberating. Exploration helps in the development of coping strategies and saying something like . . . *Tell me what is the worst thing for you – at the moment?* . . . stops us from assuming that we know and understand that person's problem before we have thoroughly explored it. Sometimes, people and families have differing goals, or make different choices, causing family tensions and conflict to arise. Respectful and compassionate negotiation between the parties will allow each person to say how they feel; expressing their thoughts, hopes and expectations, enabling family unity and thereby reducing tensions. This is not as simple as it may sound. It takes a great deal of time, patience, effort, tolerance and understanding.[22]

Where the relationship is therapeutic, the authentic exchange transforms care into shared experiences that can produce positive growth. Where shared meanings and experiences are positive ones, genuine caring will take place, generating caring relations for those concerned. When acknowledging the difficulties of another person, we show that we have heard and understood.

KEY POINT 6.7

The most important point is that the individual feels heard, understood and accepted in the place where *they are* at that moment in time – not where *we think* they are.

Valuing the individual, and ourselves, is the overriding concept in any relationship. Treating people with respect because they are human maintains a supportive relationship. Each person is *worthwhile*.

How can we respect those in our care?

REFLECTIVE PRACTICE EXERCISE 6.14

Time: 5 minutes
How can we show simple respect for those in our care?

This comes down to the small, perhaps seemingly insignificant things that are nevertheless important. They include the following.
➤ **Introduce** ourselves by name.
➤ **Ask** each individual how she or he would like to be addressed.
➤ **Remember** the individual's name.
➤ **Give full attention** – people know if we check our watch.
➤ **Do not interrupt or talk over the individual.**
➤ **Do not assume you know what the individual will say** – do not finish the individual's sentence.
➤ **Do not assume you know best** – help the individual to make his or her own choices and decisions.
➤ **Do give cultural considerations** the importance they deserve – if you do not know, ask or find out.

> **KEY POINT 6.8**
>
> The ethical foundation of the caring relationship is grounded in a sincere respect for the dignity of human life.[23]

LISTENING

As part of the communication process, listening is at the heart of therapeutic caring. The focus must be on what the person is telling us, both by their verbal and non-verbal language. It is only by truly listening, clearing our mind of our own concerns and thoughts, that we will hear clearly what is being said. If we feel anxious about what we are going to say or do next, or we are not mindfully relaxed, we will fail to hear and to see how we can help. Sometimes, the best option is to do nothing. We will often not have a solution. This does not mean that we do not make a response to what we have heard. Having no solution is not the same as having no response; responses may be more profound than answers.[24] Even when we have no answer to questions posed, always something can be done, such as *being there*. Questions can be talked about and explored, even if not answered with finality – using the words:

➤ **How** – do you feel you are coping at the moment: how have you coped in the past?
➤ **Why** – did you cry just then?
➤ **What** – does this mean for you?

People value us for our *presence*, just as much as for our knowledge and our skills:

> **Case study 6.3**
>
> Frank was very ill. He no longer wanted or needed to talk. Management of his physical, emotional, spiritual and psychological symptoms had been a priority. He had done all his talking in the last few months. Was there a need to visit? What could reasonably be achieved at this stage? He was settled and stable. I asked the family how they felt about further visits. Were further visits needed? Would they be too intrusive? Their response was: 'You may not be needed, but you are wanted and we would value it, so yes please.'

PHYSICAL CONNECTEDNESS

How and where we sit in a room makes a difference to how we interact with the people present. Can we see each other properly? Can we give appropriate eye contact? Sitting close to someone reduces physical barriers and enables the use of appropriate touch. Holding a hand while we listen says . . . *we are here and we understand* . . . standing at the foot of the bed or by the door *does not*.

Listening is a skill, which takes *time*. It is time well spent and is the basis for a relationship of mutual trust and support. When we are busy, it is easy to concentrate on *doing* rather than *being*, and often easier to do a task, rather than *sit* with pain and distress. Closely linked to the tenet of holistic care, listening is characterised by a climate of trust and a sense of being with the person, rather than merely the performance of caring tasks.[25]

KEY POINT 6.9

If we do not ask, we will not know. We should not underestimate the value of listening.

Case study 6.4

John had worked as a mercenary, working almost alone. It had been a solitary life and one where he had ended many lives. His own life was now coming to the end. John carried an enormous amount of unexpressed guilt. I asked him what he found the most helpful. His response was ... *'Being listened to!'* ... *'You are like a little bird. You fly in, sit calmly on my bed, listen to all my worries and problems. Then, you go. And I feel better!'*

REFLECTIVE PRACTICE EXERCISE 6.15

Time: 5 minutes
- Reflect on the possible distractions to listening.
- Consider both external and internal distractions.
- Think about your own feelings, attitudes and behaviours.

The art of compassionate caring requires us to be still and to listen. Sometimes people will time the asking of questions when they sense you have no time to answer or to explore. You have your hand on the door ready to go; you have children to meet from school or you are on a busy ward and another person is in need of attention. Rather than answering in haste, say that you will explore that at a later date or time. It may be better to take time for reflection and come back to the person when you can give full attention to the matter.[26] However, we must make sure that we do revisit that situation as soon as possible, even if that means returning later in the day.

When we are really ourselves, as authentic beings, and when we truly listen, something happens. Listening is *not* a passive exercise ... we have to act on what we have heard.

KEY POINT 6.10

The use of silence gives us time to reflect and think about what is needed.

REFLECTIVE PRACTICE EXERCISE 6.16

> **Time: 5 minutes**
> • Think about what it means to be authentic and to have an authentic relationship.
> • How could this enhance your practice?

One of the consequences of a caring relationship is the trust gained for each party; both in their own ability to relate effectively in the help-seeking situation, and to each other as fellow human beings.[9]

SUPPORT FOR OURSELVES

Working in intensive situations with both individuals and families in the palliative care-mental health setting creates demands on us. We have to find ways to support and maintain our own integrity. We must have belief in our own worth. Formal and informal supervision from peers will enable difficult issues to be worked through.

Supervision should be actively pursued, demonstrating commitment to improving practice and providing the very best service to the people we work alongside. It provides the opportunity for us to reflect deeply on our practice and ourselves and explore what is happening in our relationships with others. This openness is the prerequisite for true learning and for the relationship with people to be in any sense therapeutic. The ability to 'simply' sit with painful or distressing feelings is the mark of a competent professional. Understanding the need for, and the value of, silences means they are no longer threatening and we can provide a reassuring presence for people who are struggling.

CONCLUSION

> **KEY POINT 6.11**
>
> Those in our care are our teachers – if we are open, there is much we can learn.

Learn to have the courage to accompany others as they experience unknown and often scary territory. Engaging fully in the supervision process, either on a one-to-one basis, or within the group setting, is one way of doing this. This leads to greater understanding of ourselves and gives meaning to the way in which we act. In understanding our own failings and vulnerabilities, we learn how to move forward, creating a caring relationship with others.

Caring for individuals in distress needs *knowledge, skills, attention to detail, respect and compassion* for our fellow human beings. It also requires respect for their *dignity*. The *attitude* to work both professionally (empirical knowledge) and from the heart (aesthetic knowledge) must be one that creates a deep sense of compassion. It is working from the heart that enables therapeutic relating to take place.

REFERENCES

1 Berg WK, Wacker DP, Cigrand K, *et al.* Comparing functional analysis and paired-choice assessment results in classroom settings. *Journal of Applied Behavior Analysis.* 2007; **40**: 545–52.

2 Hem MH, Heggen K. Being professional and being human: one nurse's relationship with a psychiatric patient. *Journal of Advanced Nursing.* 2003; **43**: 101–8.

3 Peplau H. Interpersonal relations: a theoretical framework for application in nursing practice. *Nursing Science Quarterly.* 1992; **5**: 13–8.

4 Strand L. *Fra kaos mot samling, mestring og helhet. Psykiatrisk sykepleie til psykotiske pasienter.* [From chaos to wholeness and empowerment. Professional care of psychotic patients.] Oslo, Norway: Gyldendal; 1990.

5 McMahon R, Pearson A. *Nursing as a Therapy.* 2nd ed. Gloucester: Stanley Thornes; 1998.

6 Muetzel PA. Therapeutic nursing. In: Pearson A, editor. *Primary Nursing: nursing in the Burford and Oxford Nursing Development Unit.* London: Croom Helm; 1988.

7 Rogers C. *Dialogues.* London: Constable; 1990.

8 Davies B, Oberle K. Dimensions of the supportive role of the nurse in palliative care. *Oncology Nursing Forum.* 1990; **17**: 87–94.

9 Marck P. Therapeutic reciprocity: a caring phenomenon. *Advances in Nursing Science.* 1990; **13**: 49–59.

10 Kirby C. The therapeutic relationship. In: Basford L, Slevin O, editors. *Theory and Practice of Nursing: an integrated approach to caring practice.* 2nd ed. Gloucester: Nelson Thornes; 2003.

11 Lendrum S, Syme G. *Gift of Tears: a practical approach to loss and bereavement in counselling and psychotherapy.* Sussex: Routledge; 2004.

12 Taylor BJ. Ordinariness in nursing. In: McMahon R, Pearson A, editors. *Nursing as a Therapy.* Gloucester: Stanley Thornes; 1998.

13 Benner P. *From Novice to Expert: excellence and power in clinical practice.* Menlo Park, CA: Addison-Wesley; 1984.

14 Skilbeck J, Payne S. Emotional support and the role of clinical nurse specialist in palliative care. *Journal of Advanced Nursing.* 2003; **43**: 521–30.

15 Seymour J, Ingleton C, Payne S, *et al.* Specialist palliative care: patients' experiences. *Journal of Advanced Nursing.* 2003; **44**: 24–33.

16 Martocchio BC. Authenticity, belonging, emotional closeness, and self representation. *Oncology Nursing Forum.* 1997; **14**: 23–7.

17 Barker P, Buchanan-Barker P. Mental health in an age of celebrity: the courage to care. *Medical Humanities.* 2008; **34**: 110–14.

18 Rinpoche S. *The Tibetan Book of Living and Dying.* Gaffney P, Harvey A, editors. London: Rider; 1992.

19 Cassell EJ. *The Nature of Suffering and the Goals of Medicine.* Oxford: Oxford University Press; 1991.

20 Twycross R. *Introducing Palliative Care*. Oxford: Radcliffe Medical Press; 2003.

21 Simpson M, as cited in: Twycross R. Death without suffering? *European Journal of Palliative Care*. 2005; **12**: 14–17.

22 Benner P, Wrubel J. *The Primacy of Caring: stress and coping in health and illness*. Menlo Park, CA: Addison-Wesley; 1988.

23 Kirby C. The therapeutic relationship. In: Cooper J, editor. *Stepping into Palliative Care: relationships and responses*. 2nd ed. Oxford: Radcliffe; 2006.

24 Lunn L. Having no answer. In: Saunders C, editor. *Hospice and Palliative Care: an interdisciplinary approach*. London: Edward Arnold; 1990.

25 Canning D, Rosenberg JP, Yates P. Therapeutic relationships in specialist palliative care nursing practice. *International Journal of Palliative Nursing*. 2007; **13**: 222–9.

26 Houtepen R, Hendrikx D. Nurses and the virtues of dealing with existential questions in terminal palliative care. *Nursing Ethics*. 2003; **10**: 377–87.

TO LEARN MORE

- Barker P, editor. *Mental Health Ethics: the human context*. Abingdon: Routledge; 2011.
- Cooper J. *Stepping into Palliative Care: relationships and responses*. 2nd ed. Oxford: Radcliffe; 2006.
- Dignity in Care Network. Available at: www.dignityincare.org.uk/ (accessed 19 April 2012).
- Hurley J, Linsley P, editors. *Emotional Intelligence in Health and Social Care: a guide for improving human relationships*. London/New York: Radcliffe; 2012.
- Jeffrey D. *Patient-centred Ethics and Communications at the End of Life*. Oxford: Radcliffe; 2006.
- Kirby C. The therapeutic relationship. In: Basford L, Slevin D, editors. *Theory and Practice of Nursing: an integrated approach to caring practice*. 2nd ed. Gloucester: Nelson Thornes; 2003.
- Lendrum S, Syme G. *Gift of Tears*. 2nd ed. London: Routledge; 2004.
- McMahon R, Pearson A. *Nursing as Therapy*. 2nd ed. Cheltenham: Stanley Thornes; 1998.
- NHS Confederation. *Commission on Improving Dignity in Care*. Available at: www.nhsconfed. org/priorities/Quality/Partnership-on-dignity/Pages/Commission-on-dignity.aspx?utm_ campaign=MMH+Solus+14B&utm_medium=ezine&utm_source=Ezines (accessed 19 April 2012).
- Rinpoche S. *The Tibetan Book of Living and Dying: a spiritual classic from one of the foremost interpreters of Tibetan Buddhism to the West*. Gaffney P, Harvey A, editors. London: Rider; 2008.

ACKNOWLEDGEMENT

The author is grateful to the publisher for granting permission to adapt the chapter: Cooper J. The therapeutic relationship. In: Cooper DB, editor. *Intervention in Mental Health–Substance Use*. London/New York: Radcliffe; 2011. pp. 8–21.

CHAPTER 7

Hope and coping strategies

Jo Cooper, David B Cooper

COPING STRATEGIES

'Coping: A process by which a person deals with stress, solves problems and makes decisions . . .'[1]

REFLECTIVE PRACTICE EXERCISE 7.1

Time: 20 minutes
Consider and reflect on:
- What do you think the person experiencing serious ill-health and/or a terminal illness has to cope with? Include physical, psychological, emotional and spiritual elements.
- What do you think their fears might include?
- How do you cope in times of difficulty?

Compare your feelings with your answers:
- Do they differ?
- If so, how?

Following a diagnosis of physical and/or psychological health problems – including terminal illness – people face the enormous challenge of a threat to their world and may use many different and varied approaches to reduce emotional distress. Each individual travels a unique life journey. The way in which we cope with ill-health depends on past experiences, characteristics and personality. Each person responds differently to difficulties and copes in his or her way.

Although there are many different strategies to aid coping, four primary psychological responses have been identified[2] that can be grouped into four themes (*see* Figure 7.1):

1 Denial.
2 Fighting spirit.
3 Acceptance.
4 Hopelessness.

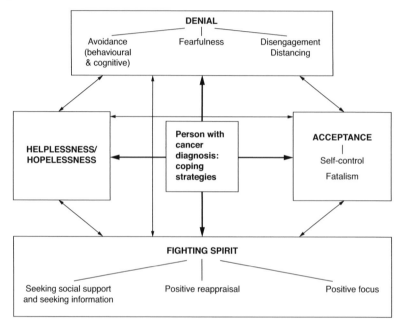

Figure 7.1 People with cancer diagnosis – coping strategies

When dealing with coping strategies, it is essential to remember that the concept of coping is a dynamic and fluctuating process[3] and people use a wide range of coping strategies, depending on the situation. It is important not to permanently place the person into any one coping strategy, as each individual is unique in his or her response and attitudes may change over time.

DENIAL AND ACCEPTANCE AS COPING STRATEGIES

Case study 7.1

Jen (51) had a long-standing history of bipolar disorder and had recently been diagnosed with late stages of metastatic breast cancer. It had spread to her bones and liver, despite aggressive chemotherapy. She was married to Jim, and had two teenage sons. Her mother had died two years previously with lung cancer, and had experienced a painful death from bone metastases. Jen began having vivid, power-ful and unpleasant dreams. These centred on the destructive elements of her illness, her loss of control and her fear of becoming a burden to her family, particularly her husband. Jen was distressed by her dreams and felt confused and muddled by their content. There was no order to them and she was unable to verbalise any of her fears and feelings to her family. She was trying to protect them from her own fears. Jen was trying to cope with the inevitable losses that she was facing.

REFLECTIVE PRACTICE EXERCISE 7.2

> **Time: 10 minutes**
> Consider and reflect on:
> • How would you help Jen cope with her intense feelings and muddled thoughts?

Helping Jen explore her story

The key skill required when helping Jen is *listening* to her story. Listen to . . .
➤ her fears
➤ observe her body expression
➤ ask simple, explorative, questions:
  − How do you feel about . . .?
  − How are you coping with . . .?
  − What happens to you when you feel that you cannot cope?
  − What is the worst thing – for you – that could happen . . .?

This encourages Jen to think and reflect on her difficulties and explore how she is feeling and coping. By *attentive listening*, we understand:
➤ how Jen is coping
➤ what she is struggling to cope with.

It is important to acknowledge Jen's distress, grief and difficulties, so that Jen knows she has been *heard*. Feeling listened to and being supported underpins the person's ability to cope.

> **KEY POINT 7.1**
>
> • Practical problems do not always have practical solutions.
> • It does not matter if we do not have the answers.
> • The answer is in the help and support that we can give.

Helping Jen

Because Jen found it hard initially to say how she was feeling, she was encouraged to paint what she saw in her dreams. She did this at home, using simple watercolours. This helped to give some order and structure to her thoughts, making it easier to explore and verbalise them. She was able to talk through her pictures, deciphering for herself each theme and the meaning it had for her. Over several weeks, Jen made some sense of her feelings and felt able to speak freely about her fears. Through gradual progression Jen discovered:

➤ **she was fearful of losing her family** – by being a burden to them
➤ **loss of body integrity** – she felt overweight and ugly
➤ **loss of her mother**
➤ **her own fear** – of a painful death
➤ **loss of independence** – her job, and loss of status
➤ **loss of her role as a mother** – being denied the joys and sorrows of watching her children mature into adulthood
➤ **loss of sexual intimacy** – with her husband
➤ **realisation that she was coping by denying** – her death and the effect this had on her and the family.

What about Jen's family?

Including Jen's family in discussions around their own fears, and how they are coping, is important. This will not only help and nurture them, but support Jen in knowing that her family feels supported.

Acceptance and action

Jen slowly began to accept the inevitability of her death but occasionally used denial to create some normality in her life. She planned a family holiday for the summer [*hope*], but was also able to talk with Jim about the realities of their situation, and plan her funeral; choosing the hymns and the music. However, Jen remained unable to talk to her sons, other than superficially.

There could be an assumption here that once acceptance has been achieved, this is permanent and stable.[4] However, generally this is not the case.[5,6] People who are seriously ill or dying may use denial as a sole defence or they may exhibit elements of partial denial at different times during the dying process. Often partial denial is used, fluctuating with acceptance, as in Jen's situation.

So is denial good or bad?

Denial, avoidance and distancing are ways of providing self-deception, protecting the person from stress.[7] This buys time, allowing Jen to have periods of normality. It is important to explore denial, in case it is concealing emotional, spiritual and psychological distress, as it was for Jen. An *area of uncertain certainty* exists between open acknowledgement of death and the desire to deny it.[8] This has been termed *middle knowledge*, and can occur at critical transition stages, for example, when a person experiences setbacks or descends towards death.[4] Therefore, the individual:

➤ has accepted the facts of their illness
➤ is facing imminent death
➤ but has the need to occasionally resist the finite nature of their situation.[4]

REFLECTIVE PRACTICE EXERCISE 7.3

> **Time: 20 minutes**
> Consider and reflect on the following:
> - Have you witnessed people using denial?
> - How did you view denial then?
> - Have you felt, or been told by another professional, that denial is a negative coping strategy?
> - What are your thoughts on denial now?

What can you do?

Denial, as a coping strategy, can be a source of concern to professionals. Historically, denial has been viewed as a negative method of coping. It has been felt that people, in order to accept their situation realistically, should be prepared to discuss sensitive issues around their death. However, not everyone wants to openly acknowledge their illness, its implications and their death, and they should be given the right to choose whether or not to disclose.

Talking about chronic and distressing ill-health or dying is not communicated at a single encounter, more as a series of interactions with individuals and families which nurture understanding, acceptance and coping over time.[9] Open communication takes time and skill.

KEY POINT 7.2

Disclosure is best led by the person – not by the professional.

Helping the individual to uncover his or her feelings and fears is important in maintaining mental well-being. Negative feelings, such as anger and fear, *can be helped.*

FIGHTING SPIRIT AS A COPING STRATEGY

> **Case study 7.2**
> John (66) had a long-standing history of depression, alcohol and drug use and was diagnosed with advanced lung cancer. Supportive treatment in terms of symptomatic relief was offered. John had no family and lived in a hostel for people experiencing substance use problems. He had little in life, no family or material assets, but he felt he had *everything* to live for, and wanted to survive.

Exploring John's story

John accepted the full implications of his illness and accepted the fact that he would die (acceptance). However, at the same time John was determined to *fight*. He would say:

> 'I won't let the cancer beat me, I'll try everything to get better . . .', 'I want to make it to my 70th birthday . . .'

. . . and on another day . . .

> 'I've had a good life . . . what's left is a bonus.'

Maintaining hope

John was able to maintain a positive outlook and viewed his cancer as a challenge . . . he had lived with challenges throughout his life. His attitude was optimistic and he generally had very little distress. Initially, his hope was that the future would bring a *miracle cure*, or that the doctors had '*got it wrong*' [*false hope*]. However, over time, as John deteriorated, his hope [*realistic hope*] was for a death without pain. John began to accept the inevitability of his death. He confided that he hoped that he would not be judged for what he described as *leading an amoral life*.

John's coping strategy of fighting spirit enabled him to cope with life's stresses, protecting against fears and anxieties. He was not overwhelmed by distress, even though this was not entirely absent. He wanted information and support and engaged in open communication about his situation.

HOPELESSNESS AS A COPING STRATEGY

Case study 7.3

Sarah (58), who has a history of depression, was diagnosed with oesophageal cancer. Despite chemotherapy and the offer of substantial professional and family support, she felt overwhelmed by her situation. She was immobilised by her circumstances and unable to make any effort to cope or adjust and abandoned hope from the outset. Her family felt that she had everything to live for. She had a devoted husband, Peter, two adult daughters, a large house, and was financially secure. She and Peter holidayed abroad twice a year; they kept horses and she taught disabled children to ride. Although Sarah accepted chemotherapy, she felt that it was futile. She was unable to talk about her fears or concerns and was anxious and depressed, a sense of hopelessness contributing to the development of depression. Sarah became dependent on her family and did not actively seek knowledge or information about her condition.

Helping Sarah

To those caring for Sarah it felt as though she was unhelpable, leaving them with a sense of helplessness; mirroring some of Sarah's own feelings.

REFLECTIVE PRACTICE EXERCISE 7.4

Time: 10 minutes

Consider and reflect on:

- Why do you think Sarah felt hopeless?
- What would you do to enable a less traumatic situation for Sarah?

It is not unusual for individuals using this coping strategy to *give up*.[10] Sarah chose never to disclose her fears: only to say that she perceived her cancer as a punishment and expressed a loss of hope in her future. She blamed herself for her illness and felt guilty when her treatment failed. However, in a caring relationship, our role is one of enabling – looking towards how blame is attributed, and directing interventions towards correcting misconceptions. There may have been instances in which lifestyle had contributed to the cause of cancer. It is only by listening that we can begin to help, smoothing the way forward. The role is one of facilitation and exploration and the art and skill of our practice is about supporting as things become difficult.[11,12]

We cannot change events for Sarah. It is difficult to know how to promote hope in a person close to death. However, respecting individuality can help to facilitate hope.[12] This may activate positive coping, leading to a stable sense of well-being. Being alongside Sarah, smoothing the way forward and not abandoning her just because she was unable to respond, meant that we were able to form a caring relationship with some degree of trust being maintained for both parties.

Assessing, approaching and caring

KEY POINT 7.3

On-going assessment and review of coping behaviours and their impact on the individual and family are cardinal in enabling compassionate and understanding care and attention.

If provision of care and attention is to be humane, compassionate and perceptive, then listening and responding are pivotal skills. However, on-going assessment and review must go hand-in-hand as essential components to approaching, engaging and caring.

It is uncertain whether maintaining hope in the face of advanced disease is a form of denial or a distinct coping strategy in itself.[13] Hopes for the future are an integral part of our emotional well-being, whether or not we are experiencing ill-health. However, the need to maintain hope influences the amount of information sought and is an important strategy in helping people to cope with the knowledge of their ill-health.[9]

HOPE
Above we have explored some of the various coping strategies we use; here we turn to how the professional can enable *hope*.

What is hope?
Hope is at the centre of our being and spirit. It can be:
➤ our religion
➤ our story or journey
➤ our love of nature
➤ our trust of a friend
➤ a precious moment in time.

Hope is whatever is meaningful to us – whatever helps us cope with our ill-health and dis-ease. Hope is intertwined with goal achieving, which gives us some kind of reward and pleasure. Therefore, the professionals' role is pivotal to enable the individual to identify hope, and think about the possibilities.

How do we enable hope?
Enabling [*facilitating*] hope is about identifying things in the present, goals to aim for that are achievable. To give false hope by identifying hope that is not practical or achievable is destructive. The individual, family and professional relationship must be open and honest, sharing what can be done, and what cannot be done. Hope is about considering possibilities.

KEY POINT 7.4

It is a waste of all we know to work in the insular belief that all individuals are the same.

It is essential to:
➤ *meet* the individual, family and your minds at the same point
➤ work *with* individual and family to identify hope
➤ work *with* individual and family to achieve their chosen goal(s) – *hope*.

Hope is at the heart of coping[13] and one can only hope if the goal is realistic. The key points of hope have been identified as:[13]
➤ hope is a realistic desire for something good in the face of uncertainty
➤ hope is not about denial or optimism
➤ hope changes as the ill-health progresses

➤ a trusted, listening ear is the most helpful support . . . not someone who offers false reassurance.

So why is hope so important?

Hope has been described as:

> . . . an inner power or strength that can enrich lives and enable individuals to look beyond their pain, suffering and turmoil . . .[14]

Categories and sub-categories identified to hope-fostering and hope-hindering include the following.[11,12]

Hope-fostering

➤ love of family or friends
➤ spirituality/having faith
➤ setting goals and maintaining independence
➤ positive relationships with professionals
➤ humour/light-heartedness
➤ personal characteristics
➤ uplifting memories.[14]

Hope-hindering

➤ abandonment and isolation
➤ uncontrolled pain and discomfort
➤ devaluation of personhood
➤ inability to visualise any meaningful future.

Bringing about exploration

Through assessment, exploration of hope – and how it can be enabled – commences. It is a process of continual appraisal . . . open to change and/or abandonment as the identified needs dictate.

Hope is integral to the psychological needs and well-being of the person and family. Understanding and enabling hope improves the quality of care, and life. Respect and courtesy[14] are important; conversely, poor communication and failure to acknowledge the needs of the individual are destructive and detrimental.

Therefore, *how* do we identify and explore hope? The following checklist might be useful:

➤ identify events that might bring hope
➤ recognise problems in achieving hope that are likely to be experienced
➤ assist the individual in the process of acknowledging, exploring and understanding barriers to hope
➤ appreciate the individual's perception of hope and its barriers
➤ consider together the options available
➤ facilitate the individual's achievement of the chosen goal [*hope*]

➤ acquaint the individual with services and facilities available to attain the goal [*hope*]
➤ be non-judgemental
➤ provide maximum professional intervention
➤ provide maximum understanding and support
➤ keep to your word
➤ keep goals [*hope*] realistic and achievable
➤ explore what is and what is not achievable to avoid building false hope
➤ speak truthfully
➤ be open to possibilities:

. . . ask exploratory questions, e.g.
➤ What does hope mean to you?
➤ Tell me about your hope.
➤ What sort of thing do you hope for?
➤ If you could identify a source of hope for yourself, what would it be?
➤ What things cause you to lose hope?
➤ What helps you to maintain hope or maybe makes you feel hopeful?[14]

Where do we go from here?

Once the individual comes to a place in his or her mind where she or he can take charge of life, then the professional can encourage the move to action. The acceptance that hope does not mean a cure, or that all will be well, but that life is good regardless of the conclusion is a step forward. To achieve this, the professional needs to support the individual to a point where she or he can:
➤ identify where she or he is now and what expectation she or he has for the future
➤ acknowledge what ill-health will bring
➤ take time to reflect on what she or he knows and does not know
➤ identify where support and care will come from and how to access this.

Where do I come in?

A good starting point is to look at each day and explore what is necessary and what is achievable – this could be a simple task like shopping. It is helpful to assist the individual to concentrate on life as if it were '*normal*': what would she or he usually do in terms of daily tasks or recreational activities? The emphasis is on what can still be done and not on what cannot be done. If the individual enjoys dancing or golf, whilst it may not be possible to fully participate as the illness progresses, it may be possible to slowly reduce the activity rather than stop altogether or participate from another perspective. It is not about giving up in anticipation of ill-health and/or death but looking at maintaining the normality of life as long as possible and making gradual reductions to accommodate ill-health.

The family

People are able to deal with pain, loss of independence and relationships by maintaining hope. Having hope extends to the family as much as to the individual. For them, maintaining hope is important in terms of helping the person to achieve each daily goal [*hope*] and for themselves to achieve their hope. To do that, each family member needs to identify where she or he is in relation to self and the person, working together in an environment where each can share worries, hopes, questions and answers. It is important for the family to understand and appreciate that they can offer something to their loved one, be that shopping with the individual, washing hair or, in the later stages of the illness, bathing or massaging.[11]

Recognising that hope is there

KEY POINT 7.5

Hope means many things to many people, each having his or her own interpretation.

It can be said that without hope there is no life. Life does not stop because one becomes ill, it merely changes the perspective on life, and with that, the individual needs to find a way to keep life rewarding until there is no life. Therefore by:
➤ being supportive and caring
➤ being *with* and meeting the person and family at the point where *they are*
➤ keeping pain effectively managed
➤ openness
➤ developing trust
➤ exploring and developing what the individual really wants from the time that is left . . .

. . . the professional can make a difference – enabling hope – to the end-of-life. It is a constant pressure not to give *false* hope, therefore keep it:
➤ accurate
➤ real
➤ honest . . .

. . . for the individual, family and yourself. Assisting the person and family to find hope is rewarding.

KEY POINT 7.6

Being human is what caring is about.

Acknowledging that hope is not the same as a promise means we have nothing to fear in encouraging it.[11]

CONCLUSION

People with advancing ill-health confront the dilemma of a shortened life and face issues of existentialism. We have a prime role in offering opportunities to the individual and family for open exchange and disclosure of concerns . . . respecting their right to choose not to disclose.

Helping the individual to identify something positive in their life, such as close family relationships, visits from grandchildren, the love of a special person, may help to promote coping and renew *hope*.[15] A healing relationship between the professional and the individual can occur when *hope* is mobilised.[16] We have a powerful influence on how people respond to their ill-health; both in *what* we say and by *how* we say it.

The uniqueness of each human being means that coping style is specific to that individual and should be supported and respected as that person's method of getting through his or her illness.

Often, there is little to offer but ourselves, and our often unspoken understanding that we have no answers to suffering and pain. Providing comfort and attentive and thoughtful listening to the person and their family without the offer of immediate solutions are frequently all that we have to give – and all that is needed.

REFERENCES

1 Anderson KN, Anderson LE, Glanze WD, editors. *Mosby's Medical, Nursing and Allied Health Dictionary*. 5th ed. London: Mosby; 1998.
2 Greer S, Morris T, Pettingale KW, *et al.* Psychological responses to breast cancer and 15 year outcome. *Lancet.* 1990; **335**: 49–50.
3 Payne S. Coping with palliative chemotherapy. *Journal of Advanced Nursing.* 1990; **15**: 652–8.
4 Copp G, Field D. Open awareness and dying: the use of denial and acceptance as coping strategies by hospice patients. *Nursing Times Research.* 2002; **7**: 118–27.
5 Copp G. *Facing Impending Death: experiences of patients and their nurses.* London: Nursing Times Books; 1999.
6 Field D, Copp G. Communication and awareness about dying in the 1990's. *Palliative Medicine.* 1999; **13**: 459–68.
7 Russell GC. The role of denial in clinical practice. *Journal of Advanced Nursing.* 1999; **18**: 938–40.
8 Weisman AD. *On Dying and Denying: a psychiatric study of terminality.* New York: Behavioural Publications; 1999.
9 Johnston G, Abraham C. Managing awareness: negotiating and coping with a terminal prognosis. *International Journal of Palliative Nursing.* 2000; **16**: 485–94.
10 Mahon SM, Cella DF, Donovan MI. Psychological adjustment to recurrent cancer. *Oncology Nursing Forum.* 1990; **17**: 47–52.
11 Penson J. A hope is not a promise: fostering hope within palliative care. *International Journal of Palliative Nursing.* 2000; **6**: 94–8.
12 Herth K. Fostering hope in terminally ill people. *Journal of Advanced Nursing.* 1990; **15**: 1250–9.
13 Current Learning in Palliative Care (CLIP), 15 minute worksheet. Psychological needs: 1.

Fostering hope. In: Regnard C, Kindlen M, Jackson J, *et al.*, editors. *Helping the Patient with Advanced Disease: a workbook*. Oxford: Radcliffe Medical Press; 2004.

14 Buckley J, Herth K. Fostering hope in terminally ill patients. *Nursing Standard*. 2004; **19**: 33–41.

15 Mahon SM, Casperson DM. Exploring the psychosocial meaning of recurrent cancer: a descriptive study. *Cancer Nursing*. 1997; **20**: 178–86.

16 Benner P. *From Novice to Expert: excellence and power in clinical nursing practice*. California: Addison-Wesley; 1984.

TO LEARN MORE

- Boss P. *Loving Someone Who Has Dementia: how to find hope while coping with stress and grief.* San Francisco: Wiley.
- Buckley J, Herth K. Fostering hope in terminally ill patients. *Nursing Standard*. 2004; **19**: 33–41.
- Groopman J. *The Anatomy of Hope*. London: Simon and Schuster; 2004.
- Holland JC, Lewis S. *The Human Side of Cancer: living with hope, coping with uncertainty.* New York, NY: Harper; 2001.
- Kinnaird B. *The Promise of Hope: coping when life caves in.* Nashville, Tennessee: Abingdon; 1981.
- Owain Hughes T. *Finding Hope and Meaning in Suffering.* London: Society for Promoting Christian Knowledge; 2010.
- Penson J. A hope is not a promise: fostering hope within palliative care. *International Journal of Palliative Nursing*. 2000; **6**: 94–8.

ACKNOWLEDGEMENT

The authors are grateful to Radcliffe Publishing for permitting adaptation of the chapter: Cooper J, Cooper DB. Hope and coping strategies. In: Cooper J, editor. *Stepping into Palliative Care 1: relationships and responses*. 2nd ed. Oxford: Radcliffe Publishing; 2006. pp. 69–80.

CHAPTER 8

Spirituality

Je Kan Adler-Collins

REFLECTIVE NOTE

> As you travel through this personal journey on spirituality, spend time, think deeply and reflect on your own spiritual journey and what this means for you.
>
> While this chapter concentrates on the end-of-life, the same principles can be applied to the individual whose life is about to be changed from 'wellness' to permanent 'illness' and her or his family, with the accompanying stigmatisation and traumatic anger.

INTRODUCTION

Welcome to this chapter on spirituality, one in which I offer the reader some thoughts drawn from many sources and many cultures. Some people hold deep and committing views and opinions about what spirituality is and is not. In my case, I offer my thoughts of spirituality through the lens of my life. I have been studying spirituality and palliative care for 25 years and in these studies that I have carried out in Asia are the influences of different types of Buddhism, shamanic practices and ideas from Chinese traditional medicine. Buddhist healing techniques that came from Thailand, Cambodia, Vietnam and Korea are synthesised to a new dynamic of my own understandings. As such, I acknowledge the words of Masters, teachers, practitioners, past, present and future with a fathomless debt of gratitude. Buddhist belief does not hold with the Western understanding that an individual owns knowledge, rather that the individual is a guardian of the knowledge and practice in its incompleteness and impermanence.

I have travelled extensively throughout Asia researching and practising end-of-life care. Through these journeys I have come to realise how little I know about death and dying other than what I have observed. Spirituality is a complicated issue and I am keenly aware that the spoken word is not the received word.

Moreover, I know the dangers embedded in the production of labels to offer the reader. I am writing this chapter with extreme caution; caution in the sense that what I am offering is just my simple understanding at the time of writing. It is not a grand narrative or a model text written in stone. It is grounded in the compassion I share with all who suffer, are still suffering, and have suffering to come. It is my hope that these few words will assist readers to question themselves and their practice with loving eyes in order to bring compassion to the end stages of their own or another's life. My understanding is by no means perfect, complete, or accurate. It is, I believe, a living dynamic and, as such, this chapter opens a window through which the reader is invited to enter the discussion about spirituality and its place within palliative care and mental health.

Much of my thinking is grounded in the teaching of Buddhism, which has taken many forms, twists and turns over the centuries. The form of Buddhism that I practise believes that the Buddha is internal; we are all born Buddhas. All I need to do is wake to its presence in every cell of my being and that the realisation of what might actually *be* can be achieved in this lifetime. The body is not an external object, reinforcing that the Buddhist teacher exists within all of us at every level of our being. We are taught that the Buddha mind can awaken even at a cellular level, and there is no separation between what we truly are. The true mind, for ease of understanding, is referred to in this text as the inner mind and the outer mind is the constructed mind that we use to construct and engage with our perceived reality. It is our outer mind that causes thoughts of separation, ego, individualism, and that gives rise to suffering.

In many ways, I see myself as a pilgrim or traveller seeking to understand what I am, as I question the value of experiences I have gained in life so far. I was born in Western culture and socialised in Western ways of thinking. Death has always been an end; something to be feared and not talked about. Spirituality, so it appeared, was always channelled by someone in authority, usually a priest, and always appeared to involve a godlike power in passing judgements from a book of rules in which heaven and hell were places for good and bad people after death. Who decided what was good and what was bad depended entirely on the cultural norms and the ability of those in power to police and enforce them. For many people in today's society, spirituality is not very high on the agenda, as daily living, with its trials and tribulations, is hard enough to face. Religion for many with all the deaths it has caused, and is still causing, through its wars, appears to be spiritually bankrupt, offering little to those seeking a greater understanding of things spiritual. For others religion is a complete solution to the question of what happens to us after death. Usually implying that only those who believe what they believe can achieve or enter this next dimension of plenty and everybody else is excluded . . . as not being part of the élite. As a Buddhist, I believe in reincarnation and that we can have many lives. Expressing such beliefs openly in my social context often results in my being dismissed as being unstable emotionally and mentally for being stupid enough to believe that spirituality is at the essence of our humanness. Such a view brings forth suffering on a global scale and fuels conflict which can be sustained in everyday life. However, when faced with a rapidly approaching death, the certainty of the outer mind starts to crack as logic tells it that it will soon be gone from existence with the death of its host whom it has controlled and dominated for all its existence.

I believe we need to look more closely at death as part of life, investigate it more carefully to empower the seeker to see the spiritual knowledge and understandings that can come to us from varying sources, belief systems and cultures. This enables us to embrace the real meanings of life and death. To this end, we need to look at what is meant by spirituality and spiritual care, learning how it can remove the fearfulness that so many experience when talking about death in general and their own or loved ones in particular.

Death is a fact, one of the very few we know to be a certainty in an uncertain chaotic world, and, as such, demands of us a measure of focused attention and a joyful exploration, rather than a morbid fixation or obsession or even denial. Death should neither be romanticised nor trivialised. In Buddhist teachings, life and death are seen as one whole. Once you have finished the life of life you move into the life of death. There is nothing negative about the experience; it is just the beginning of another chapter of continuous chapters of birth, death and rebirth.

IMPERMANENCE

Impermanence is a core feature of understanding that everything in the known universe is in a stage of on-going change. Modern science has its own ideas as to how and when the universe will end. Many credible scientific theories exist about the possible demise of mankind, be it at our own hand in war, through pollution or by triggering global changes. Another theory is that of the earth being hit by a meteorite and another extinction event being triggered. It has happened before and gave rise to our evolution and the demise of the dinosaurs; it is predicted to happen again. From the moment of the Big Bang and the expanding universe held within it, its own demise runs on a time frame beyond our comprehension. What has been seen for centuries as permanent and fixed – our existence – is now seen as impermanent and evolving, and such evolution does not carry a guaranteed place for humanity.

Impermanence plays an important part in assisting people to cope with the death and dying experience and the relief of the fear that they suffer. Everything around us is changing; everything is in a constant flux of motion. At the second of our birth, our death moves closer. We need to embrace change moving towards the opportunities it presents us in understanding ourselves. If we become attached to something, we try to hold on to it and bring it closer to us because we are fearful in our insecurities that if we let it go, we will be alone. Often, the same applies to death. We are so attached to life and fearful of death that we hold on to life and struggle against death. Acceptance of what things are in the moment and enjoying them in the moment frees us from attachment. Realising the true nature of impermanence, and living it in your heart, allows for the growth of compassion, where you can see that all things are embracing life through the process of dying. It is happening at a cosmic level with the birth and death of stars and universes. Sometimes, such insights make us feel sad because, in a world of life, we are surrounded by death; we can experience such sadness. This sadness comes not from the process of dying, rather from the understanding that so many people are attached to life and such attachment will bring about untold suffering. If we spend all our lives trying to secure material wealth, benefits, position and status, a great proportion of our energy is focused on keeping what we have struggled to obtain. We become focused on the material and no matter how much we want to keep it, the material will decay. If not the material, then certainly we will, for we leave this life, as we arrived, with nothing material, but experience and knowledge. It matters not if you were King or President, a Chief Executive of a Fortune 500 company or the person that cleans the toilets in a train station for a living. Death is the equaliser. Such a process is not without its price and that price is the loss of or disconnection from our spirituality. For, as we reflect on the meaning of reality and permanence, we soon start to understand that everything is related in highly complex relationships or networks to everything else in the universe. These relationships are dynamic as is our relationship with life and death. True spirituality, I suggest, is being aware that we are interdependent with everything, everyone. Our smallest, least significant thought, word and action have real consequences throughout the universe. Our actions and deeds ripple across space and time like those of stones dropped into a pond. We are responsible for all our actions, thoughts, words and deeds. I have often thought over the years about this and part of me asks the question: *Is there something beyond impermanence? Is something actually more stable, a hidden core perhaps?* I changed the way I thought and the way I live my world life and the values I hold in my spirituality. Consequently, I find that my outer mind keeps teasing and taunting me just outside of my ability to articulate it, or to make sense of it. It makes me think I am foolish, delusional, bordering on stupid. Yet I cannot shake the sense that contained within death is actually deathlessness? Could this be the mind as it truly is?

REFLECTION AND MINDFULNESS

When we are faced with our own mortality – with the diagnosis of terminal illness – it is only natural that we become highly reflective. Such reflection in the initial stages may not bring about any form of peacefulness. I have found in my work – and for myself – that the use of meditation assists the individual coming to terms with his or her death. We spend our lives seeking to improve our lot, filling our lives with the pursuit of material possessions, in competition, making money, forming power relationships and generally trying to hold our own, in what seems sees a hostile world. Meditation offers the opportunity of bringing the mind back home. Meditation means many things to many people. In my research with end-of-life care in a Buddhist hospice in Thailand, we found that after only nine minutes of focused meditation, the body's chemistry changed, and there was a remarkable reduction in stress-producing markers in human saliva. While it is reassuring to have confirmation from science, the practices of meditation have been known to be beneficial for centuries. Some people require formal sitting instruction, or leadership, whilst for others it is a more natural approach grounded in relaxation.

The mind spends most of its time in a state of chaos – shattered into various aspects and elements of constructed self – and resists strongly any effort to bring it into any form of cohesion. Calming the mind is the basic step towards mindfulness and is so simple in concept, yet we make it so difficult to achieve in practice. We do not need to understand meditation to do it; teaching it to ourselves, and the individual and family within our care offers the opportunity for that person to move into calmness through the gentle practice of this exercise.

MOVING MEDITATION
Example meditation technique

> **KEY POINT 8.1**
>
> As with any form of meditation, the practitioners' intention is important.

In this meditation, sit comfortably with your palms facing down on your thigh. Slowly and carefully, start to focus your attention on your breath, breathing deeply through the nose taking the breath into your abdomen. Hold your breath there for a few seconds. Try not to breathe by expanding your chest. In Buddhist belief, the focus of energy appears to be somewhere in the abdomen. When you breathe out, imagine that you are blowing a feather. Allow the air to move slowly – in a controlled manner – out through the mouth. Imagine that your mind is a grain of sand on the beach, taking no shape or no particular form. Very slowly focus your mind on your right hand. Take a deep breath in . . . and as you breathe in . . . imagine your right hand is like a flower first thing in the morning slowly opening and greeting the sun, and as the flower opens, the palm of the hand moves upward. In the next breath in, slowly and carefully, the hand should feel light and soft – without thinking, the hand will start to rise – and as it rises move it slowly towards the front of the chest . . . level to your heart. Place the right hand on your heart and relax into your breathing. Now focus your mind on the left hand and repeat the actions you took for the right hand. Keep this movement going and co-ordinate it with your breathing. Place the left hand on top of the right hand in front of your heart. Relax in the moment and focus on your breathing. Bring your mind to your right hand and slowly allow the right hand to slide down the abdomen and come to rest on your thigh, palm facing upwards – slowly and carefully focus on breathing – as you breathe in, the palm turning over like a closing flower. Now focus your mind on your left hand and repeat the actions undertaken for the right hand. You have just completed one cycle of moving meditation. With practice, this meditation can help you calm the chaos in your mind and bring the mind home.

Once comfortable in your meditation practices, whatever they are, a sense of peacefulness will enter your life, your heart and your mind. With this sense of peacefulness comes a great relief and release and the individual can start to bring her or his mind towards reflecting on the issues he or she faces . . . such as fear, anxiety, worry and attachment. In the practice of mindfulness in meditation, which can be either moving or sitting, active or passive, deep insights can be achieved. Reflection brings about changes in consciousness and we become open to the relationships and connections of everything. When, in normal life, do we notice a sunrise or sunset, the feel of the wind on our skin, of rain, of hot or cold, with different types of variation shades and reflections of the surroundings? We soon start to realise how blind we have been and how blessed we are to have the chance to move towards seeing the mind as it really is. I believe, as many spiritual practices teach, that there exists within each of us an essence of goodness that is completely incorruptible, like a clear blue sky. The outer mind is a confusion cloud just like clouds in the sky. Look for the blueness and light that will help you understand the reasons that the clouds are formed. These clouds have a relationship with the sky because they are formed in elements that can only exist in the sky, and yet they leave no mark even after the blackest of storms and once it has passed, blue sky shines clearly through. Such thinking has assisted me through many storms . . . no matter what the outside world is doing, with events that I cannot control, producing a storm, in my inside world I realise that perhaps I am causing my own storms and blinding myself, clouding my own sky.

When this understanding is lived in daily living and practices, the deepest blissful state of peace becomes the norm. Often I am asked what the best method is for meditation. The answer is simple, none! Each of us has to find our own way through simplicity, not complexity. Many people are unsatisfied with such an answer and feel that there has to be a system, or technique, or a most correct way. Systems, techniques and correctness are in themselves traps created by our own mind. Everything is as it should be and we start to wake up when it is our time to do so, once awoken we become seekers, seeking to understand the connected relational dynamics that we are part of, not separate from. For many people such an awakening is often when they are told that they are going to die.

THINKING ABOUT DEATH

There are two certain major shocks in our life. The first is the shock of our birth. We leave a comfortable environment . . . one of warmth and security, and are pushed, often quite dramatically, from security into insecurity. Birth trauma is starting to be researched in greater depth. Researchers are starting to recognise how the first few moments of life can lay down critical patterns that stay with us for a lifetime. The first hour of birth is full of changes for the mother and the child.

The second shock is that of our death. Again we leave a world of security, created by ourselves, and are faced with fact of death – the end of our life – and by being a fact this becomes part of our everydayness . . . We leave our comfort with what we understand as reality, and move to another dimension . . . the unknown. However, for many people, their understanding is not so esoteric and is grounded in their reality. Few people think about death – it is always something that happens to somebody else. We tend to focus solely on living. Hence, it is a shock to the system when told that we are going to die – or indeed that we have a lifelong and life-changing illness.

Here we should spend a few important moments looking at language . . . because language embraces values. Language has energy and meaning, so often the spoken word is not the received word as although we know what we want to say, there are seeds of misunderstanding . . . misunderstanding and confusion to the listener or reader. The listener or reader listens or reads with their own understanding of the spoken word, and their own beliefs and truths.

The words *'terminal care'* came from medicine and signify a stage when the doctor acknowledges (sadly, this acknowledgement is often belated and there is often a failure in communicating this to the individual or family) that no further medical intervention can be carried out with any hope of a successful outcome. Therefore, all invasive medical and surgical procedures are discontinued. Here there is a clearly defined move to palliation – the management of symptoms – physical, emotional, psychological and spiritual. No longer does the professional heal but moves to concentrate on comfort and peace for the individual and family. Slowly, such thinking and language have moved across into nursing. I believe that terminal care has no place in the phraseology of the nursing language . . . nurses care until the end of life . . . and often beyond.

Each person takes the news of his or her impending death in his or her own way. However, many will ask one question: How much time do I have? It is probably this question that causes the most suffering to both the dying person and their family. While it is never possible to be accurate, being given 'six weeks' to live by the professional does not mean the individual has to conform to the time line. Yet the family, and some individuals, do conform, so resources and emotional effort are placed into a time framework that quickly collapses when the person does not die 'to order'.

Emotional dependency that has been invested in a loved one will soon be removed. Often those left behind feel angry, deserted, let down and/or lost. All recipients of such news suffer from varying degrees of shock . . . expressed in their own unique way. Some people become enraged that death is interfering with life plans; others are fearful, quiet . . . and some hysterical. Some are all businesslike and practical; making lists of what they have to do . . . others fall apart. No one knows how he or she will react until they have experienced receiving this news.

END-OF-LIFE

Earlier I stated that we are dying from the moment we are born, which is hardly helpful for those seeking advice on how to cope with their own, or someone else's, death. It may seem difficult to understand that there are clear and distinct stages of dying that we need to discuss for a few moments.

While dying is a solitary process for the individual who is dying, in most cases – but not all – the person belongs to a family or community. When death approaches, the individual may become reflective, unconcerned with the hustle and bustle of daily life and living. For at a certain level we believe that the body is getting ready to die. Once the dying person has come to terms with their impending death – if in fact they do – they then have to deal with all the issues that are projected on them by surrounding family, friends and colleagues. Depending on their belief system and culture, customs are observed as part of the social dying process. These are often grounded in the belief systems of religion. Wherever possible, every effort needs to be made to find out what the wishes of the dying person are. In addition, a certain degree of frank and clear communication is needed between the individual, immediate family – though we must respect the wishes of the individual as to who in the family should be involved – professionals and carers. There is a bureaucracy attached to dying that cannot be avoided. If there is the time, legal matters such as the will need to be addressed.

Those who are burdened with a lifetime of accumulated material wealth often struggle with how or to whom they should disperse such wealth, and in so doing, attach themselves further to suffering. (A Buddhist understanding of life well lived is to give away to all those in need. Such selflessness creates merit and removes any chains that could hold the individual during the final stages of the dying process.)

Human dynamics and relationships are always complex issues at the point of dying. Often estranged spouses and/or broken families will make an effort at reconciliation and forgiveness. I believe this is an important step towards the building of compassion, both in the dying individual and all who are parts of the dying process, for we do not die in a vacuum. To die angry, bitter and full of rage produces negative karma (action, seen as bringing upon oneself inevitable results, good or bad, either in this life or in a reincarnation[1]) that follows across into the next life of the dying person and is left behind in the lives of the living as an unresolved energy. Close friends, and especially immediate family, need to understand that their loved one is dying. Their acceptance of this, even though it produces grief, arising from attachment, allows the dying process to be free from unnecessary and – I believe – selfish emotional attachments. Telling somebody to be positive when that person is dying makes no sense, while encouraging positive thinking for the living is just prolonging the suffering. However, to encourage a positive acceptance of the natural order of things can reduce suffering and help bring the mind home, and in so doing, assist in the achievement of a calm, peaceful mind. One of the most remarkable things I see in my work is that people find it so difficult to talk to dying people. People change – almost as though they are afraid that death might be catching. Perhaps such feelings arise from having our mortality reflected back to us. It is always someone else who dies, and when we actually know someone who is dying, death becomes closer . . . more real.

Sympathy, while a natural emotion, can also be a very demeaning one. Dying people do not need too much sympathy. It is more important to encourage people to be natural, to relax, and to enjoy the remaining time together. For many, silence is uncomfortable and many people feel the need to fill space with noise. Learn to understand that silence is in itself a very important space for listening. The hospice in Thailand (where this author also works) is one of the happiest, most joyful and noisiest places I know. The humour shown is reflected in laughter, dance and singing. There is no sitting around just waiting passively for death; there is an active engagement with the final moments of life. Yet at the same time, we are mindful that some people are suffering, and in that suffering, their anger can be projected to the professional without any warning. Anger is part of the process arising from fear, and not directed at the professional personally . . . but it can feel personal. The individual at the end-of-life, and their family, are our teachers and I thank each person from the depth of my heart for showing me the manner of death I would like.

I remember a great teaching from my teacher . . . an Abbot in Thailand. I was with a person whose last days were truly horrific; she was fighting for every extra minute of life. Her pain was beyond measure, yet there was no analgesia. I was outraged at the suffering. The Abbot could see my anger and distress clouding my mind and heart, and gently taught me about enlightenment. The suffering and pain were part of the process grounded in fear. Enlightenment, the Abbot said, can come with the final breath. I, with my Western-trained medical thinking, could not reconcile the ethics of my training with the belief system of spirituality. I told the Abbot this and he gently said that the problem was mine and that I was thinking like a nurse with my outer mind, rather than as a monk with the true mind. The Western approach to pain in the dying process is to use analgesics to bring relief, and the final moments of an individual's life are often spent in a drug-induced coma. This clouding of the mind is seen by many cultures to be a thing that should be avoided. Many believe that by teaching breathing techniques and meditation, the body is stimulated to produce its own endorphin response by embracing the pain, rather than moving away from it. The body's endorphin response allows the mind to be clear and, as such, the coming home of the mind is greatly facilitated.

This highlights the need for the professional to be mindful of the wishes of the individual and family in how they – not we – wish to end their life. I am completely aware that the above is part of my belief system. For many outside such belief, a comfortable death where pain relief is given is the route of choice. I believe that a combination is good; *medication* and *meditation*, and I believe that the individual should make the choice through informed consent.

REFLECTION AT THE END-OF-LIFE

If we are given the blessing to know that we are dying and have time to prepare, as opposed to being subjected to a sudden death by trauma, reflection can be both a blessing and a curse. Often the individual reflects on the life they have lived, depending on the belief system of the dying person. The person can become deeply distressed, as they see themselves facing the unknown. Guilt is a powerful emotion when you think that you are facing some sort of judgement and your eternal soul is in danger. Great compassion is needed in the listening process, allowing the individual to release whatever they need to release. The listener should render no judgement, nor is what is heard ever to be repeated.

In my life, I have made many mistakes and as I become older, I see that these mistakes were opportunities for me to learn to be a better, more conscious individual. Much of the guilt that was installed in me at the Catholic orphanage, in which I was raised, has been finally understood for what it is. I chose to serve my fellow man in my imperfect way, to the best of my ability and consciousness at the time of my doing. I understand that my consciousness will change as I learn more. I no longer 'beat myself up' but embrace the chance to learn and thank my teachers. These are my personal beliefs, not those of a dying person. It is not my place to try to convert a vulnerable mind to my way of thinking. When asked, I prefer to stay in the belief set of the individual. Yet if asked I will tell the truth – my truth – as I understand it.

TELLING THE TRUTH

I live and predominantly work in Japan and, as such, I am and always will be an outsider to the culture. I was deeply shocked when I found that the practice of not telling the individual that they had a terminal condition was the norm and not the exception. Nurses who are seeking to be seen as professionals with a responsibility to advocate for those in their care are in conflict with some practices of the medical profession, and in some cases, in conflict with the families. It is not unusual for the family to decide that the individual does not need to know.

Having a cancer is not something that can be hidden. Most of us know when there is something wrong in our bodies. We frequently leave it until it is too late to be successfully removed. Even the busiest of individuals understand in the quietness of the moment that something is wrong. Such thinking is confirmed by the sudden change in how family members treat and speak to them. I remember one person telling me:

> 'I feel so sorry for my daughter, who has not told me I have terminal cancer, she bears my dying as her burden; it is like a wall between us. So I pretend not to know, to ease her suffering. Yet my own heart cries for the loss of our limited time together. We pretend to each other that nothing has changed and everything has.'

Telling the truth is sometimes harder than it seems, for I believe that there are many truths and the truth is a fluid state of understanding. When I learned from my teacher that enlightenment can come in the last breath, I started to think about the people I wanted to thank and ask forgiveness from and the people I needed to thank and forgive. We lose contact with those we love and those we see as abusers or hurtful to us. In many cases, we are the ones that have hurt others. I have found that teaching a simple de-cording exercise often gives the individual the chance to bring about spiritual closure. I believe that the true mind – my blue sky – is connected to all true minds.

To find peace is to die without any attachment or regrets. The following meditation is often helpful for people as it allows you to forgive and to be forgiven.

DE-CORDING

Resting quietly, sit in the meditation position, if possible, with your back as straight as possible. Half close your eyes and place the focus about 10 cm in front of your nose. Breathe in through your nose and bring your breath deep within your abdomen, hold each breath for a count of four and gently release your breath out of your mouth. Place the tip of your tongue in the centre of your hard palate where there is a Tsubo pressure point that helps clear the mind.

Place your mind in a clear blue sky and gently feel yourself dissolving into the blueness. Within the teachings of your belief system ask for Gods, Guides, Angels to guard, guide and protect you, and keep you balanced, within the mind as it truly is. Look deeply into the sky and a face will appear; you will know the face. Greet the individual and surround them with the deep blue light of the mind as it truly is. Bless them, thank them and ask their forgiveness for any wrongs or suffering you may have caused them. Feel the deep love and compassion that is part of the mind as it truly is and gently forgives them for any perceived wrong or suffering they caused you and joyously let them go into the blueness of the mind as it really is. Continue with this process as each new face will appear and you release them and you from the karma.

At the end of this process, your mind will be at peace, for many of the people whom you feel hurt you . . . were your teachers, part of this life's karmic plan, likewise the individuals you hurt chose you as their teacher, and you offered them the same chance to learn forgiveness and compassion. For me this understanding shows me just how interconnected we truly are with everything in this dimension.

THE ENVIRONMENT AND THE DYING PLACE

Inspired by dreams, I moved to Japan in 2000 to set about building a place in the mountains that could be used to offer the Japanese a place to die as Japanese. This may seem strange but in Japan, my living context, the pressure is most certain to be Western. However, something is deeply wrong as the truly unbelievable number of suicides every year in Japan shows. Spirituality is forbidden in any public forum. After the end of the last war, the code of Bushido, the warrior code, was the target of the Allies so that, never again, would they have to face the kamikaze mindset. In Western society, spirituality seems to have become disconnected from our lived lives. Offering the chance to those who seek it is a way to help nurture, with love and compassion, those who have lived in spiritual hunger.

In Japan, the idea of hospice care is very limited and often revolves around a ward being set aside for terminal patients, or a side room. Some hospices exist in Japan but they are few. I wanted to create an environment in which traditional values were observed where people who had lived and worked as salaried women and men all their lives could die surrounded by peace, nature and the elements. Hospitals are not good places to die; they are, however, convenient, as the modern society has no place for the dying . . . all efforts are focused on the living.

Communities and families continue to break up and caring for a dying family member at home is not encouraged. Hospitals are busy, noisy places with strange smells and sounds, full of the negative energy of sickness and pain. There are often conflicting issues for a hospital to deal with. These can include the care, the cost of care, and getting medical colleagues to give up trying to manage or medicalise death and the dying process. Where possible, each individual should be allowed to go home to die . . . and should be supported in this wish. For this to happen, many societies need to take a closer look at investing in our spirituality alongside that of the material. It makes sense for, one day, every one of us will be there.

It is my sincere hope that the writings above – inspired by all the teachers that have entered and still enter my life – will help readers seek their own answers as I have sought mine. Should you feel drawn or have the need to discuss or talk further, I would be honoured to listen.

REFLECTIVE PRACTICE EXERCISE 8.1

Time: 20 minutes
- Reflect on what you have read and what you have understood.
- Has reading and reflecting on this chapter helped you to uncover your own spirituality?
- If you have found your spirituality, how has this influenced you?
- If you have not found your spirituality, why do you think this is? What do you need to do to advance your knowledge and understanding?
- Has this chapter given you inspiration and encouragement to help explore spirituality and the existential issues of those in your care and their families?

REFERENCE

1 Dictionary.Com. Available at: http://dictionary.reference.com/browse/karma (accessed 21 April 2012).

CHAPTER 9

All of me: embracing sexuality as a dimension of care

Agnes Higgins

INTRODUCTION

One of the primary goals of palliative care is to provide total care and improve quality of life of the person and their family. Although the World Health Organization's (1990: 182)[1] definition of palliative care (*see* Box 9.1) includes the concept of 'active total care' of the person and family, sexuality as a dimension of care is frequently forgotten or pushed into the proverbial closet.[1] In the context of palliative care for people experiencing serious and enduring mental health problems there is another layer of silence. However, for many people experiencing life-limiting illness and serious and enduring mental health problems, sexuality is a vitally important aspect of life. Thus, the challenge for professionals is to break the cycle of silence and taboo that persists around sexuality to provide true person- and family-centred care. The aim of this chapter is to explore the impact of life-limiting illness on the sexual expression of people experiencing serious and enduring mental health issues, and to provide some guidance for professionals in responding to their needs.

BOX 9.1 Definition of palliative care

'Palliative care is the active, total care of patients whose disease is no longer responsive to curative treatment. Control of pain, of other symptoms, and of psychological, social and spiritual problems is paramount. The goal of palliative care is the achievement of the best possible quality of life for patients and their families'.[1]

REFLECTIVE PRACTICE EXERCISE 9.1

> **Time: 5 minutes**
> How would you define the following terms:
> * sexuality?
> * sexual function?
> * gender identity?
> * sexual orientation?

SEXUALITY: THE CONCEPT

Sexuality is an individualised and personal concept that is unique to each person. Consequently, it cannot be easily defined or categorised.[2] Sexuality represents complex interactions between the biological, genetic, social, psychological, cultural and spiritual dimensions of a person. It encompasses:

> ➤ biological sex – whether we are born male or female
> ➤ gender identity – the psychological sense of being male or female
> ➤ sexual orientation – an emotional, romantic, sexual or affectionate attraction to individuals of a particular sex
> ➤ social gender role – the extent to which people conform to what is regarded in our society as feminine and masculine behaviour.[3]

The Pan American Health Organisation and World Health Organization (PAHO/WHO) provide a broad definition of sexuality (*see* Box 9.2).[4] This definition emphasises the all-encompassing nature of sexuality and highlights that it is more than engaging in sexual activity or reproduction and is as much about having friends as it is about having a lover.[5]

KEY POINT 9.1

Sexuality encompasses feelings, values and ideas as they relate to gender identity, sexual orientation, roles and relationships.

Sexuality is intimately bound up with the person's self-concept, self-esteem and body image and is shaped and influenced by wider social, historical, cultural, religious and political structures. Thus, sexuality or expression of sexuality is not a fixed and static state, but a dynamic evolving lifelong process that fluctuates and changes as the person ages and matures. It is an aspect of one's being which exists across the lifespan, whether one is single or coupled or in opposite and/ or same-sex partnerships.

BOX 9.2 Definition of sexuality

'Sexuality refers to a core dimension of being human which includes sex, gender, sexual and gender identity, sexual orientation, eroticism, emotional attachment/love and reproduction. It is experienced or expressed in thoughts, fantasies, desires, beliefs, attitudes, values, activities, practices, roles, [and] relationships. Sexuality is a result of the interplay of biological, psychological, socio-economic, cultural, ethical and religious/spiritual factors. While sexuality can include all of these aspects, not all of these dimensions need to be experienced or expressed.'[4]

SEXUAL DIVERSITY

Western sexuality is shaped by heteronormativity, with society viewing same-sex relationships as less valid and more superficial than heterosexual relationships.[3] Professional anti-gay bias (*see* Box 9.3) and the invisibility of lesbian, gay and bisexual identities within healthcare frequently result in lesbian, gay and bisexual (LGB) people receiving sub-optimal care and experiencing direct or indirect discrimination when they use health services (*see* Chapter 3). Research which explored LGB people's experience of the mental health services suggest that many have a deep distrust of the psychiatric service and do not feel safe to be 'out' in the mental health service because of insensitive and discriminating practices, in the form of homophobia and heterosexism from professionals and other individuals using mental health services.[6,7] Lesbian, gay and bisexual people may also be concerned as professionals sometimes cast their sexualities within the realms of deviance and pathology.[8] Research also suggests that LGB people face particular issues in palliative and end-of-life care, such as lack of recognition of same-sex relationships.[9,10] There is a need for professionals to challenge anti-LGB prejudice both within themselves and within the services. In addition, professionals need to demonstrate that their practice is inclusive of LGB people by asking open and inclusive questions that do not assume heterosexuality; by being respectful and supportive when a person 'comes out'; by ensuring that documentation, assessment forms and information leaflets use language which is inclusive of LGB people and their families; and by displaying gay and lesbian literature on bereavement and support groups.

BOX 9.3 Characteristics of professional anti-gay prejudice

- Presuming individuals are heterosexual.
- Pathologising, stereotyping and stigmatising lesbian, gay and bisexual people.
- Failing to empathise with or recognise the health concerns of lesbian, gay and bisexual people.
- Denigrating any non-heterosexual form of behaviour, identity, relationship, family or community.
- Attempting to change a person's sexual orientation.[3]

SEXUALITY AND LIFE-LIMITING ILLNESS: CHANGING NATURE OF EXPRESSION

It is important to remember that sexuality is not destroyed by a diagnosis of life-limiting illness, such as cancer or motor neurone disease. However, the expression of sexuality may be significantly altered. Research on sexuality within the mental health and palliative care literature is sparse, highlighting a distinct lack of knowledge and provision of care in this area. Research that has explored sexuality in palliative care contexts clearly indicates that for people experiencing life-limiting illness, the expression of sexuality continues to be an important part of people's lives, even in the last weeks and days of life.[11,12] Although the expression of sexuality changes over time from sexual intercourse to kissing, hand holding and touching, participants in Lemieux *et al.*'s[12] study spoke of its importance within their lives, and highlighted how the lack of privacy, shared rooms, intrusions by professionals, and size of beds were barriers to their expression of sexuality.[12]

> **KEY POINT 9.2**
>
> Of particular concern for participants in a number of studies was the failure of professionals to provide sufficient information or counselling. Consequently, people were left to cope alone with many unanswered questions and concerns.[11,13]

REFLECTIVE PRACTICE EXERCISE 9.2

Time: 10 minutes

Acknowledging one's own views and discomforts about sexuality is an important first step in learning how to recognise and respond to the people in your care. Therefore, before reading any further, please consider your own practice in the light of Boxes 9.4 and 9.5.

- How many of these beliefs do you hold about people experiencing serious and enduring mental health problems that have life-limiting illness?
- What strategies do you use to manage your discomfort when addressing sexual issues in the practice?

BOX 9.4 Beliefs and views

- Sexual issues are too private and personal to discuss.
- Sexual concerns are minor problems for people experiencing mental health issues and life-limiting illness.
- Sexual issues are unimportant compared with people's struggle with ill-health.
- People are too ill to discuss sexual concerns.
- If a person has a concern or problem they will ask for help.
- Discussing sexual issues will cause the person anxiety or embarrassment.

- People do not want to talk about sexuality issues with professionals.
- People want solutions to their problems and concerns, so if there is not any treatment, it is cruel to bring it up.
- People might misinterpret my exploration or questions as a sexual advance.
- If I discuss sexuality issues with people, members of the team may think I am being voyeuristic and nosey.
- Talking about sexual issues could make the situation worse as they may reveal past traumas that they had forgotten.
- Sex is only for healthy young people and this person is too old.
- People who have life-limiting illness are grateful to be alive and are not interested in sexual expression.

BOX 9.5 Strategies used to manage discomfort around sexuality

- Ignoring cues or not responding to cues that suggest the person wants to talk.
- Using technical/clinical language to discuss sexuality issues.
- Avoiding eye contact with the person.
- Looking busy or focusing on physical care.
- Objectifying issues in a matter-of-fact manner – talking about issues from a clinical rather than emotional and feelings perspective.
- Joking about sexual issues.
- Giving advice or false reassurance – 'Everything will be all right, so don't worry'.
- Immediately referring the person to another healthcare professional so you do not have to discuss the issue.

BARRIERS TO ADDRESSING ISSUES OF SEXUALITY IN PRACTICE

Professionals are not immune to the wider societal discourse around sexuality that emphasises shame, taboo and embarrassment, resulting in what Elias[14] termed the 'the socially generated restrictions on speech'.[14] In addition, society tends to associate sexuality with the young, healthy and beautiful and tends to misunderstand or ignore the sexual needs of people who are older, disabled and, indeed, those who have been diagnosed with a life-limiting illness. Research suggests that although professionals perceive that they have a role in supporting and counselling in the area of sexuality, overall sexuality issues are ignored, minimised or poorly addressed by professionals working alongside people who experience mental health issues or with people experiencing life-limiting illness. Professionals tend to adopt a passive waiting stance that puts the onus on the person to raise issues for discussion.

This non-involvement can arise for a number of reasons, including lack of knowledge and skills, discomfort and feelings of embarrassment. Research suggests that healthcare professionals also hold a number of beliefs that prohibit them from proactively engaging with people in relation to sexual concerns. It may be assumed that because of serious and enduring mental health issues, a discussion about sexuality is irrelevant because the person is unlikely to form a relationship. However, it needs to be remembered that the expression of sexuality does not require a partner. In addition, there is often an assumption that sexuality equates to sexual intercourse and function, which is frequently reinforced by publications that focus on a person's ability to perform sexual intercourse after the diagnosis of a life-limiting illness. However, sexuality is also about touch and feelings of belonging.

Cultural myths such as those that claim older or sick people are no longer interested in sexuality and intimacy or the presumption that people's preoccupation with survival or death will overshadow their desire for intimacy or relationships acts as barriers to open communication. Lack of time, lack of privacy, and beliefs that people will ask for help, or that discussing sexual concerns is the exclusive domain of trained therapists are also factors inhibiting professionals.[15-18] The culture of the healthcare environment also perpetuates an ignoring stance. The fear of transgressing professional boundaries or of being perceived as a 'deviant' or stereotyped as a 'nympho' by the healthcare team often inhibits professionals. In the context of mental health issues, professionals fear that they may 'open a can of worms', especially if the person reveals past sexual traumas.[19,20]

Consequently, professionals distance themselves from people at a time when they feel most vulnerable, thus compounding their feelings of isolation and loneliness. Strategies used by professionals to manage their discomfort include:

➤ avoiding eye contact
➤ ignoring cues or questions
➤ objectifying issues in a 'matter-of-fact' manner
➤ using clinical terminology and joking about issues in a dismissive way.[21]

KEY POINT 9.3

These beliefs and practices are in sharp contrast to the holistic and proactive ethos of palliative care where potential problems are actively enquired about, anticipated and, where possible, prevented.

REFLECTIVE PRACTICE EXERCISE 9.3

Time: 15 minutes

Addressing issues of sexuality in practice requires that professionals have some knowledge of the impact of life-limiting illness and treatments on sexual expression. Before you read any further, please consider the following.

● Given the expansive nature of the concept of sexuality, consider how a diagnosis of life-limiting illness might influence the person's sexuality.

● Consider your response under the following headings: physical, psychological, emotional, social and spiritual dimensions of sexuality.

IMPACT OF LIFE-LIMITING ILLNESS AND TREATMENT ON SEXUALITY

The impact of a life-limiting illness and its treatment on the person's sexuality is unique to that person and will be influenced by a number of factors (*see* Box 9.6). The causes of sexuality changes are both physical and psychological. Physical causes are due to the impact of treatments and disease on anatomical structures, nerve endings and hormone levels; and psychological are due to the impact of the disease on body image, self-esteem and mood.

BOX 9.6 Factors influencing changes in sexuality

- cancer treatment – surgery, radiotherapy, chemotherapy
- degree of tissue or organ loss/damage – sexual and non-sexual organs
- tumour location
- person's beliefs and attitudes about sexuality, body images, fertility and sex
- person's age
- nature of the person's mental health issue
- strength of the person's coping mechanisms, relationships and supports (*see* Chapter 7).

Treatment of life-limiting illnesses often requires a multimodality approach, including a combination of surgery, radiotherapy and drugs. All of these treatments can alter the person's body image, fertility, sexual desire, sexual satisfaction, sexual frequency and sense of attractiveness (*see* Table 9.1). In a number of studies involving people with cancer, people reported experiencing a decline in sexual desire, in the frequency of sexual activity and in sexual satisfaction, as well as alteration in body image and decreased feelings of sexual attractiveness.[22-29] While acknowledging that surgery and radiotherapy are continually improving, most of the sexual problems experienced by people resulted from damage to the anatomical sites associated directly or indirectly with sexual activity, including the autonomic nervous system, endocrine system and vascular compromise of the genitals.[30]

Psychotropic drugs such as antidepressant, antipsychotic and anticholinergic drugs have many adverse side effects which severely impact on the quality of life and sexuality of the person.[31,32] In addition, chemotherapeutic agents and hormone therapy used in the treatment of cancers can have significant effects on sexuality and sexual functioning.[33]

The physical body is an all-encompassing filter through which people experience the world and their lives. The body is central to perceptions of self, identity and relationships. Ill-health does not have to affect sexual organs to affect sexuality and sexual functioning. Surgical procedures resulting in amputation, changes in patterns of elimination and neurological damage can all influence the person's sexuality. Following surgery, people are often left with mutilating scars and absence of a body part that was not only an expression of gender, sexuality and sensuality, but also an important part of the ideal self. In addition to the side effects of medication that directly impact on sexual desire and function, chemotherapeutic agents may cause other changes to the body, such as hair loss, weight loss or weight gain, mucositis, fatigue, nausea, anorexia and vomiting. The fatigue, nausea and anorexia that accompany many of the treatments can profoundly change how the person experiences both their body and the world around them. Research suggests that following mutilating surgery (such as mastectomy, colectomy, laryngectomy and penectomy), people experience great difficulty in coming to terms with changes in body image, body sensation and body odour, resulting in feelings of shame, stigma, embarrassment, rejection and isolation. The breasts, like other organs such as the penis or uterus, are imbued in symbolism and social meaning. Therefore, the loss of organs, as well as other bodily changes, can leave people viewing their bodies as less attractive to themselves, as well as to current or prospective partners.[34-36]

People with life-limiting illness get little time to grieve (*see* Chapter 14) and adjust to a new self as they experience profound body image changes on an on-going basis. In an attempt to protect themselves from the possible pain of rejection and to manage the distress and stigma, they may withdraw from relationships and other friendships; thus, when social and physical contact is most needed, they may be less likely to receive it. For some people, changes in body image and sexual expression may be perceived as a punishment for past actions or thoughts, dominating their perception of themselves and influencing how they react to and interact with others.

The frontal lobe of the brain is important for the regulation of insight and feedback regarding socially appropriate behaviour. Tumours of the frontal lobes are thought to remove the moral-ethical restraints that control behaviour, resulting in decreased impulse inhibition. This may lead to indiscriminate sexual behaviour, such as improper sexual remarks or gestures and other antisocial sexual behaviour that may be considered 'inappropriate' to the time, person or location. Such changes can cause immense distress to the person and disrupt relationships between the person, partner, family and the health professionals. It is important that professionals do not interpret the behaviour as a 'symptom' of the person's prior mental health issue and that they provide support to the person and the family.

In a society that is becoming increasingly intolerant of any imperfections or deviations from what is considered the 'normal' body, navigating this terrain is challenging for people who experience mental health problems. All of the changes add to the burden of distress experienced by the person and may cause a decline in self-esteem and sense of attractiveness. If we consider the stress vulnerability coping-model of mental ill-health, both the diagnosis and the changes associated with the ill-health and treatment may worsen the person's mental health problem as they add another layer of stress and vulnerability to the person's life. However, responding to issues of sexuality with people experiencing serious and enduring mental health problems can be challenging. People experiencing mental distress may not understand the diagnosis or the changes associated with the treatment because of poor explanations by professionals at the time of diagnosis or during the subsequent care period. Therefore, professionals should not assume that issues have been discussed by the professionals prescribing the treatment or in their previous hospital experience. However, the information given should be in line with the person's needs and wants, as some people may not be interested in receiving information or may not wish to discuss issues of sexuality.

TABLE 9.1 Impact of treatments on sexuality

Treatment	Men	Women
Surgery	• infertility • dry orgasm • weak orgasm	• infertility • vaginal dryness • reduced vaginal size • painful intercourse due to adhesions and scarring
Radiotherapy	• temporary or permanent erectile dysfunction • irritation to the urethra causing pain during ejaculation and maturation • infertility	• vaginal stenosis • vaginal fibrosis • atrophy of vaginal mucosa • infertility
Psychotropic medications (antidepressants and antipsychotics)	• erection difficulties (difficulty in achieving or maintaining an erection, including morning or nocturnal erections) • ejaculatory difficulties (reduced ejaculatory volume, retrograde ejaculation, delayed ejaculation painful ejaculation or total inhibition of ejaculation) • gynaecomastia • galactorrhoea • breast discomfort • weight gain • fatigue • sedation	• desire and arousal problems (decreased sexual desire, decreased sexual excitement) • poor vaginal lubrication • diminished or delayed orgasm or anorgasmia • menstruation changes (irregular menses, amenorrhea or mennorrhagia) • gynaecomastia • galactorrhoea • breast discomfort • weight gain • fatigue • sedation
Chemotherapy	• ejaculation problems	• premature menopausal symptoms • vaginal dryness • desire and arousal problems
Hormone therapy	• decline in sexual interest and sexual satisfaction • reduced force of ejaculation • decreased orgasmic sensation • hot flashes • weight gain and breast swelling/growth • loss of ability to enjoy erotic dreams	• premenopausal symptoms, such as vaginal dryness, vaginal atrophy, hot flashes, increased UTIs or vaginal infections

CARING FOR THE PHYSICAL BODY: TOUCH

As ill-health advances and physical health deteriorates, the person's capacity to manage their bodily functions lessen, and tasks such as feeding and bathing, which were performed independently from a young age, will no longer be possible without some assistance. The loss of control over the physical body and the increasing dependence on family or professionals for activities of daily living can be a profound threat to the person. In addition, having people violate social norms and conventions around touch may pose formidable psychological challenges to the person and professional. If the person has difficulties with people entering or trespassing into their personal space they may find being touched in areas that have only been touched previously by the person themself or by others during intimate moments very traumatic.

Using touch as a medium of communication is important at this time, as touch can provide reassurance, comfort, relieve pain and ease a person's sense of isolation.[37] Touch, however, is only therapeutic if it is offered within the context of respecting the person's uniqueness, dignity and wishes, and if it is respectful of the person's space, needs and cultural background. Mental health professionals are in an ideal position to explore with the person the degree of touch they are comfortable with, as well as their concerns and wishes around being touched. Professionals need to combine both instrumental and expressive touch. While instrumental touch is functional, utilitarian, and part of the touch used when engaging in the procedural or 'tasks' of care, expressive touch can enhance the professional's ability to develop rapport and emotional connection, while also communicating care, interest, comfort, recognition and reassurance. By combining both types of touch, professionals can maximise the possibility that physical care is provided in a manner that does not objectify the person's body and maintains a sense of personhood and personal worth.

MULTIPLE TRAUMAS AND MULTIPLE GRIEF: MOURNING PAST LOSS

Many losses affect sexuality during the dying processes (*see* Chapter 13). Many people experiencing serious and enduring mental health problems will have experienced multiple traumas and losses that contributed to their mental health problem or as a by-product of their mental health problem. A diagnosis of a life-limiting illness will not only trigger a grief reaction to current losses, such as loss of body image, identity, sexual function and control of the physical body, but it may also trigger a grief reaction that involves revisiting and mourning other past losses and traumas associated with sexuality and sexual expression (*see* Chapter 14).

The social exclusion and marginalisation that arises from the stigma associated with mental health problems may have limited people's active participation in all aspects of life, including how they experienced and expressed sexuality. People who experience mental health problems report becoming cautious about relationships and especially intimate relationships, fearing that disclosure will result in rejection.[38,39] Others may have been fearful of engaging in relationships because of the sexual side effects induced by the psychotropic medication. Consequently, the person may never have experienced an intimate relationship and mourn what they may perceive as an 'un-lived life'.

Experiencing a serious and enduring mental health problem may have made it difficult for couples to maintain lasting intimate and sexual relationships; thus depriving the person of the opportunity to have a long-term relationship or become a parent, while others may have lost their partner and other roles due to breakdown in relationships. Moreover, research suggests that people experiencing serious and enduring mental health issues are at high risk of losing custody of their children.[40–43] In addition, a number of people may have experienced losses that they have kept hidden and secret, such as termination of pregnancies or adoptions. Research suggests that people who experience serious and enduring mental health problems, especially women, may have experienced increased levels of sexual exploitation and sexual coercion, and may have engaged in casual sexual encounters during periods of ill health or may have traded sex for some material gain. People experiencing serious and enduring mental health problems, both women and men, also report higher rates of sexual abuse and repeated victimisation compared with those without a diagnosis.[44,45] Consequently, in addition to the losses associated with the life-limiting illness and its treatment, the person may need to grieve losses associated with sexuality that may have remained hidden and unspoken because of stigma, self-hatred and shame.

Partners, carers, family and sexuality
It is noteworthy that attention to the needs of the families is embedded as one of the core principles of palliative care within the WHO definition.[1] When a person is diagnosed with a life-limiting illness, it is not just the person who experiences the grief and loss. Distress reverberates throughout the family and the social network. Family and friends may not know how to talk to the person, fearing that they will cause upset or worsen mental health issues; consequently, there may be avoidance, misunderstanding and unease among family and friends. Questions like, 'Can I talk to them? Mention it? Touch them? Hug them?' may become an issue. Some friends and family members may find it too difficult to continue any level of closeness, being unable to face the pain of being around the person. In many contexts, what people want is an opportunity to tell their story, to grieve their loss and for somebody that will give witness to their pain and difficulties (*see* Chapter 14).

Partners who have previously enjoyed an intimate or sexual relationship with the person may find that their sexual relationship diminishes for reasons other than the physical and psychological changes associated with the disease or the treatment. The person and the partner may have a number of fears and anxieties about initiating a sexual or intimate relationship (*see* Boxes 9.7 and 9.8).

BOX 9.7 Barriers to person experiencing life-limiting illness initiating sexual relationship with partner

- Concern that illness is contagious.
- Concern that they are not attractive or look and smell ugly.
- Concern that person only attracted to them out of pity.
- Fear that making love will hurt or worsen symptoms.

BOX 9.8 Barriers to partner's initiating sexual relationship with person experiencing life-limiting illness

- Fear of hurting the person.
- Fear that love making will sap the person's energy.
- Fear that the person could die during love making.
- Fear that if they touch or caress the person he or she thinks they are being lustful and inconsiderate.
- Guilt about making love when partner is facing a life-limiting illness.
- Fear that they will worsen the person's self-esteem if person cannot maintain an erection or achieve orgasm.
- Difficulty seeing the person they are providing intimate physical care for as sexual.
- Concern that professionals will think them selfish and inconsiderate.

Partners may also find the sexual relationship diminishes due to the physical exhaustion of taking on a carer role, the repositioning of the person as an asexual 'sick person' and beliefs that desiring or having a sexual relationship is inappropriate or unacceptable with a person who has a life-limiting illness.[46–48] As unconditional love is rare, this avoidance of intimate relationships may feel like rejection to the ill person, reinforcing their own view that they are damaged and no longer sexually desirable or attractive.

Research suggests that both cognitive and behavioural changes are important in successfully adapting to sexuality changes post cancer.[46,49] Those who successfully adapted and accepted changes were people who redefined sexual activity away from the 'coital imperative', and incorporated alternative practices that had been marginalised in favour of coital sex.[46,49] Research involving people without a mental health issue suggests that the person may find it difficult to discuss sexual changes and fears with their partner.[23] For people experiencing mental health issues, these difficulties may be exacerbated. Therefore, both the person and the partner may benefit from having time to discuss how they might continue to have an intimate relationship, which may involve renegotiating sexuality and intimacy to include non-coital intimate acts, such as caressing, cuddling, massage and mutual masturbation. In addition, they may also require support to grieve the loss and talk about their concerns and feelings of disappointment, anger, loneliness and sadness. As the person's health deteriorates and the body starts to change at a significant pace, maintaining physical closeness through touching and stroking the person's body may become the most important means of communicating presence, tenderness, affections and love.

BEREAVEMENT AND DISENFRANCHISED GRIEF

> **KEY POINT 9.4**
>
> Support of partners and family members during bereavement is central to good-quality palliative care and an important part of the professional's role.

The loss of a loved one is considered to be one of the most stressful life events that a human being can experience. During this time, people experience a range of emotions such as anger, guilt, anxiety, helplessness and sadness and require support to identify and express feelings related to their loss. The intensity of emotion and pain felt at this time is normal and should not be pathologised.

Bereaved gay or lesbian partners may be particularly vulnerable at this time as research indicated that many LG people experience the pain of 'disenfranchised grief', and are deprived of the rituals of 'communal sorrow' and other social/psychological supports that are present for heterosexual people.[8,10] Professionals need to acknowledge the significance of the LG person's loss, not just of a friend but of a partner and lover, and demonstrate a willingness to develop the communicative space necessary to talk about their loss and provide appropriate bereavement support services. For some people this may mean a preference for attending a gay or lesbian bereavement counsellor or attending services provided by gay and lesbian support groups.

REFLECTIVE PRACTICE EXERCISE 9.4

> **Time: 5 minutes**
> - How frequently do you discuss sexuality issues with the people you care for, including family members?
> - How frequently do the team you work within discuss sexuality issues of the people they care for, including family members?

SUPPORTING EXPRESSIONS OF SEXUALITY IN PRACTICE: MULTIDISCIPLINARY APPROACH

Evaluating changes in the person's sexuality, assessing reactions and coping patterns, identifying specific problems, meeting and supporting the person's physical, emotional and spiritual needs, as well as meeting the information and support needs of the person's family and significant others is not the prerogative of any one discipline, but an important dimension of holistic care provided by the whole multidisciplinary team of mental health and palliative care professionals. There are a number of frameworks for assessment and intervention provided within the literature, such as those outlined in Box 9.9.

BOX 9.9 Frameworks for assessment and intervention

PLISSIT[50]

P: Give people **permission** to discuss.

LI: Provide **limited information** relevant to person's concerns.

SS: Give **specific suggestions** about sexual activity.

IT: Provide **intensive therapy** if required.

ALARM[51]

A: Activity

L: Libido

A: Arousal

R: Resolution

M: Medical information – impact of ill-health and treatment

BETTER[52]

B: **Bring up** topic.

E: **Explain** that your concern is related to quality of life.

T: **Tell** person you will find appropriate resources.

T: If **timing** not appropriate, acknowledge the person can ask for information at any time.

E: **Educate** person about side effects of treatments.

R: **Record** assessment and interventions.

Irrespective of which model is used, it needs to be remembered that to engage in a conversation on issues of:

➤ love
➤ intimacy
➤ desire
➤ sexual needs
➤ sexual frustrations
➤ masturbation
➤ altered body image
➤ feeling of being mutilated
➤ feeling of being less desirable
➤ frustration at the loss of physical and psychological intimacy
➤ fears of not being perceived as attractive

. . . requires that professionals use their skills of:

➤ listening
➤ empathy
➤ presence
➤ emotional connection.

Communication with the person is not so much about what we tell the person but what we allow the person to tell us. Therefore, the voice and story of the person need to be central to the caring process and the therapeutic relationship developed needs to be anchored in 'being with', 'engaging with' and 'caring with' the person, which acknowledges the shared humanity that exists between the person and the professional. Although Box 9.10 provides some areas for consideration within the discussion, listening and bearing witness to the person's story need to take priority.

KEY POINT 9.5

The therapeutic and emancipating value of story telling and talking frankly about feelings and experiences should not be underestimated.

BOX 9.10 Areas for discussion

- Person's understanding of sexuality and comfort with discussing intimate issues.
- Person's understanding of diagnosis, prognosis and dis-ease/ill-health trajectory.
- Person's understanding of impact of treatments on body image and sexual expression.
- Nature of relationships with partner/significant others prior to diagnosis.
- Impact of life-limiting illness and treatments on relationships with partner/significant others.
- Person's feelings and emotions in response to changes in sexual expression:
  – body image
  – sexual desire
  – sexual function
  – roles
  – relationships.
- Person's coping patterns.
- Level of support available from significant others, professionals and services.
- Person's fears and concerns for the future.
- Person's wishes and hopes for the future.

Central to making it easy for the person to tell his or her story is the ability to live on the edge of 'not knowing', tolerating the anxiety and feelings of discomfort this creates within, while at the same time creating a context for telling through 'natural curiosity', gentle prompting, reflecting and the asking of interesting questions. Box 9.11 provides some examples of prompts and interesting questions that may be used to facilitate exploration and further discussion.

BOX 9.11 Prompts and 'interesting questions'[53]

- Would you mind saying a little more about that?
- How did that make you feel?
- What sense did you make of . . .?
- Did anything make it better or worse?
- What do you think might help?
- How do you think I might help?
- How do you think your partner might feel?
- As a couple, how would you normally sort issues?
- Would you normally talk to your partner about issues?
- Who would normally initiate conversation on sensitive issues?
- Would you like to talk to your partner?
- Would you like help in planning how to raise the issue?
- Some people have questions regarding . . . If you would like to talk, we can talk about . . .
- Other people in similar situations have said the physical expression of their sexuality has been affected by their illness. Would you like to discuss this . . .?

Professionals need to be consciously alert to the inherent power differential within relationships and fine-tune their self-reflective skills so they become critically aware of the preconceptions and biases that they may impose on the person's experience. They need to actively encourage people to challenge professional interpretations and articulate their preferences for care, so that the outcome is a mutually agreed-upon plan of care that is based on adequate information and discussion. Box 9.12 provides some issues for consideration in relation to creating a context for open and sensitive dialogue.

BOX 9.12 Issues to consider

- Acknowledge that the person may be uncomfortable.
- Give person permission not to respond.
- Relate your questions to the person's health status.
- Proceed from less sensitive areas to more sensitive areas.
- Be respectful of the person's rights to control content and pace.
- Be open and non-judgemental about myths and sexual practice.
- Use language that the person understands.
- Avoid language with a heterosexual bias.

- Consider the person's religion and culture. Consider the environment in terms of affording privacy and comfort.
- Make sure you have time to explore and discuss issues.

While including issues of sexuality within the horizons of practice requires a proactive approach, it must be remembered that people choose with whom they are most comfortable about discussing and disclosing sexuality issues.

KEY POINT 9.6

Members of the team need to create and support a culture that is open and willing to discuss sensitive issues. In this way, information will be shared between team members and the team member whom the person has chosen to talk to will be supported.

No one person within the team will have all the knowledge and skills required to respond to every eventuality. Therefore, professionals need a team that models a willingness to seek help and feedback on challenging clinical situations. A team that is not afraid to discuss sexuality in an open and non-hierarchical manner is more likely to seek specialist advice and refer people to specialist medical, surgical and sexual counselling interventions if required.

CONCLUSION

People with pre-existing mental health problems who develop a terminal illness and require end-of-life care are possibly among the most underrepresented and deprived populations in our society.[54]

KEY POINT 9.7

One of the primary goals of palliative care is to improve quality of life, by adding *life-to-days* as opposed to days to life.

In the words of Saunders (1989: xix)[55] the aim of palliative care is to enable the person to . . .

> live until they die . . . performing to the limit of their physical and mental capacity . . . where ever possible.[55]

As sexuality is a fundamental and enduring aspect of life, it follows that professionals should proactively address this aspect of the person's humanity and human experience. At present, the burden of responsibility seems to be on the person to initiate discussion, while professionals hide behind excuses of a lack of knowledge, training, or communication skills.

> **KEY POINT 9.8**
>
> This passive waiting stance is not in keeping with the proactive, holistic philosophy that underpins palliative care.

Professionals need to develop the knowledge, skill and confidence to create an atmosphere and context that encourages people to express their sexuality, raise their legitimate concerns and grieve the losses they are encountering on a daily basis. Indeed, Yaniv (1995: 71)[56] is of the view that . . .

> because most people are embarrassed and hesitant and only a very few are desperate enough or assertive enough to approach [professionals] for help, [professionals] should take the initiative.[56]

To do otherwise is to ignore the essence of what it is to be human.

REFERENCES

1 World Health Organization. *Cancer Pain Relief and Palliative Care.* Technical Report Series 804. Geneva: WHO; 1990.

2 Stausmire J. Sexuality at the end of life. *American Journal of Hospice & Palliative Care.* 2004; **21**: 33–9.

3 Higgins A, Allen O. *Gay, Lesbian and Bisexual People: a good practice guide for mental health nurses.* Dublin: Irish Institute of Mental Health Nursing and GLEN; 2010. Available at: www. iimhn.org/conference_2010.asp (accessed 21 April 2012).

4 Pan American Health Organisation/World Health Organization. *Promotion of Sexual Health: recommendations for action.* Proceedings of a regional consultation convened by Pan American Health Organisation (PAHO), World Health Organization (WHO) in collaboration with the World Association of Sexology. Antigua, Guatemala: Pan American Health Organisation/World Health Organization; 2002.

5 Higgins A. Sexuality and gender. In: Barker P, editor. *Psychiatric and Mental Health Nursing: the craft of caring.* London: Hodder Arnold; 2008.

6 Robertson A. The mental health experiences of gay men: a research study exploring gay men's health needs. *Journal of Psychiatric and Mental Health Nursing.* 1998; **5**: 33–40.

7 McFarlane L. *Diagnosis Homophobic: the experience of lesbians, gay men and bisexuals in mental health services.* London: PACE; 1998.

8 Almack K. End-of-life needs of lesbian, gay and bisexual older people. *End of Life Care.* 2007; **1**: 27–32.

9 Katz A. Gay and lesbian patients with cancer. *Oncology Nursing Forum.* 2009; **36**: 203–7.

10 Glacken M, Higgins A. The grief experience of same sex couples, within an Irish context: tacit acknowledgement. *International Journal of Palliative Nursing.* 2008; **14**: 297–303.

11 Ananth H, Jones L, King M, Tookman A. The impact of cancer on sexual function: a controlled study. *Palliative Medicine.* 2003; **17**: 202–5.

12 Lemieux L, Kaiser S, Pereira J, Meadows LM. Sexuality in palliative care. *Palliative Medicine.* 2004; **18**: 630–7.

13 Katz A. The sound of silence: sexuality information for cancer patients. *Journal of Clinical Oncology.* 2005; **23**: 238–41.

14 Elias N. *The Civilising Process: the history of manners*. Oxford: Basil Blackwell (Translated into English by Edmund Jephcott in 1978); 1939.

15 Saunamaki N, Andersson M, Engstrom M. Discussing sexuality with patients: nurses' attitudes and beliefs. *Journal of Advanced Nursing*. 2010; **66**: 1308–16.

16 Higgins A, Barker P, Begley C. 'Veiling sexualities': a grounded theory of mental health nurses responses to issues of sexuality. *Journal of Advanced Nursing*. 2008; **62**: 307–17.

17 Guthrie C. Nurses' perceptions of sexuality relating to patient care. *Journal of Clinical Nursing*. 1999; **8**: 313–21.

18 Kotronoulas G, Papadopoulou C, Patiraki E. Nurses' knowledge, attitudes, and practices regarding provision of sexual health care in patients with cancer: critical review of the evidence. *Support Care Cancer*. 2009; **17**: 479–501.

19 Cort E, Attenborough J, Watson JP. An initial exploration of community mental health nurses' attitudes to and experience of sexuality-related issues in their work with people experiencing mental health problems. *Journal of Psychiatric and Mental Health Nursing*. 2001; **8**: 489–99.

20 Higgins A. *'Veiling sexualities': a grounded theory of mental health nurses responses to issues of sexuality*. Dublin: Trinity College Dublin; 2008.

21 Meerabeau L. The management of embarrassment and sexuality in health care. *Journal of Advanced Nursing*. 1999; **29**: 1503–7.

22 Wilmoth M. The aftermath of breast cancer: an altered sexual self. *Cancer Nursing*. 2001; **24**: 278–86.

23 Maughan K, Heyman B, Matthews M. In the shadow of risk. How men cope with a partner's gynaecological cancer. *International Journal of Nursing Studies*. 2002; **39**: 27–34.

24 Kylstra W, Leenhouts G, Everaerd W, *et al.* Sexual outcomes following treatment for early stage gynaecological cancer: a prospective multicenter & nbsp study. *International Journal of Gynaecological Cancer*. 1999; **9**: 387–95.

25 Bourgeois-Law G, Lotocki R. Sexuality and gynaecological cancer: a needs assessment. *Canadian Journal of Human Sexuality*. 1999; **8**: 231–41.

26 Navon L, Morag A. Liminality as biographical disruption: unclassifiability following hormonal therapy for advanced prostate cancer. *Social Science & Medicine*. 2004; **58**: 2337–47.

27 Bertero C. Altered sexual patterns after treatment for prostate cancer. *Cancer Practice*. 2001; **9**: 245–51.

28 Pontin D, Porter T, McDonagh R. Investigating the effect of erectile dysfunction on the lives of men: a qualitative research study. *Journal of Clinical Nursing*. 2002; **11**: 264–72.

29 Manderson L. Boundary breaches: the body, sex and sexuality after stoma surgery. *Social Science & Medicine*. 2005; **61**: 405–15.

30 Saravosky R, Basson R, Krychman M, *et al.* Cancer and sexual problems. *Journal of Sexual Medicine*. 2010; **7**: 349–73.

31 Higgins A, Nash M, Lynch A. Antidepressants-associated sexual dysfunction: impact, effects and treatment. *Drug, Health Care and Patient Safety*. 2010; **2**: 141–52.

32 Higgins A, Barker P, Begley C. Neuroleptic medication and sexuality: the forgotten aspect of education and care. *Journal of Psychiatric and Mental Health Nursing*. 2005; **12**: 439–46.

33 Mercadante S, Vitrano V, Catania V. Sexual issues in early and late stage cancer: a review. *Support Care Cancer*. 2010; **18**: 659–65.

34 Fitch M, Gray R, Franssen E. Women's perspectives regarding the impact of ovarian cancer: implications for nursing. *Cancer Nursing*. 2000; **23**: 359–66.

35 Smith D, Babaian J. The effects of treatment for cancer on male fertility and sexuality. *Cancer Nursing*. 1992; **15**: 271–5.

36 Avis N, Crawford S, Manuel J. Psychosocial problems among younger women with breast cancer. *Psycho-Oncology.* 2004; **13**: 295–308.

37 Gleeson M, Higgins A. Touch in mental health nursing: an exploratory study of psychiatric nurses' views and perceptions. *Journal of Psychiatric and Mental Health Nursing.* 2009; **16**: 382–9.

38 McCann E. Exploring sexual and relationship possibilities for people with psychosis – a review of the literature. *Journal of Psychiatric and Mental Health Nursing.* 2003; **10**: 640–9.

39 McCandless F, Sladen C. Sexual health and women with bipolar disorder. *Journal of Advanced Nursing.* 2003; **44**: 42–8.

40 Dipple H, Smith S, Andrews H, *et al.* The experience of motherhood in women with severe and enduring mental illness. *Journal of Social Psychiatry and Psychiatric Epidemiology.* 2002; **37**: 336–40.

41 Chernomas WM, Clarke DE, Chisholm FA. Perspectives of women living with schizophrenia. *Psychiatric Services.* 2000; **51**: 1517–21.

42 Joseph J, Joshi S, Lewin A, *et al.* Characteristics and perceived needs of mothers with serious mental illness. *Psychiatric Services.* 1999; **50**: 1357–9.

43 Miller LJ, Finnerty M. Sexuality, pregnancy, and childbearing among women with schizophrenia-spectrum disorders. *Psychiatric Services.* 1996; **47**: 502–6.

44 McGee H, Garavan R, de Barra M, *et al.* The SAVI report: Sexual Abuse and Violence in Ireland. A national study of Irish experiences, beliefs and attitudes concerning sexual violence. Dublin: Liffey Press in association with Dublin Rape Crisis Centre; 2002.

45 Bohn D. Lifetime physical and sexual abuse, substance abuse, depression and suicide attempts among Native American women. *Issues in Mental Health Nursing.* 2003; **24**: 333–52.

46 Gilbert E, Usher J, Perz J. Renegotiating sexuality and intimacy in the context of cancer: the experience of carers. *Archives of Sexual Behavior.* 2010; **39**: 998–1009.

47 Boehmer U, Clarke J. Communication about prostate cancer between men and their wives. *Journal of Family Practice.* 2001; **50**: 226–31.

48 Holmberg S, Scott L, Alexy W, Fife B. Relationship issues of women with breast cancer. *Cancer Nursing.* 200; **24**: 53–60.

49 Reese J. Coping with sexual concerns after cancer. *Current Opinions in Oncology.* 2011; **23**: 313–21.

50 Annon J. The PLISSIT model: a proposed conceptual scheme for the behavioural treatment of sexual problems. *Journal of Sex Education Therapists.* 1976; **2**: 1–15.

51 Andersen B. How cancer affects sexual functioning. *Oncology Nursing Forum.* 1990; **4**: 81–8.

52 Mick J, Hughes M, Cohen MZ. Sexuality and cancer: how oncology nurses can address it BETTER. *Oncology Nursing Forum.* 2003; **30**: 152–3.

53 Higgins A, Barker P, Begley C. Sexual health education for people with mental health problems: what can we learn from the literature? *Journal of Psychiatric and Mental Health Nursing.* 2006; **13**: 687–97.

54 Davie E. A social work perspective on palliative care for people with mental health problems. *European Journal of Palliative Care.* 2006; **13**: 26–8.

55 Saunders C. Care of the dying: the problem of euthanasia. *Nursing Times.* 1976; **72**: 1049–52.

56 Yaniv H. Sexuality of cancer patients: a palliative approach. *European Journal of Palliative Care.* 1995; **2**: 69–72.

TO LEARN MORE

- Apfel RJ, Handel MH. *Madness and Loss of Motherhood: sexuality, reproduction and long term mental illness.* Washington DC, London: American Psychiatric Press, 1993.

- Ellison N. *Mental Health and Palliative Care: literature review*. London: Mental Health Foundation, 2008. Available at: www.mentalhealth.org.uk/content/assets/PDF/publications/mental_health_palliative_care.pdf (accessed 21 April 2012).
- Heath H, White I. *The Challenge of Sexuality in Health Care*. London: Blackwell Science, 2002.
- Saravosky R, Basson R, Krychman M, *et al.* Cancer and sexual problems. *Journal of Sexual Medicine*. 2010; **7**: 349–73.
- Whipple V. *Lesbian Widows: invisible grief*. New York: Harwood, 2006.

CHAPTER 10

Assessment

John R Ashcroft

INTRODUCTION

The World Health Organization defines palliative care as:

> . . . an approach which improves the quality of life of patients and their families facing life threatening illness, through the prevention, assessment and treatment of pain and other physical, psychosocial and spiritual problems.[1]

REFLECTIVE PRACTICE EXERCISE 10.1

Time: 10 minutes

Consider your own practice area:
- How frequently do you provide palliative care to individuals experiencing serious and enduring mental health problems?
- Think carefully – has this been a conscious or unconscious act?

The concept of palliative care has evolved and it is becoming increasingly apparent that the approach used in palliative care need not necessarily be for people approaching the end of their life.

KEY POINT 10.1

The term 'palliative care' is the alleviation of suffering regardless of the availability of cure or the stage of illness.

It is intended that through the relief of symptoms the individual and their family can achieve the best quality of life possible.

SELF-ASSESSMENT EXERCISE 10.1

Time: 5 minutes
What would you consider to be the key principles in mental health care?

Mental health nursing students frequently argue that they engage in the key principles of palliative care[2] and the similarity in philosophy between palliative care and mental health practice has been described and includes:[3]
➤ person-centred practice
➤ relationship-based connectedness
➤ a belief in compassionate, holistic care
➤ respect for autonomy and choice
➤ quality-of-life issues
➤ family as the unit of care
➤ the need for a democratic and intra- inter-discipline work team.

SELF-ASSESSMENT EXERCISE 10.2

Time: 10 minutes
• What skills, including interpersonal skills, are needed to 'find out' all about (assess) an individual so you can really help them?
• Think about 'who' the person is, not what diagnosis he or she may have.

ASSESSMENT IN SERIOUS AND ENDURING MENTAL HEALTH

Assessment has been described as the cornerstone of effective mental health practice[4] and there is evidence to suggest that the assessment process itself can be therapeutic.[5]

REFLECTIVE PRACTICE EXERCISE 10.2

Time: 10 minutes
• Reflect on the above statement.
• Write down how you think the assessment process can be therapeutic to:
  – the individual
  – you as the assessor.

Upon presentation to mental health services, assessment is often focused on determining current symptoms in order to make a 'diagnosis'. An individual may be seen by a number of professionals and be asked about the history and duration of their symptoms, in addition to receiving mental and physical examination.

SELF-ASSESSMENT EXERCISE 10.3

Time: 5 minutes

Whilst acknowledging the above is useful and necessary information for the professional, how helpful is it to the individual who may be distressed, frightened, angry, withdrawn?

Psychotropic medication may be prescribed and/or psychosocial intervention arranged. The success or failure of treatment is often determined by the reduction or continued presence of the initial presenting symptoms. Laing[6] termed this approach the *medical model*, an approach to disease that aims to find medical treatments for diagnosed symptoms *in the presence of evident pathology*.

In most medical specialties, physical examination and investigation will typically precede diagnosis. With the exception of physical trauma and infectious diseases, the exact cause of disease is often unknown, unclear, or believed to be multi-factorial. However, even if the cause of disease is unclear, pathology, in terms of the physical manifestations of the cause, is usually evident before a diagnosis is made and treatment initiated. Examples include hypertension, many cancers, and neurological disorders. Treatment is then often focused upon symptom relief *in addition* to attempts made to reverse physiological change (e.g. inflammation).

DIAGNOSIS IN SERIOUS AND ENDURING MENTAL HEALTH

Medical diagnosis and treatment in mental health is fundamentally different from diagnosis and treatment in other specialties. Diagnosis is made based on collections of symptoms (syndromes) occurring together in a predictable manner and treatment is focused on alleviating these symptoms as opposed to tackling pathology. In this way, there is an assumption that there are underlying cause(s) for the syndromes, yet to be discovered. It was the German psychiatrist Emil Kraeplin who first coined this idea and on whose work current psychiatry classification systems (ICD-10[7] and DSM-1V[8]) are still based.[9]

SELF-ASSESSMENT EXERCISE 10.4

Time: 5 minutes

If we use a classification system to uncover problems, how can this help us to get to 'know' the 'person'?

ICD-10 and DSM-1V both acknowledge the limitations of the current classification systems and describe how professionals should consider that individuals sharing a diagnosis are likely to be heterogeneous even in regard to the defining features of the diagnosis.[7,8]

A common misconception is that the classification of mental disorders classifies people, when actually it is the disorders that are being classified. It is the individual who experiences the symptoms of schizophrenia (schizophrenia being a cluster of many possible symptoms that are regularly seen together) and all that this entails, as opposed to the person being 'a schizophrenic'.

It has been argued, given the absence of evident pathology in mental ill-health (with the exception of a number of neuropsychiatric disorders) and given that treatment essentially involves the alleviation of subjectively distressing mental states, that the application of a medical model or approach to such treatment symptoms is inappropriate.[6]

Many professionals are perturbed by the suggestion that psychiatric diagnosis is not diagnosis in the true sense of the word, believing that this suggests that mental 'ill' health, as a concept, does not exist. However, it should be noted that the absence of the clinical and physical manifestations of disease is not synonymous with the absence of ill-health.

Health has been defined as:

> . . . a state of complete physical, mental, and social well-being not simply the absence of disease or infirmity.[10]

The presence of mental health symptoms, therefore, are sufficient evidence of 'ill' health.

SUBJECTIVE EXPERIENCE

KEY POINT 10.2

Remember that what the assessing professional deems as important may not be so to the individual presenting with symptoms.

The assessor may be attempting to illicit psychopathology (i.e. abnormal experiences, cognition and behaviour) in an attempt to make a diagnosis, whereas the person experiencing symptoms wishes to convey their subjective experience and distress. The objective description or label may be the same yet the subjective experience completely different. The philosophical concept of *qualia* refers to the subjectivity of perceptual experiences and the near impossibility to relay that experience verbally to others.[11] Although we label colours as red, green or blue, for example, how can I be confident that my blue is your blue?

In this context reality is determined through an individual's thoughts and their subjective perceptual experiences as opposed to objective observation. The same may be applied to subjective emotional experiences. Any two individuals with identical objectively described mental health symptoms, and indeed identical expression of these symptoms, may have completely different subjective experiences.

> **KEY POINT 10.3**
>
> The approach to each person needs to be tailored towards his or her individual needs rather than simply aimed at alleviating the symptoms as listed in any categorical diagnostic classification system.

THE PALLIATIVE CARE APPROACH TO SERIOUS AND ENDURING MENTAL HEALTH

> **KEY POINT 10.4**
>
> Although palliative care is typically reserved for individuals with terminal illness, it could be argued that given the treatment of most medical disorders involves the alleviation of symptoms as opposed to cure, all disease could be treated using a palliative approach.

However, financial and time constraints often mean that treatment is focused upon alleviation of presenting symptoms even though physical illness is likely to have impacted on other aspects of the individual's life, particularly if illness has been chronic. Similarly, it is appreciated that mental health symptoms do not take place in isolation and an eclectic, holistic, person-centred approach to assessment is essential. An understanding and appreciation of this connection are paramount if measures are to be put in place to improve quality of life of an individual experiencing serious and enduring mental health symptoms.

SELF-ASSESSMENT EXERCISE 10.5

> **Time: 5 minutes**
> How would you assess what the quality of life is for the person, and what this means for him or her?

An individual experiencing serious and enduring mental health concerns and dilemmas may remain in contact with mental health services for years if not decades. Throughout this period the person may receive a number of diagnostic labels and it may be assumed (falsely) that the original diagnosis was inaccurate. However, if the limitations of the current diagnostic classification system are recognised (i.e. that the diagnosis of psychiatric disorders is a *descriptive* process and makes no reference to the cause of illness) it is to be *expected* that diagnosis will change over time in accordance with the individual's needs and variable presenting symptoms.

A diagnosis based on *cause* would be less likely to change over time. As cause of mental ill-health is usually unknown, this is used as a rationale for employing alternative models and treatment approaches to mental health symptoms. Medical diagnosis and assessment often describe an individual's presentation *at one point in time*, i.e. in cross-section. Although possibly helpful in relaying information to other professionals, a particular diagnostic label is at best incomplete and may possibly, at worst, be stigmatising. Thus, additional information is required to gain an understanding of the unique problems of the individual experiencing serious and enduring mental health symptoms.

A longitudinal assessment is preferable to determine the impact of symptoms on various facets of a person's life over often significant periods of time. Therefore, the person-centred approach recognises that – regardless of diagnosis – an individual will have different needs at different phases of her or his ill-health.

KEY POINT 10.5

Families and carers require considerable support throughout and will have variable needs themselves.

Therefore, assessment needs to reflect this and is a continuous and on-going dynamic process.

ASSESSMENT

What is the aim of assessment?

Ultimately, the purpose of assessment is to find out what needs to be done to improve an individual's quality of life and to determine how this is best done in relation to the unique circumstances of the individual being assessed.

The assessing professional aims to
➤ gather information about the:
  − person
  − family
  − illness
  − associated problems[12]
➤ identify factors associated with the health problems[12]
➤ highlight a person's coping strategies and to explore their strengths and weaknesses.[12]

REFLECTIVE PRACTICE EXERCISE 10.3

Time: 15 minutes

Think about how you find out the above information.
• Do you assess a person using a questionnaire, filling in or ticking appropriate boxes?

- Do you ask the person a series of questions, making notes about what you feel is important?
- Do you ask a few leading questions, and then listen carefully to the person's story?
- If you write down any assessment details, do you give a copy to the person?
- Do you do something else?
- Which method do you feel would help you and the individual the most – and why? Think of the long-term consequences.

When should assessment occur?

Key recommendation 2 of NICE guidelines states that:

> . . . assessment and discussion of patients' needs for physical, psychological, social, spiritual and financial support should be undertaken at key points (such as at diagnosis; at commencement, during and at the end of treatment; at relapse; and when death is approaching).[13]

Where should assessment take place?

The assessment may be lengthy, depending upon the complexity of issues discussed and the person's ability (or desire) to relay information. Therefore, measures should be taken to ensure that assessment takes place in a private yet safe and comfortable environment. Assessment does not have to be completed all at once. Tailor the length of the assessment to the individual's needs. Assessment is an on-going procedure and not a 'one-off' exercise.

SELF-ASSESSMENT EXERCISE 10.6

Time: 5 minutes
How could the environment be manipulated in order to make it therapeutic (therapeutic environment)?

Distractions and unnecessary interruptions should be avoided. The assessing professional should book sufficient time in their diary for assessment to take place. Too much allocated time is preferable to not enough.

KEY POINT 10.6

Clock watching does not encourage an individual to engage with the assessment process. To gain a person's trust, that individual needs to feel that they are listened to, and their story is important.

A rushed assessment when an individual is made to feel that another issue is pending is unlikely to be productive.

Who should perform the assessment?

It is of paramount importance that the assessor is a professional with an appropriate level of knowledge of serious and enduring mental health problems, the many manifestations of such problems, and the various potential impacts. The assessor needs to be competent in key aspects of the assessment process and must have developed the skills needed.

REFLECTIVE PRACTICE EXERCISE 10.4

Time: 5 minutes
- How could you develop and improve your own skills of assessment?
- What changes do you need to make?

This has huge implications in terms of an individual's first contact with services and triage. A lack of expertise and experience in the assessor at this point could lead to people experiencing mental health problems not being recognised as needing assistance.

What assessment skills should be developed?

Empathy

The concept of empathy is a clinical instrument that needs to be used with skill to measure another person's internal subjective state using the observer's own capacity for emotional and cognitive experience as a yardstick.[14] Empathy should be distinguished from sympathy which implies that the observer *feels sorry for* the observed. Of course the two are not mutually exclusive although sympathy may impact on the assessor's ability to empathise.

The assessor's ability to understand a person's experience from the person's point of view – *empathy* – is preferable as an assessment skill to imagining how the assessor would feel in the same situation – *sympathy*).

> 'You never really understand a person until you consider things from his point of view . . . until you climb into his skin and walk around in it.'[15]

An understanding of non-verbal communication

Non-verbal communication can be used to infer the subjective emotional state and thought processes of an individual. Examples include the following.

➤ **Facial expressions** – e.g. smiling, frowning.
➤ **Gestures** – e.g. waving, pointing.
➤ **Paralinguistics** – refers to vocal communication that is separate from language, e.g. tone, volume, inflection, pitch.

➤ **Body language (gestures, posture, eye gaze)** e.g.:
  – avoidance of eye contact or an excessive held gaze may be significant
  – pointing may be evidence of aggression
  – a slumped, withdrawn posture may signify low mood.
➤ **Proxemics** – refers to personal space and is often dependent on culture, gender and social situation.[16]
➤ **Haptics** – refers to communication through touch. When used in a socially appropriate situation, touch may be used to communicate affection, sympathy or fear, for example, although when used in the wrong context it may suggest overfamiliarity.
➤ **Appearance** – dress sense, hairstyle, hair colour, cleanliness, presence of tattoos may all be considered a means of non-verbal communication, particularly if there is a radical change in behaviour over a period. The on-going continuous nature of assessment will make it possible to notice such changes.

We all make use of verbal and non-verbal communication in our personal lives, often on an unconscious level. The assessor should be aware, however, that non-verbal communication and gestures can vary considerably between cultures (*see* Chapter 3 and below on cultural consideration). In addition, it should be noted that mental ill-health and its treatment can have a huge impact upon non-verbal communication *within* a given culture. For example, individuals experiencing side effects of Parkinsonism secondary to the use of antipsychotic medication often have a paucity of facial expression and spontaneous movement. Moreover, individuals diagnosed with dementia, or who have suffered traumatic brain injury, may have paralinguistic changes with alteration in prosody (intonation).

Communication is a two-way process

The professional who is *aware* of his or her non-verbal conversational ability has a potentially extremely effective tool for use in the establishment of rapport, trust and the therapeutic relationship.[12] Thus, it may be beneficial in this regard to:
➤ maintain a relaxed body posture
➤ use appropriate eye contact
➤ maintain physical 'openness'
➤ use appropriate relaxed facial expressions
➤ nod head in encouragement.[12]

Appropriate use of silences

➤ Allows time for the assessing professional and individual to collect their thoughts.
➤ May encourage less communicative individuals to 'open up' and provide information (*see* Chapters 2, 3 and 6).[12]

Active listening

➤ Assists in creating a therapeutic relationship (*see* Chapter 6).
➤ Enables the individual to begin to share their world.
➤ Allows an individual sufficient time to talk and complete statements before further questions are asked or comments are made.[12]

How long should assessment take?

> **KEY POINT 10.7**
>
> As long as it takes.

The on-going nature of assessment allows for information to be gathered over more than one session.

> **KEY POINT 10.8**
>
> A balance needs to be found between gathering too much information at one time with the risk of overloading an individual, and allowing insufficient time for a person to relay their story, including their fears and expectations.

What should assessment include?

Case study 10.1 – Part One

Mike, 22, has experienced significant anxiety when in social situations since his early teenage years. He has gradually become more socially withdrawn and isolated. His alcohol use has increased over recent months and he smokes 20 cigarettes a day, although this may double when he drinks. He is currently unemployed and lives alone. Mike achieved good grades at school at GCSE and A levels although he dropped out of university after two months. Mike was studying psychology and was regularly required to give presentations in tutorials and seminars. His anxiety significantly increased with consequent avoidance of situations where he was expected to speak publicly. He felt unable to discuss his situation with tutors and decided not to return after the first semester break. Mike's mood became increasingly low. After attending his general practitioner (GP) for a chest infection, Mike also mentioned his symptoms of low mood, anxiety and disturbed sleep. Selective serotonin re-uptake inhibitors (SSRIs) medication – a class of antidepressant drugs initially used to treat symptoms of depression although which are now widely used to treat a variety of conditions including anxiety, panic, obsessive-compulsive and personality disorders – was commenced and a referral made to mental health services after Mike reported experiencing increasingly frequent thoughts of suicide. After taking medication for several days, he discontinued treatment and failed to attend the appointment offered due to significant anticipatory anxiety.

SELF-ASSESSMENT EXERCISE 10.7

> **Time: 5 minutes**
> What do you need to know about Mike and his family relationships in order to really help and work alongside him?

Primary issues
➤ Descriptive terms to define Mike's symptoms, such as depression or social phobia, do not sufficiently relay the debilitating impact that these symptoms have had on his life.
➤ Mike feels that his main concerns at present are no longer his symptoms of anxiety and low mood per se but rather the impact that they have had on his personal life.

An assessment of physical health

Mike's alcohol and cigarette use had significantly increased over several months. A recent chest infection was believed to be related to an increase in smoking.

There is much evidence to suggest that those experiencing serious and enduring mental health problems have significantly increased morbidity and an increased mortality risk.[17,18] For example, there is evidence that depression may be an independent risk factor for heart disease in men,[19] an association independent of smoking status, diabetes, hypertension, and deprivation score.[19] In addition, there is a significantly increased risk of drug and alcohol use in individuals experiencing serious and enduring mental health[20] and, therefore, the physical health complications associated with their use.

Assessment of social and interpersonal relationships

Mike has become increasingly socially isolated and he has lost contact with friends he made at school. His unwillingness to attend social events has led to him no longer being invited. Although SSRI medication may well be of benefit in terms of mild alleviation of current symptoms, there needs to be an appreciation of the longer-term impact of Mike's symptoms on his life. His only regular social contacts are with members of his immediate family, although Mike also avoids family gatherings.

Although it is the individual experiencing serious and enduring mental health problems who personally experiences the symptoms, the impact of the experience will extend to the individual's family, friends and other members of their support network.

An assessment of the individual's financial situation

In Mike's particular case his symptoms have significantly affected his ability to gain employment due to his avoidance of anxiety-provoking interviews.

An assessment of the importance of religion or spirituality to the individual (*see* Chapter 8)

A person may turn away from their religious beliefs or have difficulty incorporating their experience into pre-existing belief systems. The individual may ask, 'Why me?' Alternatively, a person may find solace through their faith or particular belief.

An assessment of the impact of mental health symptoms on the individual's sexuality (*see* Chapter 9)

Medication side effects are associated with decreased libido, ejaculation difficulty, and erection difficulties in men.[21] Men in particular are often reluctant to reveal or discuss such issues, with potentially devastating consequences.

The symptoms may strain relationships and possibly lead to relationship breakdown. Confidence and self-esteem may be affected. The person may discontinue medication with a consequent deterioration in mental health. Moreover, the individual may seek to self-medicate with illicit substances or potentially harmful black-market sexual performance-enhancing drugs.

An assessment of the impact of serious and enduring mental health on psychological well-being

Serious and enduring mental health itself is a risk factor for further mental health symptoms and there is evidence to suggest that the prevalence of psychiatric comorbidity is extremely high.[22] Mike's low mood appears to have developed secondary to his symptoms of anxiety.

Although an individual may have been diagnosed with a particular mental disorder this does not render her or him immune to the development of further psychological disturbance which may, of course, itself exacerbate pre-existing symptoms.

The risk of suicide in those experiencing schizophrenia symptoms is significantly higher than in the general population,[23] and this is believed to be related to the development of depression secondary to psychotic symptoms and associated with the use of illicit substances and/or alcohol.

KEY POINT 10.9

- *All* aspects of an individual's life are closely related.
- A problem in one area is likely to lead to difficulties in another, as issues do not occur in isolation. The physical, mental and social aspects of life are often closely interconnected.
- This increases the risk that an individual experiencing serious and enduring mental health may at some point decide to attempt to take his or her own life.

Case study 10.1 – Part Two

Mike became increasingly isolated and detached himself from family members and friends who began to visit less regularly. His alcohol use continued to increase and his physical health began to suffer. On one occasion while intoxicated, he visited the local off-licence to purchase more alcohol and got into an altercation with a member of the public. The shop owner, fearful that the situation, now taking place outside of the shop, was getting out of hand, called the police. Mike had been becoming increasingly self-conscious and paranoid while out in public, although he rarely ventured outdoors other than for self-determined essentials.

The police arrested Mike, and due to his suspicious presentation, deemed that he required psychiatric assessment. He was taken to a place of safety and assessed by a psychiatrist who found Mike to be suspicious and hostile. Mike felt he had not been treated fairly, and simply wished to return home.

SELF-ASSESSMENT EXERCISE 10.8

Time: 5 minutes

What do you feel could be contributing to Mike's feelings of paranoia?

Mike expressed a belief that he was being victimised and that there was a conspiracy against him involving the police and the assessing psychiatrist. His aggressive behaviour continued. When sober, a Mental Health Act assessment was arranged and the professionals agreed that he may be experiencing a psychotic illness. Mike was detained under Section 2 of the UK Mental Health Act 1983 – a 28-day assessment order.[24]

Mike agreed to take medication on the ward, his symptoms of paranoia and anxiety appeared to resolve, and the section was rescinded. Mike was discharged with appropriate aftercare. A tentative diagnosis of schizophrenia was made. However, Mike did not feel he needed the medication and disputed the diagnosis of schizophrenia.

SELF-ASSESSMENT EXERCISE 10.9

Time: 5 minutes

What factors, other than medication, may have contributed to the resolution of Mike's symptoms?

Despite continuing to take the medication in the community, Mike relapsed on two occasions following discharge, each occasion resulting in a hospital admission.

Relapses consisted of excessive alcohol consumption associated with suspicious and aggressive behaviour. On one occasion, Mike expressed suicidal ideation.

SELF-ASSESSMENT EXERCISE 10.10

> **Time: 4 minutes**
> What could be the cause of Mike's relapse?

Mike was again discharged into the community and significant efforts are being made for him to engage in community activities through attendance at local community groups. Following referral, Mike has been attending cognitive behavioural therapy sessions focused on anxiety management and confidence building and he has found this helpful. Mike now feels that at some point he would like to return to college.

CULTURAL CONSIDERATIONS (*SEE* CHAPTER 3)

We live in a diverse, multicultural and multi-faith society. The subject of transcultural health is huge and significant literature has been written both on the subject as a whole and on issues more specifically relating to mental health. An excellent example and the most used at an international level is the Purnell Model (*see* Chapter 3). There may be considerable variation in the presentation of individuals with physical or mental health problems from different cultural backgrounds.

Although there is minimal evidence to suggest that the experience of pain varies across cultures, studies have found that the *expression* of pain does so.[25,26] This may also extend to the expression of distress in general (*mental pain*). For example, in certain cultures depressive illness may manifest as somatic symptoms, such as headache, general malaise or abdominal discomfort, rather than subjective sadness or emotional disturbance.[27]

In addition to the variable cultural *expression* or manifestation of symptoms there is the cultural *explanation* of symptoms, which may in some instances appear to be delusional. The assessing professional needs to be aware that a belief system deemed to be abnormal in one culture may be acceptable in another. A belief in magic, spirits, or demonic possession may be a culturally acceptable explanation for serious anxiety, panic attacks and obsessive-compulsive symptoms in some societies.

Historically, there has been a tendency in the UK to make a diagnosis of schizophrenia more readily in particular cultural groups such as Afro-Caribbeans.[28] Rather than representing a difference in the incidence of schizophrenia, this is likely to reflect a lack of appreciation of cultural differences. Moreover, gestures in one culture may have a completely different meaning in another. For example, in England tapping the side of the nose with an index finger is a signal for secrecy, although in Italy it is understood as a friendly warning to take care.[29]

Subculture and cultural change

Indeed, *within societies* what is deemed to be acceptable in terms of behaviour, belief and mode of communication may change over time. Culture, inclusive of verbal and non-verbal communication, is not static. In the US, homosexuality was considered to be a mental disorder until its removal as a classified mental disorder was agreed in 1973.[30] An older generation may deem the behaviour of a younger generation to be inherently rude, disruptive, or possibly immoral.

The acceptability of alcohol and substance use can be influenced by culture. For example, the use of hallucinogens is recognised as part of religious rituals in some societies[31] and the use of substances within the dance music scene is so prevalent as to possibly constitute a subculture.[32]

It may be extremely challenging for the assessing professional to evaluate an individual from a different ethnicity. The issue may be compounded if there is a language barrier, for example if the individual is a recent immigrant or an asylum seeker.

Although possibly helpful to some, a list of do's and don'ts may be overwhelming for the assessing professional, possibly leading to avoidance of key issues in some instances. However, for those who would find a list helpful as an educational tool, the **To Learn More** section of this chapter includes such a list. However, assessment tools are merely memory aids that are helpful in certain situations, thus it needs to be remembered when using assessment tools that these are aids and do not replace person-centred assessment and clinical knowledge in one-to-one contact.

The assessing professional cannot be expected to know every nuance and aspect of each culture and religious denomination likely to be encountered. However, several suggestions and recommendations may be helpful to avoid perceived misconceptions and differences in beliefs and values.

➤ **Be aware of stereotyping and avoid making assumptions**
  — If cultural differences between an assessor and an individual with mental health symptoms are not taken into account, the assessment is prone to potentially significant errors.[33]
➤ **If in doubt, ASK**
  — It is perfectly acceptable to ask how a person wishes to be addressed or whether he or she is comfortable discussing a particular topic.
➤ **Use interpreters when necessary**
  — Where language difficulties are apparent, the use of interpreters is advantageous. Where possible, the interpreter should share a cultural background with the individual being assessed rather than simply speaking their language.
  — The assessing professional should be aware of the potential pitfalls and errors in the use of interpreters.[34] Information and context may be lost in

translation through the addition, alteration, substitution or omission of detail, for example.

— The use of family members as interpreters should be avoided and ideally reserved for emergencies only. The reasons are all the same as the potential pitfalls and errors as stated below. However, they are more likely to occur voluntarily for three possible reasons.

1 The individual may be less willing to relay sensitive information to a family member than to an interpreter.

2 The interpreting family member may be unwilling to relay perceived sensitive family details and information to the assessing professional.

3 The use of minors as interpreters is unethical due to the potentially rather sensitive nature of the subject matter likely to be discussed which may be upsetting or disturbing for younger children, teenagers, or young adults.

These factors in extreme circumstances could possibly render the interpretation meaningless if important information has in effect been voluntarily censored.

In addition to recognisable mental health symptoms manifesting in different ways in individuals from different cultures, several *culture-bound syndromes* have been described.[35,36] This term refers to mental health issues that may occur only in specific cultures. Much has been written on the subject and many such syndromes have been described.[36]

Examples include:

➤ **Amok** – from the Malay, meaning to engage furiously in battle. Seen in South East Asia and associated with outbursts of aggressive and extremely violent behaviour following a period of depression or anxiety.

➤ **Koro** – seen in males of South East Asia and associated with a fear or delusion that the penis has retracted into the abdomen or shrunk and that death is shortly to occur.

➤ **Anorexia nervosa** – has been regarded by some as a culture-bound syndrome given that it is seen almost exclusively in Western cultures or in those cultures heavily influenced by Western cultures.[37]

The topic is highly controversial, however, and some argue that the mental health issues represent local variations of recognised Western disorders as defined by ICD-10[7] and DSM-IV[8] classification systems, whereas others believe that they represent discrete, culture-specific entities. Nevertheless, modern society consists of extremely diverse immigrant groups and the assessing professional may be faced with an individual displaying behaviour uncharacteristic of the indigenous culture. The benefits of an increased awareness of the concept of culture-bound syndromes are therefore clear for professionals serving an increasingly diverse population.

CONCLUSION AND PRIMARY ISSUES

➤ The term '**palliative care**' is frequently being used more and more to refer to the alleviation of suffering regardless of the availability of cure or the stage of illness.

➤ The physical, mental and social aspects of life are often closely interconnected.

➤ A problem in one area is likely to lead to difficulties in another as issues do not occur in isolation.

➤ Ultimately, the purpose of assessment is to find out what needs to be done to improve an individual's quality of life and to determine how this is best done in relation to the unique circumstances of the individual being assessed.

➤ The professional who is aware of his or her non-verbal communicational ability has a potentially extremely effective tool for use in the establishment of rapport, trust and the therapeutic relationship.

➤ We live in a diverse, multicultural and multi-faith society. There may be considerable variation in the presentation of individuals with physical or mental health problems from different cultural backgrounds.

REFERENCES

1 World Health Organization. *WHO Definition of Palliative Care*. Geneva: World Health Organization.

2 Black C, Hanson E, Cutcliffe J, *et al.* Palliative care nurses and mental health nurses: sharing common ground? *International Journal of Palliative Nursing*. 2001; **7**: 17–23.

3 McGrath P, Holewa H. Mental health and palliative care: exploring the ideological interface. *International Journal of Psychosocial Rehabilitation*. 2004; **9**: 107–19.

4 Gamble C, Brennan G. *Working with Serious Mental Illness: a manual for clinical practice*. 2nd ed. London: Elsevier; 2006.

5 Poston JM, Hanson WE. Meta analysis of psychological assessment as a therapeutic intervention. *Psychological Assessment*. 2010; **22**: 203–12.

6 Laing RD. *The Politics of the Family and Other Essays*. London: Tavistock; 1971.

7 World Health Organization. *The ICD-10 Classification of Mental and Behavioural Disorders: clinical descriptions and diagnostic guidelines*. Geneva: World Health Organization; 1992.

8 American Psychiatric Association. *Diagnostic and Statistical Manual of Mental Disorders*. 4th ed. Text revision. Washington, DC: American Psychiatric Association; 2000.

9 Bentall RP. *Madness Explained: psychosis and human nature*. London: Penguin; 2003.

10 World Health Organization. *WHO Constitution Definition of Health*. Geneva: World Health Organization; 1984.

11 Ramachandran VS, Blakeslee S. *Phantoms in the Brain: probing the mysteries of the human mind*. New York: William Morrow; 1998.

12 Adams M, Stacey-Emile G. Assessment. In: Cooper DB, editor. *Care in Mental Health–Substance Use*. London: Radcliffe; 2011.

13 National Institute of Clinical Excellence. *Guidance on Cancer Services: improving supportive and palliative care for adults with cancer. The Manual*. London. National Institute for Clinical Excellence; 2004.

14 Sims A. *Symptoms in the Mind: an introduction to descriptive psychopathology*. 3rd ed. Philadelphia: Saunders; 2003.

15 Lee H. *To Kill a Mockingbird*. London: Mandarin; 1989.

16 Hall ET. *The Hidden Dimension*. New York: Anchor; 1969.

17 Felker B, Yazel J, Short D. Mortality and medical co-morbidity among psychiatric patients: a review. *Psychiatric Services*. 1996; **47**: 1356–63.

18 Hansen V, Arnesen E, Jacobsen BK. Total mortality in people admitted to a psychiatric hospital. *British Journal of Psychiatry*. 1997; **170**: 186–90.

19 Hippisley-Cox, Fielding K, Pringle M. Depression as risk factor for ischaemic heart disease in men: population based control study. *British Medical Journal*. 1998; **316**: 1714–19.

20 Dickey B, Normand SLT, Weiss RD, *et al*. Medical morbidity, mental illness and substance use disorders. *Psychiatric Services*. 2002; **53**: 862–67.

21 Baldwin D, Mayers A. Sexual side-effects of antidepressant and antipsychotic drugs. *Advanced Psychiatric Treatment*. 2003; **9**: 202–10.

22 Kessler RC, Chiu WT, Demler O, *et al*. Prevalence, severity, and co-morbidity of 12-month DSM-IV disorders in the National Co-Morbidity Survey Replication. *Archives of General Psychiatry*. 2005; **62**: 617–27.

23 Palmer BA, Pankratz VS, Bostwick JM. The lifetime risk of suicide in schizophrenia: a re-examination. *Archives of General Psychiatry*. 2005; **62**: 247–53.

24 Department of Health. Mental Health Act 1983. Available at: www.dh.gov.uk/en/Publicationsandstatistics/Legislation/Actsandbills/DH_4002034 (accessed 22 April 2012).

25 Greenwald HP. Interethnic differences in pain perception. *Pain*. 1991; **44**: 57–63.

26 Riley JL, Wade JB, Myers CD, *et al*. Racial-ethnic differences in the experience of chronic pain. *Pain*. 2002; **100**: 291–8.

27 Ahmad K, Bhugra D. Depression across ethnic minority cultures: diagnostic issues. *World Cultural Psychiatry Research Review*. 2007; **2**: 47–56.

28 Sharpley M, Hutchinson G, McKenzie K, *et al*. Understanding the excess of psychosis among African-Caribbean population in England – review of current hypothesis. *British Journal of Psychiatry*. 2001; **178**(Suppl. 40): S60–8.

29 Morris D. *Manwatching: a field guide to human behaviour*. London: Chatto, Bodley Head and Jonathan Cape; 1977.

30 Spitzer RL. The diagnostic status of homosexuality in DSM-III: a reformulation of the issues. *American Journal of Psychiatry*. 1981; **138**: 210–15.

31 Furst PT. Flesh of the gods: *The Ritual Use of Hallucinogens*. London: George Allen & Unwin; 1972.

32 Winstock AR, Griffiths P, Stewart D. Drugs and the dance music scene: a survey of current drug use patterns among a sample of dance music enthusiasts in the UK. *Drug and Alcohol Dependence*. 2001; **64**: 9–17.

33 Bhugra D, Bhui K. Cross cultural psychiatric assessment. *Advances in Psychiatric Treatment*. 1997; **3**: 103–10.

34 Bhattacharya R, Cross S, Bhugra D. *Clinical Topics in Cultural Psychiatry*. London: Royal College of Psychiatry Publications; 2010.

35 Guarnaccia PJ, Rogler LH. Research on culture-bound syndromes: new directions. *American Journal of Psychiatry*. 1999; **156**: 1322–7.

36 Simons RC, Hughes CC, editors. *The Culture-Bound Syndromes: folk illnesses of psychiatric and anthropological interest*. Dordrecht, The Netherlands: D Reidel; 1985.

37 Banks CG. 'Culture' in culture-bound syndromes: the case of anorexia nervosa. *Social Science and Medicine*. 1992; **34**: 867–84.

38 Cooper DB. Transcultural issues and approaches. In: Wright H, Giddey M, editors. *Mental Health Nursing: from first principles to professional practice.* London: Chapman and Hall; 1993.

TO LEARN MORE

- Bentall RP. *Madness Explained: psychosis and human nature.* London: Penguin; 2003.
- International Society for the Psychological Treatment of Schizophrenias and other Psychoses (ISPS). An international organisation promoting psychotherapy and psychological treatments for people experiencing schizophrenia and other psychotic conditions. Available at: www.isps.org/ (accessed 22 April 2012).
- MIND. Mind helps people take control of their mental health by providing information and advice, and campaigning to promote and protect good mental health. Available at: www.mind.org.uk (accessed 22 April 2012).
- Read J, Mosher LR, Bentall RP, editors. *Models of Madness: psychological, social and biological approaches to schizophrenia.* New York: Routledge; 2004.
- Soteria Network. A network of people promoting the development of drug-free and minimum medication therapeutic medication environments for people experiencing 'psychosis' or extreme states. Available at: www.soterianetwork.org.uk/index.php (accessed 22 April 2012).
- Rudnick A, Roe D, editors. *Serious Mental Illness: person centered approaches.* London: Radcliffe; 2011.

CULTURAL CONSIDERATIONS[12,38]

Examples of how references and beliefs can be misinterpreted through lack of knowledge of cultural issues.

➤ When a person of Pakistan origin refers to him- or herself as being 'royal', he or she is not necessarily deluded; it means simply that he or she comes from a wealthy family. This is not a grandiose delusion in cultural terms.

➤ 'The good Lord is talking to me' is an expression often used by Afro-Caribbean people of religious background. This can be misconstrued as the individual experiencing auditory hallucinations.

➤ Peoples of Asian, East Indian, and African descent can have what appears to be bruising that is common among darker-skinned persons. For example, what appears to be bruising on a child's body or on the individual can be 'Mongolian blue spot'. Do not to jump to conclusions without adequate exploration and assessment of possible concerns.

The following list of **'Do's'** and **'Do Not's'** (Box 10.1), applies to all cultures. The list is not exhaustive; it can be used as a reference when working with individuals from any culture.

BOX 10.1 Cultural considerations – 'do's' and 'do not's'[12,35]

Name
- **Do not**:
  - use Western titles, e.g. Mr, Miss, Ms, Mrs
  - ask non-Christians for a Christian name.
- **Do**:
  - ask for family name or first name
  - ask what name the person prefers you use, e.g. Mr or Miss or first name
  - use the chosen form of address
  - avoid repetition in clinical notes; find out the correct name first rather than misuse several different names.

Language
- **Do not**:
  - assume that all ethnic groups speak English
  - assume that all minority ethnic groups do not speak English
  - use the family to interpret intimate questions
  - use the family to break bad news; the family member may avoid the issue if it is believed to be too stressful for the individual.
- **Do**:
  - avoid making assumptions by using accurate assessment procedures
  - use an interpreter who understands medical terminology; this will avoid stress for the interpreter, individual and family and avoid misinterpretation.

Religion
- **Do not**:
  - generalise about the individual's or family's religion
  - mistake religious objects or symbols for jewellery.
- **Do**:
  - remember that for Buddhist, Christian, Jewish, Hindu, Muslim and Sikh people religion may be an integral part of daily life
  - avoid incorrect assumptions; find out the different beliefs and approaches
  - record clearly and make a note of the individual's or family's wish to see or have a religious representative present
  - ask the family if the individual is not able to relay this to you
  - remember that people from many Eastern religions fast on certain days; pray at certain times; wear religious objects and symbols
  - check whether interventions or treatments will compromise any religious beliefs
  - inform the individual and family of any interventions or treatments, before commencing, to check religious beliefs
  - check religious observations with the individual and family
  - consult religious advisers or teachers to gain permission and/or to obtain exemption, to allow procedures to take place; ensure she or he explains this to the individual and family.

Diet

- **Do not**:
  - give Jewish or Muslim people pork or pork products.
- **Do**:
  - make sure that other meat offered to Muslim people has been religiously slaughtered by the Halal method (natural slaughter)
  - remember that not all Jewish people eat Kosher food (specially prepared to be pure)
  - remember not all Muslim people eat Halal meat
  - consult the individual and family about any dietary preferences
  - remember that meal times are family occasions in Eastern cultures; matters relating to family are often discussed then
  - remember that being taken out of a close family environment can be frightening and cause loneliness, which may in turn cause loss of appetite
  - invite the family to bring food and join in meal times, if at all possible; if this is not practicable, explain why.

Personal hygiene

- **Do**:
  - remember that to Sikh, Hindu and Muslim people, washing in still water is considered unclean
  - supply the individual with a jug of water and bowl and/or tap with running water and empty washbasin to allow for washing of hands, face and body
  - make exceptions if the individual is dependent
  - remember that Muslim people use the right hand for eating and preparing food, and the left hand for self-cleaning and other procedures; anyone unable to do this because of injury or health reasons will need counselling and discussion relating to ways of surmounting this problem (it may be useful to supply plastic gloves).

Modesty

- **Do not**:
  - compromise the individual's dignity and modesty.
- **Do**:
  - remember that to expose the female body to a male will cause distress in certain cultures, especially if the individual is in purdah (the duration of menstruation)
  - offer separate bays in mixed-bedded wards or, if possible, a single room, especially if the person is in purdah
  - remember that hospital gowns expose more than they cover, and therefore are often unacceptable
  - avoid exposure of arms and legs; add additional covering to protect modesty.

Skin and hair

- **Do**:
  - remember that Afro-Caribbean people's hair may be brittle or dry; add moisturiser or oil to the scalp and comb regularly

– remember to ask the individual what she or he uses for skin moisturiser
– remember that dark-skinned people are prone to keloid scarring (hyperkeratini-sation); invasive treatment will cause excessive pigmented scarring
– remember to inject or undertake invasive procedures at a site that will avoid disfigurement if possible.

Hospital procedures

- **Do not**:
  – give Jehovah's Witness people blood transfusions
  – give Muslim, Jewish and vegetarian people iron injections derived from pigs
  – give insulin of bovine origin to Hindu and Sikh people
  – give insulin of porcine origin to Jewish or Muslim people.

- **Do**:
  – give careful thought to procedures and routines before commencing them
  – remember that discussion of elimination or other intimate issues may be cultur-ally offensive
  – approach all individuals sensitively; ensure privacy, and maintain the individual's right to self-respect
  – remember that some medications, interventions and treatments may be taboo for some religious groups
  – remember that some medications have an alcohol base which may be forbidden in some cultural groups
  – remember that individuals with alcohol problems may wish to avoid alcohol-based preparations
  – be aware of all preparations likely to contain potentially taboo or offensive ingredients.

Visiting

- **Do**:
  – remember that limiting visiting to two people may cause distress in extended family cultures
  – remember West Indian, Asian and Middle Eastern families like to visit as a family
  – remember that family may include children, uncles, aunts, grandchildren, parents and grandparents
  – compromise over visiting, and numbers of visitors per individual, if possible
  – remember that open visiting is more accommodating
  – allow the family to participate in the individual's care.

Pain myths

- **Do not**:
  – believe that people from different races have a low pain threshold; this is incor-rect, e.g.
    (i) Japanese people may smile or laugh when in pain, thus avoiding loss of face
    (ii) Anglo-Saxon people may be sullen and withdrawn, portraying the 'stiff-upper-lip' image

(iii) Eastern Europeans, Greeks and Italian people express pain vocally and freely.

- **Do**:
  - remember that every individual has a different level of pain tolerance, regardless of race, colour or creed.

Death and bereavement

- **Do not**:
  - deny a family member the right to participate in last offices as this will increase the pain already being expressed and may slow down the grieving process.
- **Do**:
  - involve the individual and family in care
  - remember that Eastern European cultures like to take an active part in the care of the dying relative, especially last offices
  - remember that in certain cultures, custom and practice will need to be followed if the individual is to proceed along the continuum of life following his or her earthly death
  - ensure you are fully conversant with specific cultural requirements for death, bereavement and last offices
  - negotiate to minimise anxiety and allow some participation, when the family's wishes come into conflict with hospital policies and procedures; this will assist the grieving process
  - compromise; the individual and family have only one chance to say their goodbyes.

ACKNOWLEDGEMENT

Adapted with kind permission from:

Adams M, Stacey-Emile G. Assessment. In: Cooper DB, editor. *Care in Mental Health–Substance Use*. London: Radcliffe; 2011.

Cooper DB. Transcultural issues and approaches. In: Wright H, Giddey M, editors. *Mental Health Nursing: from first principles to professional practice*. London: Chapman and Hall; 1993.

CHAPTER 11

Pain management

Peter Athanasos, Trevor W Mitten, Rose Neild,
Charlotte de Crespigny, Lynette Cusack

CAUTIONARY NOTE

Medication of choice varies between countries. In this chapter, we use the UK model. However, the reader should take careful note that whatever their country's medication of choice, the emphasis is always on effective pain management, i.e. the right dose at the right time and via the right route.

PRE-READING EXERCISE 11.1

Time: 15 minutes
- What questions could you ask a person under your care about his or her pain?
- Have you used a pain assessment scale to assess pain?
  - Which one did you use?
  - Why?
  - Is there a better one available?
- Think of a time you, or someone close to you, were experiencing pain.
  - What steps did you take to identify the cause of the pain and to manage it?
- Review your answers at the end of this chapter to see if you have explored all approaches, or if you could have achieved more effective pain management.

INTRODUCTION

One of the biggest challenges facing health professionals is adequate pain management. It is generally accepted that severe pain is poorly treated in the general population. There may be a number of reasons for this:
➤ Prescribing professionals may not prescribe adequate amounts of opioids

for fear of respiratory depression or cognitive and psychomotor effects, e.g. when driving a car or operating machinery
➤ The prescriber may fear the development of iatrogenic dependence (i.e. causing the person to become addicted by prescribing opioids for pain). This is a relatively rare occurrence.
➤ The prescriber may fear that the person may divert their prescription opioid drugs if these are given too liberally or are in excess of requirement.[1]
➤ The prescriber may also have a poor understanding of the pharmacodynamics and pharmacokinetics of medication in the context of pain and prescribe ineffectively.[2]

SELF-ASSESSMENT EXERCISE 11.1

> **Time: 5 minutes**
> What would you consider to be the primary aims of pain management?

PRIMARY AIMS OF PAIN MANAGEMENT
➤ **good night's sleep**
➤ **relief at rest**
➤ **relief on movement** – although this may be more difficult to achieve.

Assessing pain
In pain management, the most important factors are:
➤ ask the *right* questions
➤ *listen* to the answers.

The prerequisite for good pain management is a full and comprehensive history.

An essential aid to pain assessment is the family. It is imperative that family views are sought and taken into account. The person may not wish to be seen as complaining or weak, therefore, pain may be under-reported. Moreover, it is possible for pain to be 'eased' or to disappear altogether during conversation with the professional.

The individual may experience *referred* pain in one area that originates from elsewhere. It is estimated that up to 33% of cancer sufferers have three or more pains.[3] Therefore, it is important to ask if the individual is experiencing different types of pain, as they may well have more than one. Equally, the pain experienced might not be directly related to the cancer; however, it is important to address all pain.

On-going assessment and evaluation of pain is pivotal: a continual process, not a 'one-off' exercise (*see* Chapter 10). It may be that as one pain is managed, the individual becomes aware of another. Pain may also reappear later and/or be transformed into a different type of pain.

Assessment tools

The use of pain diaries or pain assessment tools is an important part of assessment, and gives the person a sense of control. Rating mechanisms include:

➤ visual analogue scale
➤ numerical rating scale
➤ London Hospital's Pain Chart[4] – the individual draws the pain site on a body outline.

Pain assessment in populations such as cognitively impaired older adults can be difficult to assess and this can result in poor management and outcomes.[5] Examples of assessment in this group include:

➤ Abbey pain scale[6] – a structured pain assessment scale in end-stage dementia
➤ Doloplus 2[7] – a scale for the older person with verbal communication problems.

However, while assessment tools have a valuable role, they are not effective in isolation and should form part of a full verbal and observational assessment.

Assessing the unconscious person

Relatives often ask whether it is possible to tell if someone unconscious is in pain. The signs can include:

➤ restlessness
➤ frowning
➤ tachycardia.

This can be contrasted with the 'groaning' breathing sometimes evident in the last few hours, where the individual is not in pain, but has noisy respiration.

Pain awareness

Terminology is important. The person may deny pain. This may be because of adaptation to chronic pain: the individual is unable to acknowledge or verbalise its presence. Denial is a means of surviving with the pain. It is common for pain to be described as *discomfort* rather than to be directly described as pain. By asking the individual if they have a discomfort or an ache, pain may be acknowledged. Therefore, this should not be ignored but explored carefully with the individual and family.

Even though the individual's reports of pain are accepted as the most reliable indicator of how much pain is experienced, health professionals tend not to rely on self-reporting.[8] If effective intervention in pain management is to be achieved, it needs to be acknowledged that the individual knows their own body better than anyone else, and accepted that they hold the key to the problem of their pain.

Breakthrough pain

Breakthrough pain is an increase of pain that *spikes* above a baseline of controlled pain. These episodes of pain can increase markedly, and need rapidly acting analgesia – sometimes referred to as a *rescue dose* – to reduce the pain (*see* Figure 11.1).

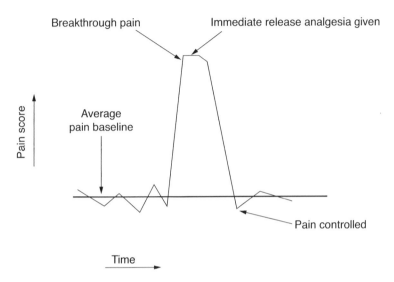

Figure 11.1 Breakthrough pain

Rapidly increasing pain

Rapid increases in pain levels may be experienced. This often occurs during the final stages of life, and is frightening for the individual and family. It often causes considerable feelings of anxiety and panic. Prompt review, a calm manner and appropriate intervention may help to allay fears and concerns. The importance of understanding that such situations can arise, and that they require prompt, effective management, cannot be overemphasised.

Analgesia may need to be increased rapidly, especially as the situation can change within the hour. Some professionals express concern at how quickly the need for pain relief increases. This can be a source of anxiety for the professional. The need for analgesia during terminal illness is often considerably greater than the level of analgesia prescribed by the professional on a routine basis. *There is no good reason for withholding adequate analgesia.* Discussion within the interdisciplinary team including the substance use services (e.g. alcohol and other drugs) will help to support the professional.

SELF-ASSESSMENT EXERCISE 11.2

> **Time: 5 minutes**
> - What non-pharmacological methods to relieve pain can you think of?
> - Have you used these to relieve pain?
> - If so, what relief did they provide?

Simple measures

Often the professional finds that the focus is on medication, which is perceived as a panacea for the relief of pain. Nevertheless, simple measures can often be effective. Simple measures are non-invasive, readily available and most importantly empower the individual, family and/or carer to feel they can do something to lessen suffering themselves. Simple measures include:

➤ **Pillows** – careful positioning and judicious use.
➤ **Heat therapy**
  — **hot bath**
  — **wheat bag** – check for allergies first as some people may develop an allergic reaction to the wheat or the bags may be impregnated with aromatherapy oils.[9]
  — **heat pad**
➤ **Massage**
➤ **Movement** – changing position and simple movements can help to reduce positional pain.

KEY POINT 11.1

- Not all pain can be completely relieved.
- It is important that the individual is supported through their pain.

ANALGESIC LADDER

The World Health Organization (WHO) analgesic ladder[10] is a useful guide to prescription of the appropriate level of analgesia (*see* Figure 11.2). This progresses from Step 1, when the use of non-opioids, e.g. paracetamol and non-steroidal anti-inflammatory drugs (NSAIDs, e.g. ibuprofen) may be appropriate. If the pain remains uncontrolled, although the maximum dose has been achieved, then progression to Step 2 follows. A weak opioid, e.g. a paracetamol with codeine combination, an aspirin with codeine combination or dihydrocodeine may be effective. These may be alternated with NSAIDs (e.g. ibuprofen) and other adjuvants as appropriate. An adjuvant (or co-analgesic) is a drug that has an independent analgesic effect or additive analgesic properties when used with opioids (e.g. NSAIDs, tramadol, ketamine, gabapentin). Step 3 drugs include the strong opioids, e.g. morphine, prescribed with or without adjuvant drugs.

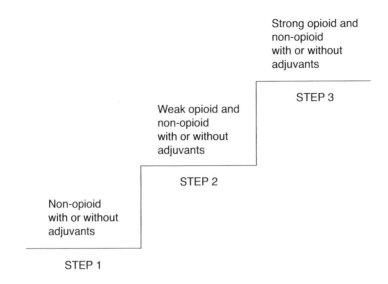

Figure 11.2 WHO Three-Step Ladder[10]

KEY POINT 11.2

- Adjuvant drugs are used to complement other drugs and to maximise pain relief (*see* Figure 11.3).
- They can be used at any step of the analgesic ladder.

A stumbling block

The main problem with prescribing analgesics is reluctance in moving from level-two to level-three drugs. Professionals, individuals and family appear concerned about morphine and describe the pain as *'not that bad yet'*, when faced with a choice of progression to such drugs. However, if the maximum dose of a level-two drug is achieved without effect, there is little evidence to suggest replacing this with another level-two drug. Level three is the logical progression if pain management is to be effective.

KEY POINT 11.3

- The WHO analgesic ladder is merely a guide to pain management. It is neither essential nor necessary to follow the ladder in all cases.
- For some people it may be more appropriate to prescribe Step 3 drugs immediately – hence the need for a thorough assessment of pain.

OPIOIDS IN PAIN MANAGEMENT

There are multiple liquid preparations of morphine. These are generally absorbed quickly (**peak plasma concentration is 15–60 minutes**),[11] and are useful for breakthrough pain, or to assess opioid need *prior* to switching to a long-acting formulation.

Oral morphine

➤ Strong opioid of choice for cancer.
➤ Regular laxative should be prescribed whenever morphine is used as constipation almost inevitably occurs.
➤ Initially, an anti-emetic may be needed if nausea or vomiting is a problem.
➤ Sedation can be a problem with large doses, though the individual does adapt to the increased dose and becomes less sedated after 3–4 days. This can recur with each dose increase.
➤ *Regular use* of morphine is much more effective than as-required doses.[12]
➤ Standard strengths in the United Kingdom (UK) are:
 − 10 mg/5 ml
 − 100 mg/5 ml
➤ Oral morphine preparations may taste sharp but can be sweetened, e.g. with a little neat blackcurrant cordial.

KEY POINT 11.4

Oral morphine – use of quick-acting preparations
● Commence morphine using a quick-acting liquid or tablet before switching to sustained-release morphine.
● Enables rapid titration to the therapeutic level.
● Oral rescue doses of liquid morphine can be offered every 30 minutes in extreme cases.[13]

Sublingual

The administration of sublingual morphine can be used in terminal stages. It may be considered where remote location or lack of other medications precludes other alternatives. In the UK, there is a tablet form of quick-release morphine called Sevredol, available as 10 mg, 20 mg and 50 mg.

Breakthrough pain

Oral doses for breakthrough pain can be offered every 60 minutes if needed.[14] The rescue dose for breakthrough pain is one-third of the 12-hourly dose of sustained-release morphine. It is important to review the effect of the morphine and the pain regularly. The dose should be increased as appropriate, taking into account all of the rescue doses taken within a 24-hour period. If additional doses are required several times during the day, consider whether the regular dose needs to be increased.[3]

KEY POINT 11.5

When pain is problematic at night, and wakes the person, increase the dose of oral morphine at bedtime.

In the UK, morphine sulphate tablets (MST), in a sustained-release formulation, are available in 5 mg, 10 mg, 15 mg, 30 mg, 60 mg, 100 mg and 200 mg strengths, and are suitable for twice-daily administration. If pain is not relieved by 90% after 24 hours, increase the dose,[3] e.g. from:

➤ 5 to 10 mg
➤ 10 to 15 mg
➤ 20 to 30 mg

In addition, consider adjuvant drugs when administering strong opioids (NSAIDs, tramadol, ketorolac, ketamine – *see* Figure 11.3).

KEY POINT 11.6

Different types of pain, e.g. bone or nerve pain, respond to different types of medication. We need to try different opioids and different adjuvants.

Opioid preparations

There are several long- and short-acting opioid preparations, as summarised in Table 11.1.

TABLE 11.1 Long- and short-acting opioid preparations

Drug	Starting dose	Indications for use
Fentanyl transmucosal-lozenge on a stick (Actiq)	200 micrograms repeated after 15 minutes if pain unrelieved	For rapid relief of incident or breakthrough pain. Good for those unable to take oral medication.
Fentanyl Transdermal Therapeutic System (TTS), (fentanyl patch)	25 micrograms every 72 hours	Stable severe pain
Hydromorphone	4 mg 12-hourly	Can be opened and sprinkled onto soft, cold food.

(continued)

Drug	Starting dose	Indications for use
Methadone	Specialist advice is needed pre-prescription	Used for severe pain, intractable cough, and opioid rotation. It has a long half-life in the body (i.e. it takes a long time to be broken down), and can accumulate to toxic levels (**seek specialist advice**). May be beneficial for neuropathic pain. For cough, a dose of 2–4 mg at night or twice daily may help.
Morcap (UK) Capsules of morphine	20 mg once a day	This is a capsule form of morphine (available in the UK) that can be opened and sprinkled onto food.
MST continus suspension (prolonged-release granules of morphine)	10–30 mg twice-a-day for opioid-naïve persons or those previously on weak opioids	MST suspension is a sachet of powder which, when mixed with water, forms a suspension of prolonged-release granules of morphine that the person drinks (available in the UK). This is useful if swallowing tablets is a problem. It can also be syringed down a gastrostomy tube. It is available in a variety of doses up to a 200 mg sachet but is difficult to mix without it forming lumps. To ensure even distribution of the mix, use 10–20 ml of very hot water as the base, and sprinkle the powder on slowly while stirring gently. Ensure the mixture is cool before administration.
MXL (sustained-release morphine)	30 mg once a day	This is a once-daily capsule preparation of sustained-release morphine (UK).
Oramorph (oral morphine sulphate)	10–30 mg 4-hourly as needed	Useful for breakthrough pain. Absorbed quickly.
Oxycodone	30 mg suppository 8-hourly	Useful for people who are unable to tolerate oral medication. This is given as a suppository, providing 6–8 hours of relief. Useful if unable to take orally and a syringe driver is inappropriate.
Oxycodone	10 mg oral twice daily	Lasts 12 hours.
OxyNorm (oxycodone capsules and liquid)	Capsules 5 mg Liquid 5 mg/5 ml	Both immediate release; last 4–6 hours.
Sevredol (immediate-release morphine tablet)	10–30 mg 4-hourly	Used for breakthrough pain. Immediate-release morphine in tablet form.

Prescribing consideration

Consideration must be given to possible adverse effects related to opioid use (Table 11.2). These may include:

➤ **possible toxic effects** – respiratory depression, prolonged QTC (a measure of the time between the start of the **Q-wave** and the end of the **T-wave** in the heart's electrical cycle) interval

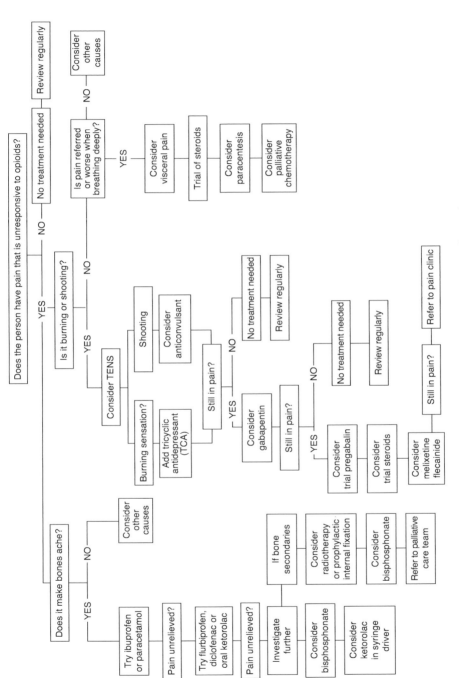

Figure 11.3 Flowchart for opioid-unresponsive pain

➤ **intolerable side effects** – constipation, nausea, vomiting, sedation – which may outweigh the benefits
➤ **renal failure** – accumulation of morphine metabolites may lead to increased sedation and respiratory depression – may need to rotate to an opioid that is less affected by renal failure (such as methadone)[15]
➤ **fear of morphine** – and an unwillingness to take the drug. This may be fear of the side effects of morphine or fear of 'becoming addicted'. Please see Iatrogenic addiction below. Alternative opioids may elicit compliance.

TABLE 11.2 Morphine side effects

Side effect	Treatment
Constipation	Laxatives, e.g. • co-danthramer (dantron, poloxamer 188) • senna • docusate
Nausea/vomiting	Anti-emetics: • cyclizine (caution: significant interaction with methadone if used) • haloperidol • metoclopramide. **Often passes after a few days so need to review.**
Drowsiness	None: passes after a few days but may recur temporarily after dose increase.
Bad dreams/ hallucinations	• infrequent – need to assess for opioid toxicity • reduce dose • add antipsychotic, e.g. haloperidol 1.5 mg three times daily • switch to different strong opioids (e.g. methadone, fentanyl, etc.)

Diamorphine profile (heroin)
➤ Chemically, diamorphine consists of two morphine molecules locked together.
➤ It is the preferred drug of choice for use in a syringe driver for subcutaneous infusion.
➤ It has a much higher solubility in solutions.
➤ It is twice as potent as morphine when administered by subcutaneous injection.[16]

OxyContin – prolonged-release oxycodone hydrochloride
A long-acting 12-hourly oxycodone tablet (**OxyContin**); 10 mg oral **OxyContin** is approximately equivalent to 20 mg oral morphine.[17] Twelve-hourly strengths range from 5 mg to 120 mg.

An immediate-relief, quick-acting liquid or tablet form (**OxyNorm**) is available.[17] There is also a rectal preparation – **Oxycodone suppositories**.

Fentanyl

The transdermal patch (**durogesic d-trans, fentanyl**) is a clear sticky patch, applied to the skin, that normally lasts three days. Durogesic d-trans is smaller and adheres better than previous patches. Fentanyl patches may cause less constipation and less of the daytime somnolence caused by morphine.[18] Transdermal patches in the UK are in five strengths:

1   12 microgram
2   25 microgram
3   50 microgram
4   75 microgram
5   100 microgram.

The patch will provide good pain relief, and seem less intrusive than the subcutaneous route. If a patch is already in place, it is unwise to rotate to another strong opioid at the end of life[19] unless pain is increasing, as the crossover period may lead to pain breakthrough. It is best to continue with the same patch.

Essential knowledge for fentanyl patch preparation

➤ Fentanyl can take from 12 to 24 hours to achieve maximum blood concentration.[12]
➤ If the person is currently receiving morphine sulphate tablets (MST), the fentanyl patch is applied with the last oral dose of MST.[20]
➤ Fentanyl patches are not suitable if pain is escalating rapidly due to slow absorption rate.
➤ It is essential that individuals with fentanyl patches are prescribed quick-release opioids for breakthrough pain.
   — This must be given in the correct dose for the patch size.
   — The dose should be increased whenever the patch size is increased.
➤ Some reports have indicated that the fentanyl patch lasts for only 2 days.[21] *The normal application period is 3 days.* If pain control is maximised at 2 days but decreases on day 3, the patch can be changed on the second day.
➤ Continual review of pain is pivotal.
➤ Counselling is essential for the individual and family throughout.
➤ Verbal and written guidance about the application of the patch is essential.
➤ Careful explanation of the potential side effects will ease anxiety and aid compliance.
➤ People *do* find the patches advantageous as the:
   — need for oral medication is reduced
   — comfort is increased
   — daily reminders relating to health may be decreased.
➤ The normal starting dose is a 12–25 microgram patch. If the person is converting from 4-hourly **oral morphine** to **fentanyl**, the **morphine** should be *continued for 12 hours* while the blood concentration achieves maximum saturation.

➤ If the person wearing the fentanyl patch is experiencing breakthrough pain, *divide the fentanyl patch by 5* (Patch/5) to give the *dose in milligrams of diamorphine administered subcutaneously.*[22] This will aid management of breakthrough pain.

Adverse effects

A small number of people experience adverse effects in the first 24 hours when switching from morphine to fentanyl patches;[20] these can include:
➤ sweating
➤ diarrhoea
➤ bowel cramps
➤ nausea
➤ restlessness.

Treatment

These adverse effects are the consequence of opioid withdrawal caused by rapid decreases in opioid dose during the changeover period. One or two doses of oral morphine will give quick relief of adverse effects.

Other fentanyl preparations

➤ trans-mucosal lozenge on a stick – for rapid reduction of breakthrough pain[23]
➤ intravenous injection (alfentanyl) – good in renal failure
➤ subcutaneous via syringe driver (alfentanyl) – for morphine intolerance.

Topical opioids

Topical opioids in a carrier gel (intrasite or metronidazole) for wound pain can be beneficial.[24–26] Topical opioids:
➤ can be helpful for a wound, e.g. pressure ulcer
➤ can be effective co-jointly with systemic opioids.[27]

One regime is **1 mg of diamorphine to 1 mg of intrasite gel** applied once daily.[28] Another is in the use of **diamorphine and instillagel local anaesthetic gel**, or with KY Jelly.[29]

KEY POINT 11.7

● Fear of seeing the wound may heighten perceived pain.[26]
● Minimise the person's exposure to seeing the wound during dressing changes – unless otherwise requested by the person.

Does adding a second opioid improve pain relief?

Inadequate pain management, with escalating opioid doses, in the presence of dose-limiting toxic effects, including:

➤ hallucinations
➤ confusion
➤ hyperalgesia
➤ myoclonus (brief involuntary twitching of muscles or group of muscles)
➤ sedation
➤ nausea . . .

. . . may be a problem in some cases. When the person requires increasing doses of a strong analgesic, benefit may be obtained from using two opioids or by combining an opioid with a non-opioid adjuvant such as tramadol, ketamine, a gabapentanoid or a non-steroidal anti-inflammatory drug.[30]

In this situation, the combination of two different opioids or a non-opioid adjuvant analgesic with an opioid may be advantageous for three reasons:
1 it may provide a multimodal coverage of a broad spectrum of pain
2 it may enable the individual agents to act in a greater than additive (synergistic) fashion
3 it may lower doses of each individual analgesic, thus may result in a lower incidence of individual adverse events.[30]

Opioid-unresponsive pain

Pains not fully responsive to opioids include the following.
➤ **Musculoskeletal** – bone pain
  — typical description:
    » aching joints – sometimes described as toothache; a pressure and/or heaviness in the bone – may be experienced in the back or hip. This is often worse on movement.
➤ **Neurogenic** – nerve pain
  — typical description:
    » stabbing
    » shooting
    » burning
    » pins and needles
    » increased sensitivity of skin
    » change in sensation.

KEY POINT 11.8

Careful and attentive listening to the description of the pain provides vital information relating to pain type.

Musculo-skeletal – bone pain

Bone pain may arise for a variety of reasons, including:
➤ osteoarthritis
➤ pathological fracture
➤ bone metastases.

The first-line drugs of choice are non-steroidal anti-inflammatory drugs. Because of their anti-inflammatory effect, NSAIDs are useful for metastatic bone and soft-tissue pains. They can be used with strong opioids[3] (*see* Table 11.3).

TABLE 11.3 Anti-inflammatory drugs

Drug	Dose
Aspirin	600 mg four times a day
Ibuprofen	200–600 mg three times a day or brufen retard (ibuprofen sustained release) two tablets daily (800 mg)
Flurbiprofen (Froben)	• 50 mg three times daily • 100 mg three times daily
Diclofenac (Voltarol)	• oral – 50 mg three times daily • oral – 75 mg twice daily • suppositories 100 mg
Ketorolac (Toradol)	• oral – 10 mg three times daily • subcutaneous infusion – 60–120 mg over 24 hours
Piroxicam (Feldene)	• oral – 20 mg once daily
Feldene melt	• dissolve on tongue

Essential knowledge for NSAID preparations

➤ NSAIDs help to control bone pain.
➤ It is worth rotating to different non-steroidal drugs if one particular drug does not work.[31]
➤ Ketorolac is a NSAID which is available in tablet form (10 mg three times daily to four times daily),[17] or by intravenous or subcutaneous injection.[32]
➤ Administration via a syringe driver is beneficial if other oral NSAIDs have failed.[33] This can be attributed to ketorolac's dual anti-inflammatory and analgesic effect.[34] The improved absorption via the parenteral route also plays a role.
➤ NSAIDs may cause gastric irritation. Thus, a gastro-protective should be considered (proton pump inhibitors – which reduce acid in the stomach, e.g. omeprazole) and H_2 antagonists (block the action of histamine and also reduce acid in the stomach, e.g. ranitidine).[35]

SELF-ASSESSMENT EXERCISE 11.3

> **Time: 15 minutes**
> - The individual in your care says the pain is burning and continuous in nature.
> - What type of pain do you think this might indicate?
> - What drug treatment might be prescribed for nerve pain?
> - What are the *Three Steps* in the WHO analgesic ladder?
> - List three non-pharmacological treatments that may help to relieve pain.
> - Identify three non-verbal indicators that the person may be in pain.
> - What are the common side effects of morphine?
> - When may fentanyl patches be indicated?

Bisphosphonates

The use of bisphosphonates in cases of bone pain is encouraging.[36] Even when individuals have a normal calcium level,[37] treatment with a bisphosphonate, e.g. – most used in the UK – pamidronate 60–90 mg intravenous (IV) every 4–6 weeks) can markedly reduce bone metastases pain. A once-a-day preparation of bisphosphonate tablet – ibandronate (Bondronat),[38,39] eliminates the need for hospitalisation for an infusion.

Radiotherapy

➤ Radiation can reduce pain in 90% of people experiencing bone pain.[40]
➤ Radiotherapy can be helpful in reducing pain from bone metastases.
➤ A single dose is often all that is required for treatment.

Strontium

➤ Injections of strontium 89 for the relief of metastatic bone pain is indicated for people with prostate or breast cancer.[41]
➤ Strontium follows the pathway of calcium, delivering local radiotherapy to the site of bone metastases.

Neurogenic – nerve pain

Nerve pain often follows nerve pathways, e.g. the facial nerve (trigeminal neuralgia) or thoracic nerve (shingles). It is not fully controlled by opioids,[42] but often responds well to antidepressant medication (e.g. **amitriptyline**, **venlafaxine** – particularly if the sensation is *burning*). Alternatively, anti-epileptic medication, e.g. gabapentin,[43] pregabalin,[44] or carbamazepine, may be considered (*see* Table 11.4).

TABLE 11.4 Drug management of neurogenic pain

Drug	Dosage/side effects
Amitriptyline	• 10–75 mg at night • can cause dry mouth, blurred vision, sedation
Venlafaxine	• 37.5 mg twice daily • increase to 75 mg after 1 week if necessary • can cause dizziness, dry mouth, insomnia, constipation
Sertraline	• 50–150 mg once daily in the morning • nausea a problem initially; also diarrhoea, restlessness, headache
Gabapentin	• 100–600 mg three times daily – slowly titrated. **NOTE: Seek advice – even if experienced.** • can cause dizziness, sedation, nausea, blurred vision
Pregabalin	• 75–300 mg twice daily • can cause dizziness, sedation, peripheral oedema

Other treatments for nerve pain include
➤ **epidural/intrathecal injection** – Epidural analgesia is directed into the epidural space of the spinal cord. The epidural space is inside the bony spinal canal but outside the dura mater membrane. Intrathecal analgesia is directed into the space under the arachnoid membrane of the spinal cord or brain.
➤ **coeliac plexus block** – The coeliac plexus is also known as the solar plexus and is a complex of nerves in the abdomen. Coeliac plexus block is the injection of local anaesthetic onto these nerves for control of pain.
➤ **chemical nerve destruction** – with phenol (also known as carbolic acid – a strong neurotoxin that can destroy nerves)
➤ **surgical nerve destruction** (e.g. cordotomy).

The flow chart (Figure 11.3) on opioid-unresponsive pain indicates considerations and actions for addressing these types of pain.

Steroids in pain management
The use of steroids in pain management needs to be weighed against the side effects of steroids. However, steroids can be effective if used appropriately. Steroids are indicated in the following instances:[20]
➤ raised intracranial pressure
➤ spinal cord compression
➤ bone pain
➤ liver capsule stretch (enlargement of the liver due to liver cancer).

Steroid use in symptom palliation
➤ reduces cerebral oedema in cerebral tumours/secondaries
➤ lowers raised intracranial pressure
➤ stimulates appetite

➤ provides euphoria and energy for special events, e.g. a wedding
➤ reduces liver capsule pain by decreasing swelling
➤ reduces nerve pain by relieving nerve compression or irritation.

Prescribing and administering steroids

Dexamethasone:
➤ is often the steroid of choice
➤ is approximately seven times more potent than prednisolone,[20] therefore fewer tablets are needed
➤ crosses the blood-brain barrier and is useful for people with cerebral tumours
➤ tablets can be crushed and made into a suspension with warm water, for ease of swallowing
➤ supplied as a sugar-free solution (Dexsol).[45]

To prevent dyspepsia/ulcers a proton pump inhibitor, e.g. omeprazole, or H_2 antagonist, e.g. ranitidine, helps protect the stomach.

Steroid adverse effects

➤ gastric irritation or ulceration
➤ water retention
➤ fluid imbalance
➤ immunosuppression
➤ steroid psychosis
➤ oral candidiasis
➤ insomnia
➤ thinning of the skin
➤ hypertension
➤ steroid-induced diabetes
➤ osteoporosis
➤ myopathy.

KEY POINT 11.9

- Steroids given four times a day can cause nocturnal insomnia.
- Once- or twice-a-day (morning and lunchtime) administration is preferable.[46]

Visceral pain

Visceral pain – i.e. pain from any internal organs, especially within the abdomen – can be:
➤ **worse on taking a deep breath**
➤ **an excruciating pain** – when an organ cannot swell to accommodate a tumour due to the presence of inflexible viscera containing the organ.

The most common example is liver pain due to metastases causing liver capsule stretch, i.e. swollen liver. This is why in physical examinations the liver is palpated. Treatment is usually with morphine and steroids (dexamethasone 4–8 mg/day[20]), to reduce peri-tumour oedema. Palliative radiotherapy or chemotherapy may also be indicated.

Non-pharmacological management of pain

Transcutaneous electrical nerve stimulation (TENS)

The use of transcutaneous electrical nerve stimulation machines has been found to be beneficial. Forty-seven per cent of people report a 50% reduction in pain intensity after treatment.[47] TENS works by blocking the transmission of painful stimuli (referred to as the gate theory) by increasing activity in the large 'A' fibres, which block activity in the smaller pain fibres. There is a concomitant release of endorphins. It is important to read – and understand – the instructions of use prior to using a TENS machine.[47]

Psychological approaches

Pain can be:
➤ physical
➤ spiritual
➤ emotional/psychological
➤ social . . .

. . . this is referred to as *total pain*.[48]

Anxiety

Recognition that anxiety can increase the intensity of pain is essential and pivotal to any intervention.[49] The individual and family need continuous assessment and restructuring of care as identified. Some people may benefit from counselling with regard to issues such as family problems, or existential or spiritual needs in addition to analgesia (*see* Chapters 6, 8 and 9).

Hope and coping strategies (see Chapter 7)

Hope and coping strategies (e.g. distraction therapy, visualisation and imagery)[50] empower the individual, and enable better skills.

Relaxation and visualisation

Relaxation and visualisation can benefit the individual and family by:
➤ promoting sleep
➤ promoting management of stress and pain
➤ reducing anxiety and depression.[51]

Pain and/or fear can cause tension, restlessness, poor concentration, and agitation. Relaxation, defined as a *state of freedom from both anxiety and skeletal muscle tension* is helpful.[50] Simple breathing exercises can promote relaxation and may be described during counselling.

Other pain management strategies

- ➤ physiotherapy
- ➤ aromatherapy
- ➤ massage
- ➤ hypnotherapy
- ➤ osteopathy
- ➤ acupuncture
- ➤ spiritual healing.

Sometimes it is necessary to use a combination of techniques and/or relaxation in conjunction with other complementary therapies to provide an effective intervention. The decision on what is best is often a matter of trial and error and based on the individual's or family's experience and wishes.

PAIN MANAGEMENT, SERIOUS AND ENDURING MENTAL HEALTH AND SERIOUS AND ENDURING SUBSTANCE USE

Within the concept of palliative care for the individual experiencing serious and enduring mental health problems it is important that we consider the needs of the individual co-experiencing serious and enduring substance use problems. The chapter continues by examining the specific and essential needs of this population of individuals.

Pain management in the opioid-maintained population

People maintained on opioids, both for the treatment of opioid dependence (addiction) and for the treatment of chronic pain, who present to clinics and general wards with acute pain conditions, are a particular challenge.[52] These people may present with a range of medical or surgical problems causing acute pain including serious illnesses, injuries and infectious diseases (e.g. hepatitis or human immunodeficiency virus – HIV). Acute pain management following surgery or due to trauma for these people may be especially problematic. In general, these individuals experience a greater sensitivity to pain and a cross-tolerance to analgesic effects of opioids as a result of their opioid dependence. This complicates treatment considerably.

There are three complications to pain management in this population.
1 **Misunderstandings** – regarding the management of acute and chronic pain.
2 **Opioid tolerance** – with opioid use, opioid tolerance develops and people require more drug to maintain the same effect.
3 **Hyperalgesia** – with the use of opioids, there may be the paradoxical development of greater pain sensitivity.[53]

SELF-ASSESSMENT EXERCISE 11.3 (ANSWERS ON P. 202)

Time: 30 minutes

Read the following case scenario carefully then answer the questions. All names are fictitious.

Case study

Lisa (38) has a long-standing history of amphetamine and heroin dependence. She has been on methadone maintenance treatment for the last three years. She fell last night and fractured her forearm on a coffee table. She was admitted to the hospital. In the morning, she began to become agitated and demanded the 150 mg of methadone she claims she has daily. However, her urine drug screen has come back negative for methadone but positive for amphetamines. Lisa is scheduled for surgery on her arm later on that day.

CASE QUESTIONS

- Why might Lisa have become agitated and demanded methadone?
- What further information do you need and where might you find it?
- What should your approach to her pain relief be?
- How would you discuss your observations and further assess Lisa?

Common misconceptions

Many misconceptions around pain management and opioid dependence arise due to common stereotypes associated with dependence. This stereotyping can lead to inappropriate or suboptimal pain management. For example, it is important to consider that physical dependence and tolerance are typical and predictable consequences of regular frequent opioid exposure. People who use opioids for chronic pain management or treatment of opioid dependence often become tolerant to relatively high doses of opioids and require even higher doses for acute severe pain. Similarly, people who are maintained on opioids for any reason become physically dependent, and if their dose is abruptly ceased, they are likely to go into withdrawal. Opioid withdrawal may significantly worsen the experience of pain and may further complicate adequate pain management.

The physical conditions of tolerance and withdrawal do not in themselves indicate psychological dependence or problematic drug use. Definitions help to clarify the relationship between physical tolerance, dependence, and pain management. Ranges of definitions are described below. Some general principles and a number of common misconceptions follow these. Specific nursing guidelines are then described.

DEFINITIONS
Dependence
Physical dependence

Physical dependence occurs when the central nervous system (CNS) has been continually exposed to a drug and upon cessation of the drug, the CNS goes into withdrawal. A rule of thumb is that the withdrawal syndrome will be the opposite of the drug's effects on the individual. For example, one of the withdrawal symptoms from a stimulant such as methamphetamine will be feelings of fatigue and possibly extended sleep. Withdrawal symptoms from a depressant such as alcohol or opioids will include agitation, sleep disruption and anxiety.

Psychological dependence

Psychological dependence is when someone has been continually exposed to a drug and, upon cessation of the drug, experiences psychological withdrawal. The person desires the drug and is preoccupied with thoughts of acquiring the drug. It may or may not be accompanied by the physical signs of withdrawal. Another definition (as well as another way to describe addiction) is the compulsion to use a drug despite knowledge that it is harmful. This process may occur with other non-drug forms of psychological dependence such as gambling or shopping.

Iatrogenic dependency

Iatrogenic dependency is where a person is treated with analgesics for a legitimate pain condition and consequently develops a dependency. People suffering from painful conditions often express concern about this. They may state 'I need pain relief but I don't want to become addicted' or even deliberately under-report their pain. However, iatrogenic dependency is uncommon following a single surgical procedure.

In some situations, iatrogenic dependence is more likely to occur. For example, an automobile accident may result in multiple traumas for a person. The person may be required to undergo a number of surgical procedures, potentially resulting in a series of recovery periods with inadequately managed pain.

The prospect of successive undermanaged pain episodes can be extremely stressful. It is more likely that the stress associated with the anticipation of undermanaged pain will be a trigger for the development of dependence than the effective use of opioids for pain management.

Pseudo-psychological dependence

KEY POINT 11.10

Pseudo-psychological dependence, in the context of pain management, is where a person appears to be drug seeking but is merely trying to ensure adequate pain relief.

The person may exhibit extremely inappropriate behaviour in their attempts to manage their pain.

They may be:

➤ involved in illegal activity such as buying opioids on the black market
➤ 'doctor shopping'
➤ displaying aggression
➤ stockpiling large amounts of opioids
➤ going to extreme lengths to manipulate professionals and friends to obtain opioids.

Psychological or pseudo-psychological dependence?

The differentiation between psychological dependence and pseudo-psychological dependence can be difficult for the professional.

With adequate pain management these aberrant behaviours should cease and the behaviour be considered pseudo-psychological dependence. If adequate pain management is forthcoming and these behaviours do not cease, then it is likely to be psychological dependence. The confounding factor is the difficulty in ascertaining if adequate pain management is being provided.[53] Failure to provide adequate pain management may increase the likelihood of progression to psychological dependence.[54]

Tolerance

Physical tolerance

Physical tolerance occurs when progressively larger amounts of the drug are required to get the same effect. Alternatively, if the amount of drug consumed remains constant, the effect of the drug diminishes. The development of physical tolerance by people on long-term opioid therapy is the central problem for effective pain management for this population. In spite of being maintained on relatively large amounts of opioids, individuals require even larger amounts of opioids for analgesic effect. Effective pain management starts by administering the dose usually required for an opioid-naïve individual, and then titrating doses upwards until adequate pain relief is achieved. Analgesics should not be withheld unless the person is becoming over-sedated or experiencing depressed respiration.

Psychological tolerance

Psychological tolerance is when progressively larger amounts of the drug or addictive activity are required to get the same psychological effect. The person has become 'used to' the drug, the behaviour or the feelings experienced. For example, if the person has a gambling problem, they may feel the need to gamble more and more to derive the same sense of satisfaction they initially felt. This may occur without physiological changes.

A person's desired psychological effect from their drug of choice may be quite different from the prescriber's intended target therapeutic effect. Some people prefer to tolerate seemingly large amounts of pain with little analgesia. Others prefer to be sedated, thus feeling the smallest amount of discomfort. Just as the physiological perception of pain may differ between individuals, there is also a significant interpersonal variation in the psychological perception of pain. This is an important factor in a person's psychological tolerance.

Differential development of tolerance

Tolerance develops more rapidly to such effects as:
➤ analgesia
➤ euphoria
➤ sedation
➤ nausea
➤ vomiting
➤ respiratory depression.

Interestingly, it develops slowly or not at all to miosis ('pinning' of the pupils) and constipation. Those maintained on methadone and buprenorphine may complain of constipation for years after commencing treatment. It is important to remember that opioid tolerance develops to the desired effects (e.g. analgesia and euphoria) as well as the undesired effects (e.g. opioid-related sedation and nausea).

Cross-tolerance

Tolerance to one opioid makes a person cross-tolerant to another opioid. It is the mechanism by which opioid substitution works. People are given long-acting methadone or buprenorphine because it stops the withdrawal syndrome associated with a shorter-acting opioid such as heroin. Similarly, benzodiazepines are administered to alcohol-dependent people to stop them going into withdrawal (alcohol and benzodiazepines act at the same receptors and so cross-tolerance occurs).

Pseudo-tolerance

Pseudo-tolerance in the context of acute pain management is where a person's level of use of a drug increases and they require an increased amount of opioid but it is not due to the development of analgesic tolerance.
  It could be due to:
➤ drug interaction – if the person starts taking a different drug, the original drug may not be as effective
➤ progression of the disease or the development of a new disease
➤ increase in physical activity.

Hyperalgesia

KEY POINT 11.11

Pain is important for human functioning.

Pain signals to the brain that certain behaviour may cause injury. During opioid maintenance, there is a relatively large amount of opioid being circulated around the body providing analgesia. The body, in an effort to provide homeostatic balance, becomes more sensitive to pain. It 'counter-balances' the analgesic effect of the opioid to maintain responsiveness to pain. Unfortunately, it commonly sensitises more than required and people maintained on opioids become more sensitive to pain, even those with high plasma opioid concentrations, compared with opioid-naïve people.

This may contribute to the development of opioid tolerance. As the body becomes more sensitive to pain, it requires more opioid to achieve a pain-free state. As stated, it is the primary complicating factor in the pain management of opioid-dependent people.

GENERAL PRINCIPLES

> **KEY POINT 11.12**
>
> There are misconceptions around the use of opioids, pain and dependence. It is crucial that professionals have a good understanding of these general principles.

Maintenance opioids do not provide analgesia

➤ There are three main factors preventing maintenance opioids from providing analgesia:
1 Methadone and buprenorphine have an analgesic duration of action of approximately 4 to 8 hours. Yet these drugs are administered and provide protection from withdrawal for 24 to 48 hours. Therefore, the period of pain relief is quite small relative to dosing periods.
2 Tolerance develops very rapidly to the analgesic effects of opioids when maintained for a period of time. The person becomes tolerant to both large amounts of methadone or buprenorphine but is also cross-tolerant to the analgesic effects of other opioids.
3 The development of hyperalgesia.[53]

Adding opioids does not cause respiratory and CNS depression

Like analgesia, tolerance to the respiratory and CNS depression effects develops quickly. For example, as the pain increases for people with carcinomas, and opioid doses are increased in consequence, there is generally no increase in respiratory and CNS depression in doses adequate to achieve pain control.

> **KEY POINT 11.13**
>
> Pain is a natural antagonist to opioid-induced respiratory and CNS depression.

Seeking relief from pain is not the same as drug seeking

> **KEY POINT 11.14**
>
> Seeking relief from pain is different from drug seeking.

A careful clinical assessment for the objective evidence of pain will decrease the chance of manipulation by a drug-seeking person and also support the administration of opioid analgesics in a person with a history of drug dependence.

Professionals often perceive opioid-dependent people with pain issues to be demanding and manipulative. In turn, opioid-dependent people, often due to a history of discrimination and inadequate pain relief, may:
➤ become distrustful of the medical community and concerned about being stigmatised
➤ fear that their pain will be undertreated or that their opioid maintenance dose will be altered or discontinued
➤ act inappropriately to get opioids but only be suffering from unrelieved pain (pseudo-psychological dependence)
➤ have good pain relief but be fearful of the re-emergence of pain
➤ fear withdrawal symptoms should their pain relief be discontinued
➤ fear a reduction in the current effective doses of opioid analgesics.

Major health effects of unrelieved pain

> **KEY POINT 11.15**
>
> Major health implications are associated with unmanaged pain.

There are major health implications associated with unmanaged pain:
➤ physical stasis (bedsores, foot drop, etc.)
➤ prolonged post-operative recoveries
➤ clinical depression
➤ cardiovascular stress
➤ increased tumour growth
➤ relapse or exacerbation of dependence issues.

> **KEY POINT 11.16**
>
> It is critical for pain to be well managed to achieve optimal overall health.

Factors affecting the pain experience
The pain experience of people maintained on opioids with chronic pain is not simply augmented by opioid-induced hyperalgesia. It is also exacerbated by subtle withdrawal syndromes. It may also be influenced by intoxication with related

sympathetic arousal and muscle tension. Sleep disturbance, mood changes and functional changes (associated with a comorbid condition such as hepatitis C) may also affect the pain experience.[53,55]

Identifying and treating co-occurring conditions which affect the perception of pain and, therefore, the successful management of the pain are of paramount importance. Important examples of frequently comorbid conditions are depression and anxiety. Both may significantly complicate the treatment of pain and dependence, but may be responsive to a range of treatments.

The dangers associated with unrestricted opioid dosing

The answer is not as simple as dosing without restriction in an effort to produce pain relief. While there are dangers with unmanaged pain, there are dangers with unrestricted opioid dosing. While opioids theoretically have no maximum ceiling, hyperalgesia (as stated), neuroendocrinological (hormone) dysfunction, and possibly immunosuppression (decreased functioning of the immune system) may occur at high doses. Respiratory depression can present difficulties in spite of tolerance (especially if the person is on other medication or consumes alcohol or another central nervous system depressant). Sedation can interfere with daily function and the processes of driving and safety around the home, and care of dependants may be affected with lethal consequences. It has also been suggested that repeated dose escalations lack incremental benefit at higher doses (e.g. more than 200 mg of morphine daily or equivalent).[1]

SPECIFIC PAIN MANAGEMENT GUIDELINES FOR OPIOID-TOLERANT PEOPLE

People with active dependency

Build trust

➤ Openly acknowledge history of dependency, and allow people to discuss fears about how this may affect pain management and treatment by the professionals.
➤ Reassure people that their history of dependency problems will not prevent adequate pain management.
➤ Respect and believe the person's report of pain.
➤ Reassure the person that professionals are committed to assertively providing effective pain relief.
➤ Aggressively treat acute pain; treatment for dependency issues is not the priority during the acute pain period.

Professional education

➤ Prescription of opioids to a person with a known dependency problem for the management of pain is not illegal or unethical.
➤ People with a dependency problem may be relatively pain intolerant.
➤ Detoxification is an ineffective short-term treatment for a dependency problem and inappropriate in the presence of pain.

Broaden the treatment plan
➤ With the person, develop a treatment contract for opioid analgesia.
➤ Request consultation from a substance-use medicine specialist.
➤ Carefully document treatment plan, including analgesic use, response, and regular reviews of efficacy of current plan.

Knowledgeably administer opioids
➤ Utilise non-pharmacologic and non-opioid analgesic alternatives (as discussed earlier).
➤ Consider patient-controlled analgesia which may decrease total opioid requirements and the drug-seeking behaviours.
➤ Choose long-acting opioids (e.g. slow-release morphine sulphate; slow-release oxycodone) with gradual onset of action and lower street value, administered under continuous scheduled dosing orders (e.g. 4 times a day – QID) rather than as-needed orders (PRN).
➤ Opioid cross-tolerance and the person's increased pain sensitivity will often necessitate higher opioid analgesic doses administered at shorter intervals.

KEY POINT 11.17

If the individual is physically maintained on an agonist (e.g. methadone), *do not* administer a mixed opioid agonist/antagonist (e.g. buprenorphine) – withdrawal may be precipitated.[53]

Individuals on opioid-maintenance therapy
➤ Continue the usual dose of methadone or buprenorphine (or equivalent).
➤ Use short-acting opioid analgesics and titrate to effect (e.g. morphine, codeine, oxycodone).
➤ Contact methadone or buprenorphine maintenance clinic or prescribing physician:
  — notify them of admission, discharge and confirm the time and amount of last maintenance dose
  — notify them of any medications such as opioids or benzodiazepines given to the person during hospitalisation because they may show up on routine urine drug screening
  — notify them of any short-term analgesia (opioid or otherwise) provided on discharge.[53]

Individuals currently abstinent
Build trust
➤ Openly acknowledge history of dependence, and allow person and professional to discuss fears of reactivation of dependency.
➤ Explain any intent to use opioids or other psychoactive medications.

➤ Respect person's right to decide whether or not to be administered opioids.

Education of the individual

➤ Explain health risks associated with unrelieved pain, including risk of relapse.
➤ Explain that the known risk for reactivation of dependency to opioids in the context of pain is small.
➤ Ensure the person understands differences between psychological and physical dependence.

Minimise withdrawal following procedure or treatment

➤ Taper opioid analgesics *slowly* to minimise emergence of withdrawal symptoms.
➤ Assess for presence of withdrawal symptoms at least 4 times daily during analgesic taper; treat symptomatically.
➤ Offer non-pharmacological and non-opioid analgesic alternatives.

Support abstinence

➤ Encourage the person to increase contact with family and/or significant other supports. Reassure person that it is acceptable to take medications for medical reasons. Offer to advise/reassure significant others if required.
➤ Request consultation from substance-use medicine specialist.
➤ Request consultation from allied health professionals to devise pain management plans to support and minimise analgesic requirements.
➤ Screen for mental health and substance-use conditions. Arrange diagnosis and treatment including referral if necessary.
➤ Include family in plan of pain care.
➤ If relapse occurs, intensify abstinence efforts; *do not terminate pain care.*[53]

Individuals on naltrexone for alcohol or opioid dependence

➤ Cease naltrexone prior to pain-producing procedures if possible. Encourage the person to seek additional support as required to maintain abstinence during this period (3–5 days), and caution opioid-dependent individuals about the risk of inadvertent overdose with relapse.
➤ In the initial 24-hour period as the naltrexone begins to wear off, the following multimodal analgesic regimes are recommended:
  − non-steroidal anti-inflammatories (e.g. ibuprofen)
  − paracetamol
  − ketamine
  − tramadol
  − regional nerve blocks/anaesthetics.
➤ **Caution**. There is experimental evidence of opioid receptor upregulation following naltrexone/opioid antagonist withdrawal. Therefore, abrupt

discontinuation of naltrexone may lead to increased opioid sensitivity and possibility of opioid toxicity/overdose with opioid administration. Increased supervision and monitoring are encouraged during this time. Dose administration in smaller increments may be warranted to allow increased surveillance.

➤ Continued administration of naltrexone will prevent the analgesic effects of regularly used doses of codeine or opioid-based analgesia.

➤ If unable to decrease naltrexone (e.g. due to emergency department admission or for an emergency surgical procedure), the following multimodal analgesic regimes are recommended:
  — non-steroidal anti-inflammatories (e.g. ibuprofen)
  — paracetamol
  — ketamine
  — tramadol
  — regional nerve blocks/anaesthetics.

➤ If pain is not managed, the individual should be transferred to a High Dependency Unit and opioids titrated. At very high doses and in combination with opioid adjuvants . . .
  — non-steroidal anti-inflammatories (e.g. ibuprofen)
  — paracetamol
  — ketamine
  — tramadol
  — regional nerve blocks/anaesthetics

. . . opioids will override antagonist effects of naltrexone and provide relief. The therapeutic window may be narrow, necessitating careful monitoring for precipitous respiratory and CNS depression.[53]

Individuals experiencing chronic pain and dependence

➤ complicated by the need to take opioids on a regular basis for the treatment of pain

➤ complicated by the lack of clear pathology underlying the pain experience

➤ complicated in that complete analgesia is not the practical goal of opioid treatment.

Treatment

➤ Address dependency issues.

➤ Use specific treatment contracts that should detail frequency of review, dispensing agreements and any specific monitoring.

➤ Define and manage physical and emotional components of pain. A range of interventions including counselling may be helpful. These interventions might be particularly important if the painful condition has caused significant life changes or loss of function, resulting in grief and loss issues.

➤ Identify and treat mental health–substance use conditions as indicated.

➤ Use holistic care including the use of physiotherapy and occupational therapy as required, addressing pain management and functional capacity. Interventions may include:
  − acupuncture
  − exercise plans
  − anxiety management
  − mindfulness training.

Assess, monitor and document

➤ Assess, monitor and document:
  − pain severity and quality
  − level of function
  − presence of adverse events
  − opioid analgesic use
  − evidence of opioid misuse
  − evaluation and plan
  − progress towards therapeutic goals.[56]

Therapeutic goals

➤ Includes the functional restoration of:
  − physical capabilities
  − psychological intactness
  − family and social interactions
  − degree of healthcare utilisation
  − drug use for symptom control.[53]

Preparing for discharge

➤ If the individual has become dependent or remains dependent, minimise withdrawal.
➤ If the individual is already physically dependent on opioids, initiate onto long-acting, substitution medications to prevent withdrawal.
➤ If detoxification prior to discharge is agreed upon, taper opioids *slowly* to minimise the emergence of withdrawal symptoms.
➤ Monitor for emergence of withdrawal symptoms at least 4 times daily, and treat aggressively and symptomatically.
➤ If the individual is discharged on opioid analgesics with limited maintenance
  − choose a single, long-acting formulation with lower street value (e.g. methadone or long-acting morphine)
  − write prescriptions for decreasing quantities of opioids for short periods of time with no repeats. Specify frequent dispensing. Clearly communicate discharge plans and medications to all community professionals.
  − specify dosing times (*not* 'as required')

— assess person's level of motivation for drug treatment and encourage entry into treatment.[53]

CONCLUSION

Collaborative practice and regular consultation among the interdisciplinary team – including the specialist palliative care and mental health teams – are important to achieve a common approach and optimise treatment outcome. Involving the interdisciplinary team throughout will ensure a consistent approach to the identified problems, improve understanding of the nature of the pain and facilitate communication.

The key to effective pain management is continuous assessment and restructuring of interventions as directed by the individual or family. The individual and family are the experts in appreciating the complexity of the pain and the best way to treat it.

The role of the family is pivotal. The family should never be excluded from pain assessment. It is difficult to overstate how extremely distressing it is to see one's partner, sibling or child in chronic, unrelieved pain. Therefore:

➤ inclusion
➤ support
➤ guidance
➤ intervention
➤ opportunity . . .

. . . to discuss how the individual feels are imperative if therapeutic intervention is to be successful.

KEY POINT 11.18

It is important to continue supporting the individual even when interventions have not proved successful. Being present and *alongside* is a therapeutic intervention, encourages the therapeutic relationship and can be powerfully healing.

Taking care of the individual and family is pivotal. However, of equal importance is that professionals need to take care of themselves. Being with someone in pain and deep distress is emotionally draining. Discussing one's feelings about the situation and seeking support, within the context of regular supervision and good management, is not a failing. It is good-quality practice and is essential if our interventions on behalf of the individual and family are to be effective.

Dependency, for people receiving opioids for dependency treatment or chronic pain, produces changes on a neurophysiological, psychological and societal level. In particular, there are the neural changes of opioid tolerance and hyperalgesia. Physical dependence and tolerance are predictable consequences of frequent opioid exposure, and alone do not indicate maladaptive behaviour.

> **KEY POINT 11.19**
>
> As a result of tolerance, people maintained on opioids will receive less analgesia from a given dose than people who are opioid naïve. Tolerant people will require higher opioid doses to manage acute severe pain.

Maintenance opioids do not provide pain relief.

Iatrogenic dependency and relapse of dependency may occur as a result of effective management of acute severe pain, but are more likely to occur with suboptimal management of pain. Suboptimal management of pain is also likely to produce a variety of pseudo-dependent behaviours in a person's effort to ensure adequate pain relief.

Good practice should demonstrate a sound understanding of the pharmacodynamics and pharmacokinetics of pain medication in the context of opioid maintenance to prescribe, monitor and assess pain in this population effectively.

> **KEY POINT 11.20**
>
> It is important that professionals do not allow concerns of being manipulated to cloud their judgement concerning the individual's pain experience and lead them to providing suboptimal acute severe pain management.

Careful monitoring and aggressive pain management will reassure the person, facilitate both physical and psychological recovery, and ensure the most effective management of both pain and dependency issues.

REFERENCES

1 Chou R, Fanciullo GJ, Fine PG, *et al.* Clinical guidelines for the use of chronic opioid therapy in chronic noncancer pain. *Journal of Pain.* 2009; **10**: 113–30.

2 Alford DP, Compton P, Samet JH. Acute pain management for patients receiving maintenance methadone or buprenorphine therapy. *Annals of Internal Medicine.* 2006; **144**: 127–34.

3 Twycross R. *Introducing Palliative Care.* 4th ed. Oxford: Radcliffe Medical Press; 1999.

4 Dudgeon D, Raubertas R, Rosenthal S. The short-form McGill pain questionnaire in chronic cancer pain. *Journal of Pain and Symptoms Management.* 1993; **8**: 191–5.

5 Murdoch J, Larsen D. Assessing pain in cognitively impaired older adults. *Nursing Standard.* 2004; **18**: 33–9.

6 Abbey J, Piller N, Debellis A, *et al.* The Abbey pain scale: a 1-minute numerical indicator for people with end-stage dementia. *International Journal of Palliative Nursing.* 2004; **10**: 6–13.

7 Doloplus. Available at: www.doloplus.com/pourquoi/pourquoi.php (accessed 23 April 2012).

8 Hanks G, Cherney N, Christakis N, *et al.*, editors. *Oxford Textbook of Palliative Medicine.* 4th ed. Oxford: Oxford University Press; 2011. p. 600.

9 Chandler A, Preece J, Lister S. Using heat therapy for pain management. *Nursing Standard.* 2002; **17**: 40–2.

10 World Health Organization. *Cancer Pain Relief.* 2nd ed. Geneva: World Health Organization; 1996.

11 Twycross R, Wilcock A, Charlesworth S, *et al. Palliative Care Formulary.* 2nd ed. Oxon: Radcliffe Medical Press; 2002. p. 174.

12 Hanks G, Hoskin P, Aherne G, *et al.* Explanation for potency of repeated oral doses of morphine? *Lancet.* 1987; **ii**: 723–5.

13 Davis M, Walsh D. Rapid opioid titration in severe cancer pain. *European Journal of Palliative Care.* 2005; **12**: 11–14.

14 Hanks G, de Conno F, Cherney N, *et al.* Morphine and alternative opioids in cancer pain: the EAPC recommendations. *British Journal of Cancer.* 2001; **85**: 587–93.

15 Vadalouca A, Moka E, Argyra E, *et al.* Opioid rotation for cancer patients: a review of the literature. *Journal of Opioid Management.* 2008; **4**: 213–50.

16 Kaiko R, Wallenstein M, Rogers R, *et al.* Analgesic and mood effects of heroin and morphine in cancer patients with post-operative pain. *The New England Journal of Medicine.* 1981; **304**: 1501–5.

17 Twycross R, Wilcock A, Charlesworth S, *et al. Palliative Care Formulary.* 2nd ed. Oxon: Radcliffe Medical Press; 2002. pp. 186–7.

18 Ahmedzai S, Brooks D. Trans-dermal fentanyl versus sustained-release oral morphine in cancer pain: preference, efficacy, and quality of life. The TTS-fentanyl – comparative trial group. *Journal of Pain and Symptom Management.* 1997; **13**: 254–61.

19 Ellershaw J, Kinder C, Aldridge J, *et al.* Care of the dying: is pain control compromised or enhanced by continuation of the fentanyl trans-dermal patch in the dying phase? *Journal of Pain and Symptom Management.* 2002; **24**: 398–403.

20 Back I. *Pain in Palliative Medicine Handbook.* 3rd ed. Cardiff: BPM Books; 2001. p. 77.

21 Gibbs M. The role of transdermal fentanyl patches in the effective management of cancer pain. *International Journal of Palliative Nursing.* 2009: **15**: 354–9.

22 Twycross R, Wilcock A. *Symptom Management in Advanced Cancer.* 3rd ed. Oxon: Radcliffe Medical Press; 2001. p. 381.

23 Hanks G, Nugent M, Higgs C, *et al.* Oral transmucosal fentanyl citrate in the management of breakthrough pain in cancer: an open, multicentre, dose-titration and long term use study. *Palliative Medicine.* 2004; **18**: 698–704.

24 Flock P, Gibbs L, Sykes N. Diamorphine-Metronidazole gel effective for treatment of painful infected leg ulcers. *Journal of Pain and Symptom Management.* 2000; **20**: 396–7.

25 Grocott P. Palliative management of fungating malignant wounds. *Journal of Community Nursing.* 2000; **14**: 31–40.

26 Naylor W. Assessment and management of pain in fungating wounds. *British Journal of Nursing.* 2001; Suppl. **10**: 33–56.

27 Zepetella G. Topical opioids for painful skin ulcers: do they work? *European Journal of Palliative Care.* 2004; **11**: 93–6.

28 Naylor W. Malignant wounds: aetiology and principles of management. *Nursing Standard.* 2002; **16**: 45–53.

29 Doyle D, Hanks G, Cherny N, (2003). *Oxford Textbook of Palliative Care.* 3rd ed. Oxford: Oxford University Press; 2003.

30 Mercadante S, Villari P, Ferrera P, *et al.* Addition of a second opioid may improve opioid response in cancer pain: preliminary data. *Support Care Cancer.* 2004; **12**: 762–6.

31 Toscani F, Piva L, Corli O, *et al.* Ketorolac versus diclofenac sodium in cancer pain. *Arzneimittel Forschung – Drug Research.* 1994: **44**: 550–4.

32 Buckley M, Brogden R. Ketorolac. A review of its pharmacodynamic and pharmacokinetic properties and therapeutic potential. *Drugs*. 1990; **39**: 86–109.

33 Blackwell N, Bangham L, Hughes M, *et al*. Subcutaneous ketorolac – a new development in pain control. *Palliative Medicine*. 1993; **7**: 63–5.

34 Micaela M, Brogen B, Brogen R. Ketorolac – a review of its pharmacodynamic and pharmacokinetic properties, and therapeutic potential. *Drugs*. 1990; **39**: 86–109.

35 Regnard C, Dean M. *A Guide to Symptom Relief in Palliative Care*. 6th ed. Oxford: Radcliffe; 2010. p. 70.

36 Johnson A. Use of bisphosphonates for the treatment of metastatic bone pain; a survey of palliative care physicians in the UK. *Palliative Medicine*. 2001; **15**: 141–7.

37 Ripamonti C, Fulfaro F, Ticozzi C, *et al*. (1998) Role of pamidronate disodium in the treatment of metastatic bone disease. *Tumori*. 1998; **84**: 442–55.

38 Body J, Deal I, Bell R, *et al*. Oral ibandronate improves bone pain and preserves quality of life in patients with skeletal metastases due to breast cancer. *Pain*. 2004; **111**: 306–12.

39 Twycross R. Wilcock A. *Pain Relief in Symptom Management in Advanced Cancer*. 3rd ed. Oxford: Radcliffe Medical Press; 2001. p. 27.

40 Osterland H, Beirne P. Complementary therapies. In: Ferrell B, Coyle N, editors. *Textbook of Palliative Nursing*. Oxford: Oxford University Press; 2001. pp. 374–5.

41 Nilsson S, Strang P, Ginman C, *et al*. Palliation of bone pain in prostate cancer using chemotherapy and Strontium-89 – a randomized phase II study. *Journal of Pain and Symptom Management*. 2005; **29**: 352–7.

42 Kaye P. (2003). *A-Z Pocketbook of Symptom Control*. Northampton: EPL Publications; 2003. p. 112.

43 Eisenberg E, River Y, Shifrin A, *et al*. Antiepileptic drugs in the treatment of neuropathic pain. *Drugs*. **67**: 1265–89.

44 Freynhagen R, Strojek K, Greising T, *et al*. Efficacy of Pregabalin in neuropathic pain evaluated in a 12-week, randomised, double-blind, multicentre, placebo-controlled trial of flexible- and fixed-dose regimens. *Pain*. 2005; **115**: 254–63.

45 Twycross R, Wilcock A, editors. *Palliative Care Formulary*. 4th ed. Nottingham: palliative drugs.com; 2011. p. 491.

46 Edwards A, Gerrard G. The management of cerebral metastases. *European Journal of Palliative Care*. 1998; **5**: 7–11.

47 Poole D. Use of TENS in pain management, part 2: how to use TENS. *Nursing Times*. 2007; **103**: 28–9.

48 Saunders C. *Hospice and Palliative Care: an interdisciplinary approach*. London: Edward Arnold; 1990. p. 27.

49 Stimmel B. *Pain and its Relief Without Addiction*. New York: Haworth Medical Press; 1997. p. 77.

50 Coyle N, Ferrel B, editors. *Oxford Textbook of Palliative Nursing*. 3rd ed. New York, NY/Open University Press; 2010. p. 172.

51 McCaffrey M, Pasero C. *Pain: clinical manual*. 2nd ed. London: Mosby; 1999.

52 Athanasos P, Smith CS, White JM, *et al*. Methadone maintenance patients are cross-tolerant to the antinociceptive effects of very high plasma morphine concentrations. *Pain*. 2006; **120**: 267–75.

53 Compton P, Athanasos P, de Crespigny C. *Opioid Tolerance and the Effective Management of Acute Pain*. Sydney: Drug and Alcohol Nurses of Australasia Conference; 2006.

54 Schnoll SH, Weaver MF. Addiction and pain. *American Journal of Addiction*. 2003; **12**(Suppl 2): S27–35.

55 Parish JM. Sleep-related problems in common medical conditions. *Chest.* 2009; **135**: 563–72.

56 Passik SD, Kirsh KL. The need to identify predictors of aberrant drug-related behavior and addiction in patients being treated with opioids for pain. *Pain Medicine.* 2003; **4**: 186–9.

TO LEARN MORE

- Basford L. Complementary therapies. In: Basford L, Slevin O. editors. *Theory and Practice of Nursing: an integrated approach to caring.* 2nd ed. Cheltenham: Nelson Thornes; 2003. pp. 569–96.
- Behavioural pain assessment scale and discussion for older patients with verbal communication disorders: Available at: www.doloplus.com/pourquoi/pourquoi.php (accessed 23 April 2012).
- British Pain Society: Available at: www.britishpainsociety.org/index.html (accessed 23 April 2012).
- Cooper J, editor. *Stepping into Palliative Care 1: relationships and responses.* Oxford: Radcliffe Medical Press.
- Cooper J, editor. *Stepping into Palliative Care 1: care and practice.* Oxford: Radcliffe Medical Press.
- Discussion of pharmaceutical and other treatment of pain: Available at: www.palliativedrugs. com/index.html (accessed 23 April 2012).
- Hanks G, Cherny N I, Christakis N.A, *et al.* editors. *Oxford Textbook of Palliative Medicine.* 4th ed. Oxford: Oxford University Press; 2011.
- Information on TENS machine settings: Available at: www.electrotherapy.org/ (accessed 23 April 2012).
- International Association for Pain and Chemical Dependency. Available at: www.iapcd.org/ (accessed 23 April 2012).
- Regnard C, Dean M. *A Guide to Symptom Relief in Advanced Disease.* 6th ed. Oxford: Radcliffe; 2010.
- Relaxation exercises: Available at: www.patient.co.uk/showdoc/27000363/ (accessed 27 February 2012).
- Smith H, Passik S. *Pain and Chemical Dependency.* New York, NY: Oxford University Press; 2008.
- Stimmel B. *Pain and its Relief without Addiction: clinical issues in the use of opioids and other analgesics.* Birmingham, NY: Haworth Medical Press; 1997.
- Twycross R, Wilcock A, Stark Toller C. *Symptom Management in Advanced Cancer.* 4th ed. Nottingham: palliativedrugs.com; 2009.
- Twycross R, Wilcock A, editors. *Palliative Care Formulary.* 4th ed. Nottingham: palliative-drugs.com; 2011.
- Wall P. *Pain: the science of suffering.* New York, NY: Columbia University Press; 2002.

ACKNOWLEDGEMENT

The authors are grateful to the editors and publishers for permitting adaptation of the following chapters.

Mitten T. Introduction to pain management. In: Cooper J, editor. *Stepping into Palliative Care 2: care and practice.* 2nd ed. Oxon: Radcliffe; 2006. pp. 16–39.

Athanasos P, Neild R, de Crespigny C, *et al.* Pain management. In Cooper DB, editor. *Care in Mental Health–Substance Use.* London/New York: Radcliffe; 2011. pp. 215–28.

ANSWER TO SELF-ASSESSMENT EXERCISE 11.3 (P. 186)

Lisa might have become agitated due to having uncontrolled pain as a result of her fracture. Her pain may be uncontrolled due to lack of analgesia or inadequate analgesia. Lisa may also be experiencing emerging withdrawal syndrome from one or both of her drugs of dependence. Information from Lisa's methadone treatment provider is necessary. This will confirm her current dose and dosing schedule, including information to confirm the last dose given and any take-away doses. Information about observed dosing will help to establish the likelihood of diversion of Lisa's prescribed methadone.

Confirmation of the results of Lisa's most recent urine drug screen will also be useful. It is important to confirm the type of urine drug screen test that was performed when Lisa was admitted to hospital as not all standard screens will detect methadone. The hospital laboratory will provide this information. It is important to be aware of any recent medication changes as some medications may significantly alter the metabolism of methadone. A serum methadone level (blood test) may be useful in cases such as this.

After Lisa's methadone treatment dose has been confirmed and confidence has been established that she is currently taking her methadone, her regular dose should be given. This regular dose will not provide any analgesia for her acute pain. Intra-operative pain relief should be given as usual and short-acting opioids should be titrated to effect. Post-operatively, long-acting opioids should be given with short-acting agents titrated for breakthrough pain. Non-opioid pain relief should also be used and may remain as part of the treatment plan as opioid analgesia is reduced after the initial effects of the injury begin to settle.

Lisa may have been receiving take-away doses of methadone and diverting these doses elsewhere. This would have resulted in a negative urine screen for methadone. If there is any doubt as to Lisa's compliance with her current methadone treatment (concern about potential diversion) overall dose may be reduced and given as a split dose. Short-acting analgesic agents should be titrated to effect. Consultation with her usual methadone treatment providers should be sought in this instance to promote restabilisation prior to discharge.

Lisa should be reassured that her pain will be treated. She should be told that it could sometimes be somewhat more complicated to treat pain in those on methadone maintenance treatment but that staff will not give up until her pain is adequately treated. An explanation of the relevance of her recent drug-use history including the illicit use of drugs and pharmaceuticals should be given alongside reassurance that any information given will be used solely to optimise her treatment.

CHAPTER 12

Managing restlessness and agitation at the end-of-life

Jo Cooper

REFLECTIVE PRACTICE EXERCISE 12.1

Time: 20 minutes

When a diagnosis of dying has been made, unpleasant symptoms such as restlessness and agitation may be experienced during the last days or hours of life.

Have you noticed restlessness and agitation in a person who is dying, either in your working environment, or in a family member or friend? Take a moment to recall the picture to your mind.

- What did you notice? Think physical, emotional, spiritual and psychological.
- How did this make you feel?
- What effect did this have on your own emotions?
- Were you able to do anything that you felt was helpful? If so, what were you able to do?
- How was the situation managed?
- What was the outcome for the person following interventions?
- Was that person's death peaceful or distressing for them?
- What was the outcome for you? For example, how did you feel after the situation had been managed (or not managed)?

INTRODUCTION

The need to explore the impact of terminal restlessness and its treatment on the family is imperative. The family is often present during the last days or hours of life prior to death. Whatever happens to the person, any action, omission or decision made will have significant consequences for the family members. Below we discuss the concerns and dilemmas raised and how we can act to alleviate these problems.

WHAT IS TERMINAL RESTLESSNESS?

The terms *terminal restlessness*, *terminal anguish* and *delirium* are often used interchangeably. Terminal restlessness overlaps with but is not necessarily identical to delirium.[2]

Terminal restlessness can be defined as the agitation and restlessness that may occur during the last few hours or days of life. Sixty-eight per cent to 88% of people may exhibit:[3]

➤ anxiety
➤ agitation
➤ impaired consciousness
➤ physical distress
➤ myoclonus (muscle jerking).[4]

Delirium – also known as acute confusional state – may be accompanied by:

➤ reduced attention
➤ memory impairment
➤ disorientation
➤ hallucinations
➤ altered perception and misinterpretation
➤ restlessness
➤ anxiety
➤ irritability
➤ noisy, aggressive behaviour.[5]

ASSESSMENT AND AIM

Assessment includes physical, psychological, emotional and spiritual dimensions. It is continuous – not a 'one-off' (*see* Chapters 5, 6, 8, 9 and 10). The aim is to:

➤ **provide** – physical and emotional comfort
➤ **maintain** – a conscious level that enables family relationships and communication, if possible
➤ **reduce** – the distress of the family.

Terminal restlessness and agitation is distressing for the person and the family, and it can be mismanaged through fear of over-sedation. Therefore, an intra- inter-disciplinary approach, skilled assessment and effective and prompt treatment are imperative and underpin palliative care.

Misdiagnosis or mismanagement may result in a poor-quality death and loss of dignity.

SELF-ASSESSMENT EXERCISE 12.1

Time: 5 minutes
List the causes of terminal restlessness.

Identifying the cause

The causative factors leading to restlessness and agitation need to be identified quickly and effectively (*see* Box 12.1).

BOX 12.1 Treatable causes of terminal restlessness[4]

- **Pain** – treat with appropriate analgesics following on-going, regular assessment; consider culture – meditation and relaxation techniques may be helpful (*see* Chapters 3 and 11).
- **Generalised physical discomfort** – e.g. relieve with gentle repositioning and the use of specialised pressure-relieving aids.
- **Bladder or bowel distension** – consider an indwelling catheter; micro-enema or suppositories to reduce constipation.
- **Breathlessness** – consider opioids to reduce the sensation of breathlessness, an electric fan, an open window, gentle breathing exercises and relaxation.
- **Nicotine withdrawal** — consider nicotine patch or Nicorette nasal spray.
- **Alcohol withdrawal** — consider diazepam.
- **Infection** – consider antibiotic for symptom management.
- **Drug induced restlessness** – e.g. opioids, antibiotics, anticonvulsants, digoxin, diuretics, NSAIDs, steroids, hypnotics – review medication and/or modify when necessary.

When assessing terminal restlessness, agitation and delirium consider the following factors:
➤ **opioids** – in 64% of cases[6]
➤ **misdiagnosis** – jeopardises quality of life[7]
➤ **cause** – may be multifactorial or not be found[2,6]
➤ **irreversible cause** – when identified it is often irreversible (e.g. liver failure or cerebral metastases, multi-organ failure)[2,6]

➤ **tests** – often inappropriate if time is short or the person is cared for at home

➤ **communication** – the person may be unable to state the cause of their restlessness (e.g. feeling uncomfortable, experiencing pain, feeling afraid).

Precipitating factors of terminal restlessness are listed in Box 12.2.[3]

BOX 12.2 Precipitating factors of terminal restlessness[3]

- unresolved psychological or emotional problems
- cerebral oedema
- heart failure
- primary brain tumour
- cerebral vascular event
- biochemical imbalance (urea, calcium, sodium, glucose)
- deteriorating liver and renal function.

As well as assessing and aiming to correct the cause of terminal restlessness or delirium, it is important to take symptomatic and supportive measures to minimise the distress caused to the person and their family.[6]

The opportunity should be taken to review and discontinue medication where necessary. Drugs frequently cause delirium and agitation. Therefore, it is imperative to check current medication. This can be addressed frequently with other members of the intra- inter-disciplinary team, and communicated to the family, together with the reasons that certain medications are being discontinued. It can be a great worry for the family if a drug which has been used over a long period of time is suddenly stopped. The family members are not only informed, but given the opportunity to ask their own questions.

KEY POINT 12.3

It is common to find more than one drug responsible for causing delirium.[6]

MANAGEMENT

Although the successful management of restlessness, agitation and/or delirium relies heavily on appropriate medication, emotional, spiritual and psychological support for the person and family is necessary and appropriate in order to reduce emotional pain (*see* Chapter 8). In addition, practical supportive measures, which have been found helpful, include:

➤ **environment** – provide a safe environment. If the person is delirious, there may be a danger to self and others.

➤ **injury** – if appropriate, a mattress placed on the floor, although not ideal,

may be a safer option in the acute situation, until treatment becomes effective
➤ **quiet** – encourage a peaceful, quiet environment
➤ **lighting** – use of soft lighting. Fears are often exacerbated at night. Low light at night promotes a feeling of safety.
➤ **noise** – reduce levels to aid sleep where possible
➤ **company** – if appropriate, reassurance that someone will stay may help to reduce anxiety. A member of the family or a friend can help to reduce distress.
➤ **massage** – gentle, simple massage using relaxing essential oils may help feelings of well-being. Essential oils, used in a vaporising burner, may provide sensory pleasure and reduce anxiety.
➤ **touch** – can be powerful; it tells someone that we care and that we are present
➤ **explanations** – give simple and clear explanations about what we are doing, and what can be done to help. The person may be able to hear us, even if they cannot respond. Giving regular updates to the family is also important, to ensure they know what to expect at each step.
➤ **reassurance** – reassure the family that this is often natural at the end of life. Families often feel responsible for the person's condition – a feeling that they have 'done something wrong'.
➤ **recuperation** – try to ensure that the family members have the opportunity for rest and take time for themselves.
➤ **observation** – increased nursing observation is essential
➤ **continuity** – staff continuity is a priority.

Cognitive interventions can apply to the person and family,[7] and can include:
➤ **communication** – simple and clear
➤ **acknowledgement** – of feelings – when we encounter the distress of another, it is easy for us to want to run away. Sitting with that distress, sometimes just saying nothing, but staying with it, is important; say what you see . . . 'I can see that watching "Mary" is making you feel very sad . . .'; this often helps to open up communication at a time when it is most difficult.
➤ **fostering a sense of control** – explain the reasons why we are doing what we do; do not leave families to guess
➤ **balancing hope and reality** – hope changes as time passes; hope for a cure and to go home may be replaced by the hope for a peaceful death (*see* Chapter 7).

PHARMACOLOGICAL THERAPY
ESSENTIAL NOTE

Drug dosages are not given in this chapter. Each individual will require specialist assessment, and medication should be titrated to the needs of the individual, specific to their medical history and situation at the time. For guidance, see **To Learn More** at the end of this chapter.

KEY POINT 12.4

Intramuscular (IM) injections are painful for people when they are frail, and should be avoided. The subcutaneous route is kinder and effective.

When agitated and distressed, people are often unable to take medication orally. The subcutaneous route is, therefore, used to provide continuous relief of suffering at the end-of-life. A syringe driver is the preferred method in the provision of medication to manage distressing symptoms, such as restlessness, agitation, pain, nausea, etc. This provides 24-hour-per-day relief and reduces the need for repeat injections.

The medication of choice for terminal restlessness without delirium is midazolam (a benzodiazepine).[2]

KEY POINT 12.5

Remember to administer an immediate (stat) dose of midazolam, subcutaneously, prior to setting up the syringe driver. This is good practice and will calm the person quickly, while the syringe driver medication takes effect.

KEY POINT 12.6

If the person fails to settle comfortably with midazolam then consider introducing haloperidol before increasing midazolam.[8]

Midazolam[5]
➤ Midazolam has a quick-onset action.
➤ Midazolam is *water-soluble* and it mixes with most of the drugs commonly given by syringe driver.
➤ In agitated terminal delirium, larger doses are sometimes necessary, especially if anxiety has been a feature, or in the case of a person who has been using denial as a coping mechanism.

➤ Tolerance may develop after the person has shown a good initial response.
➤ Continual review is pivotal to good management.

Diazepam (a benzodiazepine)[5]

Diazepam given as a suppository per rectum (PR) is useful in a crisis. An immediate dose, followed by a dosing regimen of 6–8 hourly, may be helpful.

SELF-ASSESSMENT EXERCISE 12.2

> **Time: 5 minutes**
> List the difficulties we may encounter using the rectal route when managing terminal restlessness and agitation.

Limitations
➤ Rectal administration of diazepam at home may be difficult due to the practical problems of moving and changing position.
➤ The person will need to be alert enough to give their consent.
➤ There may be problems if the person is impacted or has diarrhoea.
➤ Haemorrhoids, tumour, rectal discharge or pain may also exclude this route.[9]

Levomepromazine (phenothiazine)
➤ Levomepromazine is often used to reduce agitation.[10]
➤ Give an immediate (stat) dose prior to setting up syringe driver. This will help to settle the person, reducing symptoms promptly.
➤ Depending on the response, titrate the dose.
➤ Drug action onset – approximately 30 minutes.[8]
➤ The duration of the dose action is 12–24 hours.[8]
➤ Levomepromazine also has anti-emetic benefits.[7,8]
➤ If there is a risk of convulsions, midazolam can be added.[5]

Haloperidol (a butyrophenone)
ESSENTIAL NOTE

> If the person is already taking haloperidol for mental health symptoms it may be necessary to consider increasing the dose (adjusting or adding medication for side effects accordingly), or using an alternative medication as set out below.

➤ Haloperidol is the drug of choice for restlessness *with* delirium.[11,12]
➤ Oral haloperidol is effective in the early stages, and some people manage well with this.[2]

➤ It is usually effective in targeting:
  − fear
  − agitation
  − paranoia.[2]
➤ Haloperidol does not induce severe sedation.
➤ Communication may still be maintained.
➤ Parenteral doses are approximately twice as potent as the equivalent oral dose.[2]
➤ Haloperidol can be administered over a 24-hour period via a syringe driver.
➤ Haloperidol is useful for managing agitation and improving cognition. However, if death is likely to occur soon, this may be unachievable.[2]
➤ The causes of delirium may be irreversible in the active, dying phase.[2]
➤ If the delirium cannot be reversed, sometimes it may be necessary to use:
  − **Midazolam**
  − **Levomepromazine.**

PSYCHOLOGICAL AND EMOTIONAL SUPPORT

Although prompt treatment with the appropriate drugs remains paramount, psychological, spiritual and emotional support is implicit in relieving the distress caused by restlessness and agitation at the end-of-life.

Psychological, emotional and spiritual support should start early on in the relationship – getting to know the person, their likes and dislikes, their needs, their wants and their choices. It has to be acknowledged that his or her choice may be to avoid engagement, and to remain independent, or aloof, or in denial of his or her illness. It is important that we respect this choice, while remaining as supportive as the individual will allow.

Moreover, it is important to remember that the people we care for, their family and carers all bring their own knowledge and life experience, as do other professional colleagues, who have often known the family over the course of several years. The background detail that all of these people provide helps us in decision making, in our care process, and in deciding on the appropriate support, intervention and treatment.

KEY POINT 12.7

It is important to remember the need for emotional, spiritual and psychological support throughout.

REFLECTIVE PRACTICE EXERCISE 12.2

Time: 15 minutes
● Consider the concept of loss. This could be the loss of your job, your home, a friend or family member, a pet, the breakdown of a relationship, loss of dreams for your future. Notice the feelings that arise in you.

- Think about how you would feel if you lost something or someone precious to you. Notice the feelings that arise in you.
- What would help you most at this time?
- What might not be so helpful?

Unresolved emotional and spiritual problems

Unresolved problems and unfinished business in the person's life can cause restlessness and agitation. Spiritual pain or fear can be resistant to treatment. Spiritual or emotional pain, fear and anger may remain undisclosed and may not be communicated until physical symptoms (e.g. pain, nausea, vomiting, or breathlessness) are effectively relieved.

Emotional and spiritual problems should be explored early, if time allows (i.e. if you have established the relationship early enough), and, with the person's agreement, with the family. Unfinished business may relate to distress caused by an estranged relationship, and the person may worry about leaving this untended. The person may feel that too much time has passed and it is too late to heal the pain. Family dynamics are often complex and solutions may not always be easily found. However, often this is a time for reconciliation of relationships, forgiveness and compassion.

REFLECTIVE PRACTICE EXERCISE 12.3

Time: 15 minutes
- Try to put yourself in the position of leaving a relationship untended and feeling that you had no chance to make it right.
- What do you think you would need from others at this time, in order to help you?
- This requires you to reflect on your own mortality.

As the emotional and spiritual needs of the family may differ from those of the person who is dying, the opportunity to talk through any fears and concerns, together with – or away from – the person, should be offered. Ensuring a safe environment for such disclosure is essential. It may be necessary to arrange meetings within or outwith the home environment and it should be emphasised that this is possible. However, not every family will want this. For some, the need to focus on practical responsibilities alone will be all that they feel they can cope with. We can help by being respectful and sensitive to their chosen coping strategy.

Other professionals may be able to offer a helping relationship, e.g.
➤ counsellor
➤ clinical psychologist
➤ family therapist
➤ hospital chaplain or a specific member of the person's own church.

Non-acceptance of death

Some people are unable to accept they are dying. Acceptance of life's difficulties and pains may be something they have always denied. Denial can be a means of coping right up to the end-of-life. While supporting the person, identifying and aiming to reduce distress, there must be respect for the individual's choice. The person needs to feel safe and have the opportunity to cope in his or her own way.

Although it is important for us to acknowledge this freedom of choice, if emotional distress is not gently explored, the person is often unable to control thoughts, with unresolved fears breaking through into the confused mind with devastating results.[5]

THE FAMILY – MAKING CONNECTIONS AND SMOOTHING THE WAY

Guiding the family, making connection and smoothing the way forward and '*being with*' them through this distressing time is an essential part of caring. There are no short cuts. Attention to small detail is as important as the medication. Intra- inter-disciplinary teamwork remains implicit if we are to provide enough support. Families benefit from an intra- inter-disciplinary approach exploring the multifaceted needs of each person. Families often experience a sense of helplessness and isolation, just as we may feel helpless and impotent to help. The family may feel 'pushed away' by the person who is dying, as he or she prepares emotionally for death.

KEY POINT 12.8

We learn, mostly through our work with families, that we cannot fix problems. We can, with time, skill, attention and empathy, give sensitive and humanitarian care, even at the most poignant and difficult of times.

The use of medications to relieve restlessness, agitation and delirium will cause a certain level of sedation. Restlessness and agitation are major symptoms, which, without the appropriate drugs, will lead to a poor-quality death. Sedation should always be discussed with the family. Their views are important and should be sensitively explored. The aim is to offer clear, straightforward information, checking the family's understanding throughout. The family needs to be aware that medication will make the person sleepy, with verbal communication becoming difficult. Listen to the responses from the family, what is said, and what is not said. Give time and opportunity for each family member to express individual concerns and any problems that are important to them. The person must be given the choice (when possible) of whether or not to accept a drug which will make them less aware of their symptoms and make them sleepy. Some cultures (and beliefs? *See* Chapters 3 and 8) wish to decline all, or certain drugs, and each person is treated individually and with respect.

Whatever we *do* for the person who is dying and *how* we do it will always be remembered by the family. The individual and family listen to every word we say, and *how* we say it, which is often more important than the actual words spoken.

Family time

Families need to know that time set aside for them is important and that it is acceptable to take that time. Taking care of themselves will help them to care for the person they love. Families often feel guilty about taking this time. There is the feeling for them that 'personal time' can take them away from what they feel they *should* be doing.

Using supportive complementary therapies and attending a support group may be helpful. If the person wishes to die at home – and time permits – agencies within the family's local community may provide 'home carers', who can stay with the person while the family member shops, visits the hairdresser, or attends to their own healthcare needs. It is often difficult for the family to understand and accept that they have needs of their own. They feel frightened to leave the house, or the hospital bedside, in case that person should die when they are not there. This needs careful and gentle exploration and it is worth taking time with the family, helping them to look at their feelings around this common concern.

BEING HONEST

When a person is approaching death and is feeling afraid, colluding with them that they will get better and 'everything will be all right' is not helpful. The family may sometimes feel that it is easier to collude with the person when they feel unsure about what to say or do. Therefore, time spent helping the family to give that person open and honest feedback about what is really happening makes communication less stressful. Colluding may serve to undervalue feelings, blocking *any* useful communication, thus making 'letting go' difficult.

Try to be calm and genuine when responding. If you do not know, then *say so*. People will know if we try to 'bluff it'. Be yourself. Show that you understand and that you are there. Listen carefully to fears, concerns and questions. This helps to form a trusting and honest relationship. Clever words and phrases are inappropriate and unnecessary. The unspoken, the silence, and the '*being with*' can all offer comfort to the person and their family.

Listening is the most important skill we have to offer. If we truly listen, then something happens – *listen* and we will instinctively know what it is we need to do.

Sometimes permission needs to be given by the family, so that the person can 'let go'. This needs careful handling, with appropriate timing. The family needs to be ready and to feel that the time is right for them to say this. People often wish to hold on to what they know and love. It can be a struggle for both parties to let go. It is sometimes sufficient for the family to tell the person that it is all right for them to die.[13]

REFLECTIVE PRACTICE EXERCISE 12.4

- Think how it would be for you to give someone you love permission to die. Consider the clinical attitude, and psychological and spiritual dimensions.
- How does this make you feel?
- Have you been in this position? If so, how was the situation managed?
- Have you witnessed this situation in your working life, with a family?
- What did you learn from the experience?
- What was the outcome, for the person themself, their family, the care team?

Dying may give rise to many repressed emotions such as sadness, numbness, guilt and jealousy of those who are well.[14]

The person faces many losses; everything in fact. These feelings are normal and anger is often directed to the closest family member. It is often helpful to the family members for them to understand that being open and honest often opens up communication which may not have been possible before. Repressing these difficult emotions may lead to further pain and distress. Often just asking the person '*how*' they – the family – can help may be useful. The person is sometimes able to give the family help and guidance in meeting their needs.

REFLECTIVE PRACTICE EXERCISE 12.5

Time: 30 minutes

Case study 12.1

John was 39. His mother, Dolly, was dying. He knew this and that her expected length of survival was about 3–4 weeks. John lived about 40 miles away with his own family. Dolly was able to fully communicate with her husband and son, and she herself knew she was dying. Knowing this had helped her to plan for her death and make her own funeral arrangements with the help of her husband. What Dolly and her son John had not been able to achieve was some meaningful communication about the fact that she was dying. John had things that he wanted to say to Dolly but did not know how to say them, or how to even start this kind of conversation. They talked about everything except the things that had real meaning for him.

John approached you. He said, 'I don't know what to say to Mum, or how to say it. I want to tell her that she has been a wonderful mother and that I love her, but I just can't find the right words, and I'm scared that this will upset her. If she cries, I just won't know what to do.' He felt desperately sad and alone in his grief and guilty that he, as a grown man, could not bring himself to speak about the unspeakable.

CASE STUDY 12.1 QUESTIONS

- Picture this scenario in your mind. Really think about what John is saying and the meaning behind his words.
- How might you help John?
- What helpful responses could you make?

The way forward

John is fearful that he might upset his mother, and in doing so he may increase his own pain, which he would find just as hard to deal with.

You might want to spend some time with John, somewhere where you will be undisturbed and where he can feel easy about speaking with you. You could suggest that he has everything inside himself that is needed to speak with his mother; after all, he has found the words with you, and that he might want to start by saying to Dolly, 'I don't know what to say, but . . .'

John may want you to be present. Sometimes a third party helps to dispel the tension and some facilitation may be possible. The most important thing is to work with John in finding a way for him to express his feelings to Dolly before she dies. He needs to say them, and she needs to hear them.

In fact, John did speak with Dolly – alone. He spoke the words to her; in just the same way he had spoken them to the nurse. Dolly helped him and had things she needed to say to him. For the one week that Dolly lived after her conversation with John, words were no longer necessary. After Dolly had died, John approached the nurse, saying that he had felt a great sense of relief and fulfilment at being able to '*talk*' with Dolly. It was a simple thing to do, on the surface, but families are complex and we have no way of knowing what has gone before in the world of that family.

CONCLUSION

Terminal restlessness is a frightening experience for everyone. It represents a challenge for all those involved. On-going assessment and evaluation is central to reducing the suffering caused by undesirable symptoms. Constant monitoring, using a team approach, is needed to enable rapid, effective and therapeutic responses to any change.

Preparing the family for the possible occurrence of restlessness and agitation is generally helpful. We have to remember that some families will not want to *hear* and this comes back to us fully knowing and understanding the family. Reassurance that in all cases something *can and will be done* helps to reduce some of the inevitable anxieties. We hear so many times, from the individual and family, that *'they've told us that nothing more can be done'*! The culture in palliative care is that there is so much that *can* and *will* be done to help; to bring peace and to relieve suffering.

Being prepared for possible events leading up to death may help the person and family to cope better. If the family has some awareness and understanding that such events are a natural part of dying, and are not due to negligence in the care the family has given, this may make it easier for them in minimising the extreme distress and difficulties that can occur at this time.

> **KEY POINT 12.11**
>
> Whilst dying is part of the human condition, dying poorly ought not to be.[15]

Dying is not always peaceful. Like birth, it can be painful and protracted. However, achieving a peaceful death for people within our care should always be our aim. It is a human right. In addition, it is important to remember to take care of ourselves and of each other so that we may continue to meet the needs of those for whom we care (*see* Chapter 16).

> **KEY POINT 12.12**
>
> Regular supportive clinical supervision is a helpful way to explore and share our own feelings within the context of a challenging situation.

Keep in mind:
- **be realistic** – about what we can achieve
- **the whole picture** – consider the whole picture – its physical, psychological, emotional, spiritual and social dimensions
- **professional update** – continually update knowledge with research and evidence-based practice
- **maximum skills** – maximise the use of intuitive, factual skills and empirical knowledge
- **limitations** – it is acceptable and necessary to acknowledge our own limitations
- **clinical supervision** – working in the field of serious and enduring mental health problems and palliative care exposes us to grief, loss and distress on a daily basis. There is a need to care for ourselves, making time and opportunity to discuss not only the 'clinical', but also the emotional and spiritual aspects of the work that we do.

Embracing the above enables us to provide high-quality care and support for the person experiencing serious and enduring mental health problems, and their family. Pharmacological *and* non-pharmacological treatments have an important role in the management of restlessness and agitation at the end of life.

SELF-ASSESSMENT EXERCISE 12.3 (ANSWERS ON PP. 218–19)

Time: 20 minutes

1 How would you define terminal restlessness and agitation?
2 List three possible treatable causes of restlessness and agitation.
3 What practical support can be given to the person?
4 What is the drug of choice for terminal restlessness without delirium?
5 What is the drug of choice for terminal restlessness with delirium?

Now list what support you can give to the family and/or carer during this difficult time.

REFERENCES

1 Brajtman S. The impact on the family of terminal restlessness and its management. *Palliative Medicine.* 2003; **17**: 454–60.
2 Breitbart W, Chochinov HM, Passik S. Psychiatric aspects of palliative care. In: Doyle D, Hanks GWC, MacDonald N, editors. *Oxford Textbook of Palliative Medicine.* 2nd ed. Oxford: Oxford University Press; 1998.
3 Lawlor PG, Gagnon B, Mancini IL, *et al.* Occurrence, causes and outcomes of delirium in patients with advanced cancer. *Archives of Internal Medicine.* 2000; **160**: 786–94.
4 March PA. Hospice techniques: terminal restlessness. *American Journal of Hospice Palliative Care.* 1998; Jan/Feb: 51–3.
5 Twycross R. *Symptom Management in Advanced Cancer.* 3rd ed. Oxford: Radcliffe Medical Press; 2001.
6 Centeno C, Sanz A, Bruera E. Delirium in advanced cancer patients. *Palliative Medicine.* 2004; **18**: 184–94.
7 Brown S, Degner LF. Delirium in the terminally ill cancer patient: aetiology, symptoms and management. *International Journal of Palliative Nursing.* 2001; 7: 266–72.
8 Twycross R, Wilcock A, Charlesworth S, *et al. PCF2 Palliative Care Formulary.* 2nd ed. Oxford: Radcliffe Medical Press; 2002.
9 De Sousa E, Jepson BA. Midazolam in terminal care. *The Lancet.* 1988; **i**: 67–8.
10 Oliver DJ. The use of methotrimeprazine in terminal care. *British Journal of Clinical Practice.* 1995; **39**: 339–40.
11 Mazzocato C, Stiefel P, Buclin T, *et al.* Psychopharmacology in supportive care of cancer: a review for the clinician. *Neuroleptics Support Care Cancer.* 2000; **8**: 89–97.
12 Breitbart W, Strout D. Delirium in the terminally ill. *Clinics in Geriatric Medicine.* 2000; **16**: 357–72.
13 Callahan C, Kelly P. *Final Gifts.* New York: Poseidon; 1992.
14 Rinpoche S. *The Tibetan Book of Living and Dying.* London: Ryder; 1998.
15 Chochinov HM. Palliative care: an opportunity for mental health professionals. *The Canadian Journal of Psychiatry.* 2004; **49**: 347–9.

TO LEARN MORE

- Callanan M, Kelley P. *Final Gifts: understanding the special awareness, needs, and communications of the dying*. London: Simon & Schuster; 2012.
- Cooper J. Coping with death and bereavement. In: Basford L, Slevin O, editors. *Theory and Practice of Nursing: an integrated approach to caring practice*. Cheltenham: Nelson Thornes; 2003, Chapter 35.
- Hanks GW, Cherny NI, Christakis NA, *et al. Oxford Textbook of Palliative Medicine*. 4th ed. Oxford: Oxford University Press; 2011.
- McMahon R, Pearson A. *Nursing As Therapy*. 2nd ed. London: Chapman and Hall; 1998.
- Rinpoche S. *The Tibetan Book of Living and Dying: a spiritual classic from one of the foremost interpreters of Tibetan Buddhism to the West*. London: Rider; 2008.
- Twycross R. *Symptom Management in Advanced Cancer*. 3rd ed. Oxford: Radcliffe Medical Press; 2001.
- Twycross R, Wilcock A, Charlesworth S, *et al. PCF2 Palliative Care Formulary*. 2nd ed. Oxford; Radcliffe Medical Press; 2002.

ACKNOWLEDGEMENT

The author is grateful to the publisher for permitting adaptation of this chapter from:

Cooper J. Terminal restlessness. In: Cooper J, editor. *Stepping into Palliative Care 2: care and practice*. 2nd ed. Oxford: Radcliffe; 2006.

ANSWERS TO SELF-ASSESSMENT EXERCISE 12.3 (P. 217)

1 The agitation and restlessness that may occur in the last few hours or days of life.

2
- physical discomfort
- bladder or bowel distension
- breathlessness
- nicotine withdrawal
- alcohol withdrawal
- illicit drug withdrawal
- infection
- other drugs

3
- provision of a safe environment
- a mattress on the floor
- a peaceful, quiet environment
- use of soft lighting, with low lights at night
- continuity of carers and a familiar friend or family member to stay
- gentle massage with relaxing oils
- appropriate use of touch
- providing information and an explanation to the family

4 Midazolam.

5 Haloperidol.

Now that you have read this chapter, you may be able to think of other approaches you could use. The important thing to remember is to be you. Be genuine in your responses.

CHAPTER 13

End-of-life

Shiphrah Williams-Evans, Barbara Broome

ESSENTIAL NOTE:

> It is important that this chapter should be read in conjunction with Chapter 12, 'Managing restlessness and agitation at the end-of-life' and, indeed, in conjunction with all chapters in this book to fully comprehend the importance of care at the end-of-life.

INTRODUCTION

There is scant literature that includes discussion of end-of-life care and serious and enduring mental health and the effect on individuals and families. End-of-life care creates challenges for the individual experiencing serious and enduring mental health and their family coping with impending loss. Comprehensive care must include certain elements to address the needs of these people. The type of death is always an issue, whether it is sudden, due to a terminal illness, contains prolonged suffering over a period of years, or is related to the health decline of ageing. The individual experiencing serious and enduring mental health must be supported throughout the end-of-life. Professionals should be educated to intervene in complex situations and about the numerous challenges presented by individuals and families experiencing the need for palliative care within serious and enduring mental health.

KEY POINT 13.1

Palliative care is a concept that has utmost importance throughout the life span.

Palliative care is defined as care that is given when there is a life-altering, life-threatening, or potentially terminal diagnosis that may result in death. End-of-life experiences affect people of all ages. When we think of dying ourselves, we think of dying 'when we get old'. However, individuals in all age groups experience death and the factors that influence the dying process.

KEY POINT 13.2

For individuals who have been diagnosed with mental ill-health, dying can be even more challenging and complex.

This chapter will present case studies across the life span of individuals with a variety of diagnoses. It will outline the issues that relate to stigmatisation, family support and communications that require carefully planned strategies to navigate the path each individual proceeds on towards death.

Case study 13.1

Before birth – Sam and Louise

Sam and Louise had been sweethearts for two years prior to their marriage. However, at the age of 19, Sam decided to marry Louise, his 23-year-old girlfriend. Her family stated he was the best thing for her. Sam's parents thought he was too young, but supported his decision in the end. He was mature, had been in college for 2 years, and was a junior. He met Louise when he first came to college at age 17, and they had already been living together for a year. She had long suffered with depression and had been on medications for years. She had even had one suicide attempt that resulted in hospitalisation when she was 13 years of age. She had been on an antidepressant since that time. Louise became pregnant during their first year of marriage. She had just graduated from college and was working on her first professional job. Sam was now a senior. The pregnancy was uneventful, no signs of depression, no morning sickness, and no episodes that would question the viability of this pregnancy. As the time got closer for Louise to deliver, she was becoming more excited about being a mother. She was given a baby-shower (gifts for the new-born child) where she worked, the nursery was prepared, she had two weeks until her due date. However, one morning the professional called Sam at his job and gave him some bad news. He told him the ultrasound confirmed that the baby would not survive. The baby had anencephaly. The professional suggested that because of Louise's mental health diagnosis, the best option was for Sam to get Louise from work and bring her to the office . . . at this time, the professional would break the news to her. When they arrived at the office, the professional had a copy of the ultrasound on a screen. The professional pointed to the screen and began to sob, trying to tell Louise that her baby would not survive. Emotionally, the professional was unable break the news to her. Therefore, Sam had to take over and inform his wife; he had to do what the professional was unable to do. Sam told Louise that the child had been diagnosed with anencephaly and would not survive long. Louise became angry with Sam because they had come to the office together and he had not told her about the baby. Then she became angry because this was a situation she could not control – the loss of her child. A Caesarean section had to be scheduled, as vaginal delivery was impossible due to the undeveloped cranium. The baby was a boy . . . 6 pounds 7 ounces, 19 inches long, but no one seemed to care. The baby was placed in an area by himself . . . he was crying, and appeared like a normal new-born from the neck down. This was all so sudden . . . Sam decided he would stay with the baby until he died. Sam was not allowed to sit in the nursery, but sat by the door, outside the room, and listened to the baby for 13 hours. He did not allow Louise to witness the death of the baby or his grief, because of her physical condition following her recent Caesarean section. He sat; too petrified to move, even to go to the bathroom. He did not know how long the baby's death would take. The professionals would not look at him. They did not know what to say. He wondered if it was something he and Louise had done that caused the baby to be this way. Both sets of parents remarked, 'No child like this has ever been born in our family.' What was he supposed to do when the child died? Would a funeral have to be planned? When the baby died, no one even offered Sam a drink of water as he sobbed for the loss of his child. Sam decided to bury the child immediately without a funeral. He needed to get home and 'tear down' the nursery and get rid of the baby's things so Louise would not come home and see it. His in-laws scolded him for not having a Christian burial. Sam took care of everything, but no one took care of him. Neither parent touched or held the baby. Only Sam saw the baby.

SELF-ASSESSMENT EXERCISE 13.1

Time: 10 minutes
- What are the issues involved?
- What could have been done to avoid emotional trauma for Sam and Louise?
- Reflect on this statement from the above case study:
  - 'The professionals would not look at him; they did not know what to say.'
  - Make a note of the feelings that might have arisen in:
    » the professionals
    » Sam
    » Louise
    » you.

BREAKING BAD NEWS

In the above case study, Sam and Louise should have received the news together. The method of communication integrated the professional's uncontrolled personal feelings into the poor attempt to deliver the information. While it is admirable that the professional cares deeply for this couple, it is important that composure is retained when delivering bad news. This method of breaking bad news caused dissonance in the couple's relationship.[1] This method of delivery was based on the mother's history of poor mental health. How did the professional think the diagnosis of depression would influence the mother's actions? She had been asymptomatic during this pregnancy. The professional had a preconceived notion that, because she had a diagnosis of depression, she may react in a certain way. The professional's methodology was flawed by personal stigmatisation of serious and enduring mental health that compromised the quality of care this couple received.

There was no explanation of how death would occur or how long it would take. No encouragement was offered to bond with the child. The child was allowed to cry until he died. No professional in the nursery touched the child or rendered any care.

> **KEY POINT 13.3**
>
> The child's crying is an overt sign of terminal restlessness that went uncared for – and untreated.

SELF-ASSESSMENT EXERCISE 13.2

> **Time: 5 minutes**
> What do you understand by the term *terminal restlessness?*

There are occasions when parents know that their child will be born dead, or will die shortly after birth. Palliative care needs to be initiated with these parents to provide support. A protocol for breaking bad news needs to be followed (*see* Table 13.1). Before the birth of a child whose life will be altered by a debilitating illness after birth, and after the death of this new-born, parents need to be monitored for signs and symptoms of depression and difficulty grieving (*see* Table 13.1). They need to be supported through the process of hearing the news; throughout the dying process. Elements of this journey must be individualised for the specific person and their family.[2] Young couples should be referred for marriage counselling in that communicating with each other may be difficult. Urges to treat the event as though it never happened – hiding baby clothes, suddenly taking down the nursery, and quick burial are just a few of the things that can take place. The couple should be supported to work through these issues together. Together with the assistance of appropriately qualified professionals, a plan needs to be devised to set the stage for taking this journey with dignity. The individual experiencing mental health problems should immediately be seen by a mental health professional. In this case, if genetic counselling was in order, a referral should be made. The professional was ill prepared to deal with this situation and found the challenge overwhelming. The professionals also lacked preparation to support this young couple through the dying process of their son.

> **KEY POINT 13.4**
>
> It is imperative that an experienced mental health team exist, or be assembled quickly, to meet the challenges of these individual events and this special population.

TABLE 13.1 Breaking bad news – a protocol

Knowledge about issues	Communicating of news	Meeting needs	Strategic planning
• Know the facts related to the case and all aspects that may influence this interaction • Know related mental health diagnosis and the person or family's history of symptoms • Undertake a thorough assessment of the knowledge of person and family • Assess how much the person and family know • Assess what the person and family want to know • Assess if pathology is understood • Assess if the prognosis is understood • Assess if process of dying is understood	• Therapeutic communication is a mandatory skill • Do not allow interruptions once interaction has commenced • Assess what language is spoken • Assess if an interpreter is needed (see Chapter 3) • Assess if the person or family have a disability that will prevent them from understanding the spoken word, e.g. hearing and learning difficulties, etc. • Assess if resources are available to assure communication is clear – if not, organise these before progressing • Assess what location is best to have this type of communication • Assess who needs to be present at what time; this must be at the choice of the person and family	• Select a private environment that is conducive to the type of interaction that will take place • Ensure the environment is comfortable, light and spacious enough to accommodate the population that will be present • Provide enough professionals to be with younger family members and/or the family member with mental health problems • Have tissues ready • Employ active listening and observation at all times • Assess how the person and family need to proceed on this journey and who is needed with them – accommodate this	• Be sure the person is ready to begin this journey • Plan how you will proceed based on assessment of the person and family, and the type of news to be conveyed • Arrange for a case manager/ key worker – who will not change throughout the individual's journey – to be the focal professional for trouble shooting • Arrange appropriate time so that all family members/friends who the person wants present can be present • Review legal issues with fellow professionals, the person and the family (see Chapter 4)

END-OF-LIFE **225**

Knowledge about issues	Communicating of news	Meeting needs	Strategic planning
• Evaluate the person and family's care. Are these needs understood?	• Be sure that professionals who need to be present for support are there, e.g. case manager, social services, pastoral support, Palliative Care nurse/nurse practitioner, physician, grief counsellor, etc. • Do not become personally offended by anger – it is not about you • Understand that expression of anger may be prolonged and presented in the form of complaints about certain professionals – or may be genuinely about poor quality of care • Learn to distinguish between poor-quality care and internal anger – act on both • Be willing to modify the care for the person by removing professionals who may impede this communication process • Be aware of mental illness and watch for signs and symptoms of exacerbation • Never give false hope • Always provide facts • Keep emotions stable – the person and family need you to be stable, not emotionally compromised • Always remain empathetic and compassionate	• Allow cultural and religious expressions of shock and disbelief (*see* Chapter 3) • Allow and support anger • Respond to feelings with empathy • Respond to the person and family by telling them they can take time to process feelings before making any decisions • Encourage the person experiencing mental health problems to seek one-to-one therapy for support throughout this process • Review economic needs and provide sources that can assist to make meeting these needs and the process smoother	• Assist with needed paper work and the processing of documents using compassion, and assist the individual to develop mechanisms to cope (*see* Chapter 7) • Assist with development of realistic, attainable goals • Assemble a team of professionals who are consistent during this journey • Cost is a factor that needs to be discussed – include what is realistic for the economic resources the person and family have or may qualify for • Ensure the person and family are not alone during any part of this journey • Follow up as often as is needed by the person and family • Have a plan for end-of-life care – who will be there, who will assist and support • Have a plan for professional support, e.g. clinical supervision – and use it

Case study 13.2

Young adult

'My sister was 3 years older than me and we shared a very close sisterly bond. As a child, I always knew something was special about her, as she seemed to be very different from me in character. For example, during our teenage years, our surrogate parents were very strict on us because we were girls. My sister experienced a delusional disorder that none of us understood. She would be okay most of the time, but she would get tired of taking her medication. Then the wild behaviour would start. As a teenager, she was diagnosed with manic-depressive disorder. When my sister was on medication, she would stay at home listening to her music and reading books. When she did not take her medication, she would sneak out of the house and go to parties. She soon accepted that she needed to take the medication. Moving forward five years, my sister married her high-school beau at the age of 19. She was stable and happily married with three children, all girls. We talked on the phone practically every day. If we missed a day, one of us would race to call the other and see what had happened. One day, while in the shower, my sister noticed a lump in her right breast. This was followed up by her medical practitioner (aka general practitioner) over a period of about a year; then after a biopsy came the devastating news that she indeed had breast cancer at the age of 29. Although devastating, we knew that our mother had also died of breast cancer at the age of 28. My sister successfully underwent a radical mastectomy and completed chemotherapy and radiation. She took her medication, because she wanted to stay stable for her children. Her chemotherapy regime was modified to accommodate her medication for manic depression. The professionals never involved the family in her care. Both diseases were treated in isolation of each other. Only the medications were considered in merging treatment. Even though she knew the disease of cancer could claim her young life, her personality and habits remained the same. No matter what she went through during the surgery, chemotherapy, and radiation, she never seemed angry or bitter towards this ugly disease or us. The only thing she seemed concerned about was losing her hair; we shopped for a wig that looked so much like her usual style, it was barely noticeable that it was indeed a wig. She embraced her illness as her destiny and was only concerned about her young daughters, should anything happen to her. The treatment was deemed successful and she returned to her usual job as a warehouse clerk within about a year. All seemed well, and we continued our rituals of daily phone contact, shopping at yard sales, getting the children together to play, etc. Another year passed and all of a sudden, my sister began to complain of shortness of breath. I remember around this time, we had been shopping and she brought a navy-and-white dress, which she hung on the outside of the closet door. Noticing that it had been there for a couple of weeks, I asked her when she would wear it. She said, "I don't know . . . I think I'll save it." I also noted that she stopped wearing her wig, saying she preferred her short hairstyle. She had some symptoms of mania and her medications were adjusted. She was so afraid of what the stigma of her illness would do to her children if anyone found out, especially people in the church. She was assessed by her oncologist and told that she had a pericardial effusion (fluid around the heart); aetiology unknown. The physician scheduled her for a pericardial window, we were told that it was a 15-minute procedure and she should be fine. My sister died on the operating table at the age of 32 . . . her heart too weak to withstand the surgery and anaesthesia. Later, I would find out from my brother-in-law that my sister would not allow him to attend the last two follow-up appointments. Had her cancer returned? Did she not want us to know? We remain unsure to this day. Yes, we thought of getting her medical records – but whatever the case was, this is what she wanted and we chose to keep it that way. Losing my sister was the most devastating event of my life. I felt as if someone had cut a part of my heart out . . . I cried almost daily. Approximately two years after her death, while away on a school trip, I experienced a dream so vivid that I wonder to this day – was it a dream or some type of reality? Around this time, my brother-in-law had started to date and was considering re-marrying. I understood this, as he was a minister and had three young daughters to raise. In this dream, my sister visited me to let me know that she was okay. She possessed her same sweet, kind spirit even beyond death, but with a newfound happiness. She said to me, "I'm okay now", with the most peaceful smile I had ever witnessed. I asked her, "But what about Moofy (my brother-in-law's nickname) and the girls?" She replied, "It's alright. My heavenly father has already explained that to me." I will never forget waking up with tears all over my pillow, but with a final feeling of peace. That dream gave me more peace than any therapy, reassurance, or medication I could have ever received. Although it has now been over 23 years since my sister died, I still think and dream about this wonderful angel of a person. She is always happy, walking and talking with me or singing gospel music. I still miss her and yes, I still cry from time to time. Someone who lost a sister asked me . . . "At what point do you get over this?" My reply . . . "Never". (*See* Chapter 7.)

STIGMATISATION (*SEE* CHAPTER 5)

Stigma against serious and enduring mental health can be synonymous with discrimination.[3,4] Individuals experiencing mental health problems have been discriminated against for many reasons – none of which are acceptable. There is no all-inclusive list of reasons; however, some may be:

➤ behavioural issues secondary to pathology
➤ stereotyped forecast of impending behaviours that may be inaccurate
➤ lack of education on a variety of mental health diagnoses
➤ poorly trained and ill-prepared professionals.

Sometimes professionals will work in an area for a period of years, but they have no specific expertise in that area . . . 'it is just a job'. Society – and even some professionals – places labels on various behaviours and identifies the individuals as 'crazy' – 'nutters' – 'loonies' – 'lunatics' – 'off their rockers' – 'a slice short of a full loaf' – a 'fruit cake' . . . and other such derogatory slang stigmatising terms. When a person who does not have a mental health problem exhibits these behaviours, he or she is labelled 'mentally ill'; thereby creating a false perception of mental health problems. Indeed one 'professional' has an email address including 'nuttynutnurse' in it! It becomes a challenge for the person experiencing serious and enduring mental health problems to move past these preconceived notions. It allows society to socially isolate and place less value on the person experiencing mental health problems – and to feel this is acceptable.[5] This discredits the person experiencing the mental health problems as a person who is 'silly' – 'not right in the head' – and 'not all there'. This lack of knowledge regarding mental health can lead to an inability to achieve personal and professional goals.[4] The person will be overwhelmed by stigmas, and may omit establishing goals or trying to accomplish those goals. The professional who is ignorant of the fact that a stigma exists may accept stigma as fact and develop unrealistic goals that include stigma-induced data, thereby setting goals that cannot be accomplished.

TABLE 13.2 Types of stigma

Structural stigmatisation	Professional stigma	Familial stigma	Revenue stigma
• Limited access to treatments • No medication prescribed or available • Lack of follow-up care • Lack of housing • Diagnosed person's and family's acceptance of negatives • Feeling of shame, low self-esteem, withdrawing socially • Disability	• Ignorance • Poor level of education • Human rights violations and fear • Inability of a variety of disciplines to advocate • Dehumanisation	• Embarrassment • Ignorance • Misinformation about intimate relationships • Misunderstanding of the treatment regime • Labelling	• Employment termination – the person's employment may be terminated as a result of symptoms related to their ill-health and not to their lack of ability to perform employment tasks • Misinformation of various diagnoses • Labelling • Treating all individuals with a mental health problem the same • Limited education

The term *stigma* refers to 'a social devaluation of a person'.[6] When one is socially devolved it negatively impacts all aspects of one's life (*see* Table 13.2). Therefore, the individual and family experiencing serious and enduring mental health become accustomed to facing these obstacles in life. This leads to 'structural discrimination', for example:

➤ poor, inadequate care and/or lack of access to care

➤ lack of belief and ignorance when the person becomes physically ill

➤ questioning if the physical illness really exists

➤ minimising an illness that demands attention

➤ considering the individual to be exaggerating because they are experiencing mental health problems

➤ latent diagnosis with diseases being discovered in the late stages
➤ limited treatment alternatives and compromised recovery.

Case study 13.3

Middle age – Mary

Mary is a 49-year-old educator who had been employed in the local school system for 32 years. Her desire to teach began when she was a young high-school
student. She worked as a summer intern in the school system every year until she
graduated from college. She quickly continued with her education and obtained
a Masters degree in education. She was 21 years old at that time, and taught
until she became ill. Mary was the eldest of nine children born to young parents
(father 22 and mother 17 at the time of her birth). Neither parent had a high school
education. They raised their children using the same discipline techniques as those
used by their parents – whippings: with belts, switches, extension cords, fists and
boards. Though Mary was a long way past these beatings, she remembered some
as if they had happened yesterday. She would cry as she discussed them with her
siblings but she never discussed them outside the family. Her siblings would insist
that she 'talk to somebody' about her memories, but she declined. She did not want
to be seen as a person 'with mental illness'. She knew this could jeopardise her
job. She immersed herself in her career, attempting to drown the memories. She
worked towards and earned the highest awards in her profession. Her career – and
shopping – were her passions. She would always shop for others, not for herself.
Since she had no children of her own, she shopped for her nieces and nephews.
The parents of the nieces and nephews never had to worry about school shopping,
special occasions and Christmas, since this was Mary's favourite. She loved to
shop, thus she shopped when she had money and when she did not have money.
She had filed for bankruptcy twice in her lifetime. During her times in bankruptcy
when she could not shop (with credit cards), she began to gamble. It was a great
substitute for shopping. She could still give her winnings to others. Gambling was
against everything she had ever been taught. She could never let her co-workers
know . . . but she ended up borrowing money from friends close to her. Initially, she
never borrowed from her family, but that would change as her dependency grew.
Approximately one year prior to her diagnosis of colon cancer, she told her sister
that she was so tired that she would lie down on the bed when she got home from
work; not getting up until the next morning. She was diabetic and admitted to not
taking her medication or eating during this time. She was encouraged to go to her
primary care professional. She did see her primary care professional and requested
that she be put in hospital for tests to see what was wrong. The professional refused
to comply with that request, focusing on her diabetes and eventually suspending
her from his practice for issues with personality change that included being argu-
mentative with professionals. One year later, she found herself in an intensive care
unit (ICU) in ketoacidosis (occurs when the body cannot use sugar – glucose – as a
fuel source because there is no insulin or not enough insulin), with a blood sugar of

greater than 1200 mg/dL (normal: between 4 and 7 mg/dL before food). Six months later, she was diagnosed with stage-4 colon cancer with metastasis to the liver. She began to gamble more and have more childhood memories and frequent thoughts and fears regarding dying. To avoid working through these issues she would go to the casino. This was the place that Mary described as evoking 'no thoughts or fears of dying and no childhood memories'.[7] Mary was known to be a person of integrity in her family and in her profession. However, her addiction to gambling consumed her life. She lied to family and friends as to why she needed the money, and she did not pay essential bills to maintain her well-being, such as utilities, mortgage and car payments. This behaviour was not characteristic for her. The oncology practice that she chose for chemotherapy provided isolated care. There was no case management, no interdisciplinary care, and no concerns for her mental health. She once became brave enough, at the insistence of her family, to share with her physician that she was gambling. Her oncologist told her 'everybody has to have some fun'. A rare cry for help was missed. Gambling was seen as supported by her doctor and it was the medication she needed. Some of the family staged an intervention with her minister, which only embarrassed her and exposed her problem. The minister was ill prepared to deal with this issue even though he agreed to this intervention. Two very close friends and her sister attended. The minister referred her to his wife who was a psychiatrist who told her it was probably when her blood sugar was elevated that she gambled. The psychiatrist failed to open a case file and only saw Mary because her husband, the minister, requested she do so. No one dealt with the post-traumatic stress disorder (PTSD) or the 'serious substance-use problems' as terminal restlessness. Mary suffered needlessly. Diagnosis was never made due to the professionals' inability to correctly diagnose, and Mary's concerns about the stigma attached to mental health problems.[6-8] *Her terminal restlessness was unrecognised and mismanaged.*

END-OF-LIFE – A PERSON-CENTRED APPROACH

Case study 13.4

Bennie

Bennie was a very active child and at the age of 6 he was diagnosed with attention deficit hyperactivity disorder (ADHD). At the age of 8 he was diagnosed with a neuroblastoma, which is a common childhood tumour. Because of his ADHD with symptoms of hyperactivity, restlessness and impulsivity, his symptoms related to his tumour – such as overt psychosis – were accepted as a part of his illness. However, upon thorough investigation it was found that the psychosis was a symptom related to his cancer. It is important at all ages and especially in children to rule out physical illnesses, in the presence of emotional symptoms. At the age of 10, Bennie began to lose his battle with cancer. Even though he had experienced psychosis during much of his illness, the psychosis now caused him to have symptoms of violence. It was known his symptoms of violence were not associated with his mental health problems. As Bennie approached the final hours of his life, it was critical that he was comfortable and that his family were supported. The family needed education and training regarding the possible exacerbation of symptoms, including violence, and how they were to be managed. In addition, they also needed assurance that Bennie's symptoms – both physical and emotional – would be treated. They needed reassurance that any violence would *not* be treated as a symptom of his poor mental health but as a symptom of terminal restlessness.

KEY POINT 13.5

The process of dying presents many challenges to the individual . . . who experiences the event . . . the family and the professional.

It is important to elicit the assistance of palliative care and hospice professionals as early as possible in end-of-life care. When a person is experiencing serious and enduring mental health problems, the process may be coupled with behavioural symptoms that may complicate care. A few of the symptoms that may be displayed include:

➤ exaggerated anger
➤ uncontrolled violence
➤ manipulation of body waste.

It is important to note that a progressive lack of oxygen to the frontal lobe may be the primary cause of these symptoms. Persons without mental health problems may also experience these symptoms. However, people experiencing mental health problems who have a history of violence, and a lack of control of behavioural symptoms, appear to experience these symptoms sooner than persons without mental health problems or a history of these symptoms.[9,10] During this time, it is important that professionals do not allow stigma to influence the care and treatment of the individual. The family and significant others must be helped and guided to understand the symptoms that arise in different conditions experienced by the person. In addition, the family should be helped and guided to understand that regardless of the status of a person, neurological dysfunction may occur at the end-of-life.

KEY POINT 13.6

The primary goal is to treat the symptoms as the priority, rather than the mental health problem per se.

Health professionals and the family must use anticipatory guidance to prepare for the variety of behaviours the person may exhibit. Anticipatory guidance means to be knowledgeable regarding what to expect and to share this knowledge with those involved in the care of the person; thereby alleviating fear and anxiety that might be related to such situations.[10] If a person becomes violent, the person, family, professionals and others must be kept safe. Each individual should be treated with dignity and respect and in a safe environment. It is important that professionals and the family speak directly to the person, ensuring that a full explanation is offered as to what is taking place, even if there is little verbal acknowledgement of understanding and/or apparent comprehension. Family members may want to be present to assist with the process of calming the distressed individual. The presence of love and support from family members is comforting. In some cases, spiritual assistance may be needed. A minister, rabbi, an Islamic or Muslim preacher, Greek orthodox preacher, or other spiritual leader, for example, may be helpful in relieving spiritual distress (*see* Chapter 8). Everyone who comes into contact with the individual has a role. It is imperative that information be disseminated to all members of the professional team, the family and others associated with care *prior* to their involvement in this very personal journey for each individual. Each person will have a separate set of circumstances that demands individualised approaches to care and management.

Terminal restlessness
Terminal restlessness refers to the last days or hours of life. It involves the dying person's comfort, and support of the bereaved. At this stage, the aim includes the minimisation (management) and alleviation of the physical and mental distress experienced by the individual. Some empirical data shows that terminal restlessness can be a prolonged process involving untreated signs and symptoms of critical mental distress for the person and their family.[9,10] Mary's case study demonstrates failure to manage her distress. The failure of professionals to recognise these symptoms leads to an incomplete, complicated, prolonged grieving process for the person and those closest to them. It is critical to treat these symptoms early. However, many professionals lack the listening skills allowing them to *first listen* and then *interpret* these symptoms as delusional, psychotic, or as depression. The person and their family are left alone to struggle through without the comfort of trying to allow their mental health to maintain the baseline it has most of their lives (*see* Chapter 12).

It is possible that during the final days/hours the individual may revisit past events and that these could be unpleasant in nature, leading to agitation and restlessness. The individual might make a move to get out of bed or leave the room but when asked about this behaviour is unable to explain why or in some circumstances becomes aggressive and unmanageable. However, these are examples only, and with careful management of symptoms, using appropriate medication, this situation need not arise. Such events can be extremely upsetting for the family, who may demand that some action be taken. However, intervention in the form of correct medication may lead to the person feeling sleepy, while easing his or her 'troubled mind' and it is not uncommon for the distressed family to feel that the end of the person's life is being hastened by the medication. Thus, careful explanation around the use of medication, and its effect on the individual, is needed prior to administration of any new medication or increase of existing medication.

If the person is experiencing extreme behaviours then it may be necessary to ask the family to wait outside (both to avoid distress to them and to offer a quiet, calm environment to the individual) until the situation is managed. Such extreme behaviour can be termed 'emotional bleeding' and requires prompt response from the professional. The person is likely to be unaware of his or her actions even though she or he may appear to be awake, have their eyes open, and be speaking during this activity. Emotional bleeding is profound impairment in the frontal lobe leading to severe cognitive dysfunction that may be caused by lack of oxygen to that part of the brain as the body begins the journey towards death. Addressing symptoms early is a priority. Again, safety of the person and direct communication are imperative. This is especially important when attempting to provide medication. Though it is the professional's choice of medication, the individual should be made comfortable (at peace and with a restful mind) as soon as is possible, and careful titration of medication to manage the symptoms should be the priority. Such 'emotional bleeding' is a part of the terminal restlessness that is experienced by some at the end-of-life. For further exploration of terminal restlessness and its management, *see* Chapter 12.

Managing breathlessness

Breathlessness is a complication that needs careful management. It does not always or necessarily accompany terminal restlessness.

Breathlessness is a common symptom at the end-of-life and is very distressing for the individual and family. The primary goal of the professional is to relieve the breathlessness and provide comfort. Again, the symptoms are the priority and not the underlying mental health problem. Providing oxygen can ease breathlessness, as can opening a window, and/or using a fan to cool the circulating air, which may aid reduction of the feelings of breathlessness.

A calm presence by professionals and family is important to reduce the fear and anxiety that accompany breathlessness. Panic attacks can be common as the individual feels that he or she is suffocating and will die. Appropriate medications, such as opioids, nebulised saline and oxygen, will reduce the feelings of breathlessness.

Decreased thirst

During the last few days of life, the individual may not wish – or be able – to take fluids. This is perfectly natural and it is important not to attempt to over-hydrate the person. Good oral hygiene and moistening the lips with a moisturising agent such as Vaseline or Aquaphor can be helpful. The family needs to be aware that these comfort measures are helpful and careful explanation as to why hydration is not being attempted should be given in an empathic and caring way. If the family is aware of a preferred method adopted by the individual to moisten the lips then efforts should be made to accommodate this knowledge.

Decreased appetite

At the end of life, the person's appetite decreases. It is important that family members understand *not* to force-feed the person . . . or say anything that will make the individual feel bad about not eating. Family members need to understand that decreased appetite can occur days or weeks prior to the end-of-life. The person is not eating because they are dying. They are not dying because they are not eating. Food and eating in families have many different meanings. Help the family to understand the meaning of anorexia at the end-of-life. Family members will need to be supported during this time. Inability on the part of the family to understand this process can cause dissonance within families long after the family member's death. For example, there have been instances where members in the family will accuse others of not feeding the person or not making them eat; therefore the lack of food may have caused the person's death. Discussion of this is something that must not be omitted when helping inform the family regarding symptoms that present at the end-of-life.

Therapeutic presence

The person needs to be supported with therapeutic presence:
➤ talk normally to the person
➤ do not assume the person cannot hear you
➤ tell the person how much they are loved
➤ tell the person other information that family members feel they need to express
➤ help family members to speak with the person about things that have meaning for them
➤ ensure that no one is present whom the person does not want to have present, even if they are family – this could increase the agitation and distress of the individual.

Pain management

It is essential that pain be managed well at the end-of-life. Pain is traumatic for the individual to experience and for the family to witness (*see* Chapter 11).

The end-of-life

During the last few days or hours of life the dying process continues.
➤ **Decreased perfusion** of oxygen in the cells causes a decrease in responsiveness and skin colour.
➤ **Eyes** – the eyes begin to glass over and there is decreased eye movement. Prevent irritation and dryness by using artificial tears.

➤ **Communication** – the person gradually loses the ability to communicate with those in the immediate environment. Those in the person's environment must use caution regarding what is said during this time. Communication should consist of respectful commentary and spiritual vocalisations that the person would appreciate if he or she had the ability to communicate.

➤ **Cultural consideration** (*see* Chapter 3) – this process should include any cultural consideration upheld by the person taking this journey and their family.

➤ **Closure** – it is important to convey that the process of life closure is unpredictable and that it may take only a few minutes or that it may continue for days and weeks. Regardless of the time it takes, one should maintain therapeutic presence, and remain respectful of all elements of care needed until life closure is complete. The more prepared the family is for this journey, the more at ease family members are with the closure of the life of their loved one. The inclusion of palliative and hospice care during the process is valuable.

➤ **Last few hours** – as the process of dying deepens and progresses towards death, concerns include:
  — **physical care** – attention to detail
  — **comfort** – takes time and skill
  — **emotional support** – holding a hand; touch shows we are present
  — **spiritual support** – lessens existential distress (*see* Chapter 8)
  — **family support** – support to the family enables them to support their loved one.

➤ **Place of death** – it is important that the individual (if possible) and the family decide where the individual wants to die (e.g. at home, in a hospice or hospital), and all efforts should be made to facilitate the fulfilment of this wish. However, sadly, this is not always possible and the family needs to be supported at this time – for example, if the individual is too ill to be moved. In addition, as death approaches, the person's original choice may change; e.g. they may no longer feel that dying at home is their priority.

CONCLUSION

The dying process is one that will be remembered by family members for the remainder of their lives (*see* Chapter 14). It is critical that professionals and the family work alongside each other to synchronise the events that take place during this time to provide the best experience for all involved. With the dying person as the central focus, the end-of-life should highlight minimal suffering, avoidance of unnecessary suffering, quality symptom management techniques, family and individual support as well as care of the body.

This is the final act of caring which family members and caregivers can provide for the person. It may include care of the body, preparation of memorial events and/or sitting with the body prior to burial (*see* Chapters 3 and 11). Such wishes should be accommodated and supported by the professional.

The closer this journey comes to an end, the more the care is related to family concerns and coping. This is an opportunity for the professionals to pave the way for a healthy transition for the person and their family.

REFERENCES

1 Ferrell BR. The impact of pain on quality of life: a decade of research. *Nursing Clinics of North America*. 1995; **30**: 609–24.
2 Ro E, Clark LA. Psychological functioning in the context of diagnosis: assessment and theoretical issues. *Psychological Assessment*. 2009; **21**: 313–24.
3 Sartoris N, Schulze H. *Reducing the Stigma of Mental Illness*. Cambridge: Cambridge University Press; 2005.
4 Sartoris N. Stigma and mental health. *Lancet*. 2007; **370**: 810–11.
5 Thornicroft G. *Shunned: discrimination against people with mental illness*. Oxford: Oxford University Press; 2006.
6 Saxena S, Thornicroft G, Knapp M, *et al.* Resources for mental health: scarcity, inequity, and inefficiency. *Lancet*. 2007; **307**: 878–89.
7 Fong TW. Pathological gambling: update on assessment and treatment. *Psychiatric Times*. 2009; **26**: 20–5.
8 Personal communication. Patient's family member quotes. 3 January 2009.
9 McCasland L. Providing hospice and palliative care to the seriously and persistently mentally ill. *Journal of Hospice & Palliative Nursing*. 2007; **9**: 305–13.
10 Williams-Evans S. *Personal Clinical Experience*. 2009.

TO LEARN MORE

- Back AL, Arnold RM, Quill TE. Hope for the best, prepare for the worst. *Annals of Internal Medicine*. 2003; **138**: 439–43.
- Cooper J, editor. *Stepping into Palliative Care 1: relationships and responses*. 2nd ed. Oxford: Radcliffe Medical Press; 2006.
- Cooper J, editor. *Stepping into Palliative Care 2: care and practice*. 2nd ed. Oxford: Radcliffe Medical Press; 2006.
- Cooper J. Coping with death and bereavement. In: Basford L, Slevin O, editors. *Theory and Practice of Nursing: an integrated approach to caring practice*. Cheltenham: Nelson Thornes; 1995. pp. 664–81.
- Goffman E. *Stigma: notes on the management of spoiled identity*. Englewood Cliffs: Prentice Hall; 1963.
- Prince M, Patel V, Saxena S, *et al.* No health without mental health. *Lancet*. 2007; **37**: 859–77.
- U.S. Department of Health and Human Services (1999). *Mental Health: a report of the Surgeon General – executive summary*. Rockville, MD: U.S. Department of Health and Human Services, Substance Abuse and Mental Health Services Administration, Center for Mental Health Services, National Institutes of Health, National Institute of Mental Health; 2007.
- Wang PS, Aguilar-Gaxiola S, Alonso J, *et al.* Use of mental health services for anxiety, mood, and substance disorders in 17 countries in the WHO World Mental Health Surveys. *Lancet*. 2007; **370**: 84150.
- www.Palliativecare.com (accessed 24 April 2012).
- http://nationalcancerinstitute.org (accessed 24 April 2012).

- www.emro.who.int/aiecf/web35.pdf (accessed 24 April 2012).
- www.MentalHealth.org.uk/palliativecare (accessed 24 April 2012).

CHAPTER 14

Living with loss

Jenny Penson

'Give sorrow words. The grief that does not speak whispers the o'er fraught heart and bids it break.'[1]

INTRODUCTION

Most of us live as if our everyday lives in this world are safe, predictable and endless. This illusion of infinite time clouds our understanding of the preciousness of life and of one another. Therefore, we are deeply challenged when facing a life-threatening physical illness and equally so when facing serious and enduring mental health.

SELF-ASSESSMENT EXERCISE 14.1

> **Time: 10 minutes**
> Read the first two sentences again carefully. Try to deeply understand and appreciate their meaning and implication.
> • What feelings do they arouse in you?
> • Is this something you consider in your everyday life?

Although this chapter will focus on what palliative care may have to offer those working with people who experience serious and enduring mental health, it must be acknowledged that the practice of palliative care has gained many insights from mental health, e.g. about depression, anxiety, family conflicts and other existential concerns. Any constraints due to fear or a lack of experience can be addressed through collaborative working and education. Indeed, collaboration between the two philosophies, which takes advantage of their complementary affinities, can benefit both.[2]

The diagnosis of *dementia* is sometimes referred to as 'the new cancer' ...

a gradual process of deterioration, rather than something occurring at a fixed point in time. Good palliative care is essential but, as with a slow-growing cancer, it is not always easy to determine when this is appropriate.

> **KEY POINT 14.1**
>
> The main concern is for the quality of life of the individual and support for their family, for as long as possible, and this may involve symptom management, medication, supportive care and providing a 'safety net' to enable the family to care for their loved one for as long as possible.

> **Case vignette 14.1**
>
> Maggie and her sisters lived in the same town as their 85-year-old mother. Maggie explained that 'when my mother was diagnosed with dementia, we all thought it was the end of the world. However, we decided to share her care and to look at what she *could* do, rather than at what she couldn't. She lived life as fully as possible during those last few months. Though she's gone now, we feel good about how things went.'

Case comment

Experiences of shared love and purpose provided a good legacy for Maggie and her sisters, which can be very helpful when adjusting to bereavement. It can be useful to suggest to relatives that they project themselves into the future, to after the death of their loved one, and then ask themselves how, looking back, they would have liked things to have been.

GRIEF

Grief is the expression of loss. It is a process, a cycle of change, of completing the past and acknowledging that it has indeed passed. It is a time of discomfort and distress, of mourning all the losses and, at the same time, living with the uncertainty of what will come next. This can be a profound time of transformation. Who is it that will emerge from the ashes?

There are numerous perspectives on the grieving process. Arguably, the most widely known are those of Kubler-Ross,[3,4] Parkes,[5] and Worden.[6] It has become evident that these models can be applied not only to the process of bereavement but also to the acceptance of other difficult, and even catastrophic, life experiences.

Bereavement means 'to be robbed of something valued'. The word 'rob' suggests that what has been lost has been wrongfully taken away, leading to anger and a strong sense of injustice. It begins from the moment the person knows that their loved one is going to die. This is a pertinent definition for those whose experiences are due to serious and enduring mental health.

Although bereavement and loss are common human experiences, in the context of serious and enduring mental health there are a myriad of losses which are experienced in daily living that add to the suffering caused by the 'ill-health' itself. These will be further exacerbated by a bereavement caused by the serious ill-health and/or death of a close family member or friend.

It is well known that talking about our experiences can help when managing bereavement and loss. This can be a particular problem for those experiencing learning difficulties or serious and enduring mental health who do not have the opportunity to do this in the same way. Therefore, it is important to think about the best way to facilitate communication of that loss. Listening and allowing expression of feelings is key to facilitating grieving.[7]

DISENFRANCHISED GRIEF

This describes a major loss, which is not generally acknowledged by others. This may often be because it is hidden, e.g. AIDS or a physical illness, which is not immediately visible to others as may be the case in serious and enduring mental health. Moreover, grief may be disenfranchised when the individual chooses not to recognise it, to deny the situation due to painful feelings and not knowing how to respond. When an individual is denied the opportunity to share their feelings, they may feel disenfranchised and misunderstood. Concealing their ill-health, denying it or covering it up are all results of disenfranchised grieving.

Unrecognised grieving is also about the small losses of everyday life and how they accumulate. It is possible that these losses may not be acknowledged by the individual themself.[8] Recognising hidden sorrows, especially those connected with an imagined future, the loss of assumptions made and plans envisioned, need to be grieved over before any new dreams can be created and pursued.[9]

UNRESOLVED GRIEF

This can be a trigger for mental health problems. People need help to talk through their feelings because there may be a tendency to dissociate by blocking out painful ones. Actual losses may not always be the expected ones.

Case vignette 14.2

Lynne was a 60-year-old lady, experiencing *serious and enduring depression* who had suffered a major deterioration in her illness 10 years before. This was precipitated by the death of her father, followed only two weeks later by the sudden death of a close friend. She struggled to 'hang on to the cliff by my fingertips' and continued to go to work. Her bereaved mother showed anger and guilt and fell out with her other daughter, causing Lynne to act as the 'go-between'. Her work became more stressful and she struggled to hold on to her job. She felt unable either to confide in her closest friends or to bother her sister who had just had a baby. She became exhausted. After a year, things had improved – though Lynne still felt tense and angry with her mother – but one day there was an unexpectedly stressful incident at work and she knew she could no longer cope. 'It felt like grief,' she explained, 'I fell into a black hole.' In order to move on she needed to talk about it, to tell her story. However, this was frightening and needed to be in small manageable steps. She realised that moving on would be a slow process 'like a stuck truck in a muddy field'. She was helped by reading about the bereavement process. 'I read that you get by at the time and then later break down. That's what happened to me.'

STIGMA

An individual carries a stigma if they are unable, for any reason, to fulfil society's stereotypic criteria for 'normality' (*see* Chapter 5). Failings that are less obvious or have been concealed render the individual 'discreditable', in the sense that their identity is vulnerable. They may prefer the effort and the risk attached to trying to pass as 'normal' to the frank stigma of admitting the attribute that deviates from the norm. This behaviour can lead to a lack of sympathy and of support, which is, of itself, isolating. Feelings of being stigmatised may lead to depression, anxiety and anger, all emotions associated with bereavement.

The stigma of serious and enduring mental health may impair the achievement of personal aspirations; therefore professional practices need to be examined in terms of their effect on stigma. The loss of self-esteem and self-efficacy caused by self-stigma has been viewed as the anchor at one end of a continuum, with personal empowerment at the other end. People who believe that they have control over their lives and their treatment are less likely to experience self-stigma. When group identification is pronounced, when the individual purposefully affiliates with groups and is willing to admit their issues, they are less easily overwhelmed. This has obvious implications for practice.[10]

Living with serious and enduring mental health, e.g. a diagnosis of *schizophrenia*, leads to losses in several areas of life such as:

➤ emotional and cognitive functioning
➤ social contacts
➤ study and employment
➤ daily activities.

Feelings of meaninglessness and emptiness result from this enforced passivity. Psychotic episodes are experienced as highly traumatic because of frightening thoughts and feelings. This has been described as 'sheer hell'. The prolonged presence of symptoms plus the side effects of medication cause distress. Commonly reported perceptions of loss included faulty memories, garbled thinking and fatigue.[11]

SUICIDE

There is a specific stigma attached to death through *suicide*. The increased risk of suicide among individuals after the diagnosis of serious and enduring mental health is indicative of their suffering. Feeling powerless and desperate can lead to a suicidal state of mind. Moreover, the lack of support to families bereaved by suicide is exacerbated by their fear of talking about the nature of their loss.[12]

Case vignette 14.3

Jon was 18 years old when he was diagnosed with *schizophrenia*. His future life appeared to him to be one of a troubled path to hospitals and treatments. He attempted *suicide* on two occasions. He felt guilty about the effect of this on his parents, but also loss at his failure – again – to control his life. This was in addition to the loss imposed on him by his prevailing mental health problem. His parents, in turn, felt the loss of a son who had had such a bright future ahead of him, and the loss associated with his wish to die. Sadly, he succeeded on his third attempt. His bereavement had ended but his parents were left with the pressing questions:

- 'What should we have done?'
- 'How could we have helped him more?'
- 'Why did he have to die before us?'

They needed the help and support of a Bereavement Service but, as is often the case, there was not one available.

EXPRESSIONS OF LOSS

What I feel is so painful

Experiencing suffering is frightening. The fears are of being overwhelmed, of 'losing one's mind', the pain of being 'different'. Yet emotions are most usefully thought of as e-motions. As long as they are felt and expressed and so stay in motion, then they can pass and feelings that are more peaceful can follow. This process will be re-experienced many times, as people attend to their painful feelings at their own pace and in their own way.

I feel very alone

Feelings of loneliness involve a deeply felt sense of alienation, a yearning to belong, the experience of being isolated from others. It is the loss of self, of the idealised self ... of the person we thought we would be ... living the life we expected to live. In addition, this may involve the loss of being part of something greater than ourselves.

The erosion of a person's social network has many consequences, one of which is the almost total lack of the practical and emotional support offered by friendship. When thrown back upon family ties alone, individuals may well become more dependent and become acutely aware of being a source of concern. A huge sense of failure then ensues.

Many bereaved people find that they need to keep their grief hidden from the everyday world because others would not understand. This is especially likely to be experienced by those experiencing serious and enduring mental health.

I feel so ashamed

For many people, feeling humiliated is one of the most painful and unforgivable experiences of their lives. It is a violation of the most basic instinct to survive because we have failed to protect ourselves from one of the most painful of personal traumas. Feeling vulnerable to personal humiliation is devastating. Furthermore, the trauma of being deeply humiliated can be so consuming that the individual may fear interacting with others lest it lead to being humiliated again. It may even lead to a desire for vengeance as our reasoning mind demands some kind of justice.[13]

I do not know who I am any more

In bereavement, people usually experience a loss of identity. The question, 'Who am I?' is one we may return to many times in our lives, especially at challenging times. The loss is of the old 'you', the person you were before, the person you will never be again. The new 'you' is forever changed, and feels crushed, broken and irreparable. Kubler-Ross and Kessler[4] say that it feels as if a . . .

> terrible loss of innocence has occurred, only to be replaced with vulnerability, sadness and a new reality where something like this can happen to you, and has happened.[4]

Moreover, this is experienced by those facing serious and enduring mental health.

I am anxious all the time

Bereavement brings up many fears, especially those of vulnerability. This is due to the breach of inner security with which we live our everyday lives. The world has been found to be no longer predictable or safe and this is devastating. This deep fear is at the level of survival and, as more fears come to the surface, they feed off the first. Some of these will be very real while others may be illusionary anxieties.

I feel really angry

People do not always recognise or admit to anger. It can manifest as irritability over seemingly small things or the passive-aggressive kind of response where the anger may be masked by 'niceness'. Anger, and even rage, may be observed rather than expressed. It is often felt as a very physical thing, held in the body, e.g:

➤ in the solar plexus

> ➤ in the neck and shoulders
> ➤ expressed through headaches
> ➤ expressed through digestive upsets.

Indeed, anger directed towards oneself may lead to guilt.

EXPERIENCING LOSS

Bereaved people need support in trusting that some kind of restoration will come, bringing new insights, new beginnings, and a life with meaning and purpose. This has been aptly described as 'resurrection after loss'.[8]

Case vignette 14.4

Jane is a 45-year-old divorced woman experiencing *Obsessional Compulsive Disorder (OCD)*. This becomes worse during the winter months because of associations with cold weather. Following her diagnosis, Jane's husband left and she experienced profound grief at the loss of her relationship and of her work, culminating in the loss of her identity. What Jane needed, she felt, was 'someone to help me create some order out of the chaos of my mind'. One year later she no longer feels as if she is 'outside herself, looking in' but still struggles to express her feelings and to get into some kind of balance. All professional support she has received so far has felt 'very short-term, what I need is a long-term relationship where I can trust that I won't be abandoned'. 'A small self-help group of others recovering from similar situations would be of great benefit.'

KEY POINT 14.3

Understanding the factors that make an individual feel better is as important as understanding those that make them feel worse.[14]

PHYSICAL EXPRESSIONS

Unexpressed emotions can be held within the body. We know that emotional states such as anxiety impact on physical health and, as the mind affects the body, the state of the body also affects the mind. Many disease states such as cancer, heart disease and chronic illnesses appear to be triggered by 'stress'. For example, long-term serious depression has been shown to increase the risk of physical disease.[15] The growing body of knowledge of psychoneuroimmunology (PNI) – the study of the interaction between psychological processes and the nervous and immune systems – demonstrates this close link between illness, both physical and mental, and emotional states.

There has been little attention in the literature to how the body experiences loss and the memories associated with it.[16]

SPIRITUALITY

There is an emphasis in Palliative Care on the spiritual dimension of life (*see* Chapter 8). This is not necessarily about religious expression. Listening to a wise inner voice is healthy and normal. Such an experience may be deemed spiritual when it is meaningful, personal and constructive. This contrasts with the perception of someone experiencing *schizophrenia* where she or he may believe for a time that they *are* a religious figure, or even God. Therefore, it is necessary to distinguish between a spiritual experience and a delusional one.

Sensitive and encouraging questions that elicit thoughts about beliefs, meaning and values can be very helpful. These might include:

➤ What, if any, spiritual beliefs do you have that have supported you before in times of trouble?
➤ Have you ever had any spiritual experiences?
➤ If so, what effect did they have on you?

Professionals are often reluctant to take a spiritual history, often feeling it is unnecessary and time wasting. However, when it was suggested that psychiatrists take a spiritual history, they were 'amazed by what it revealed'.[17]

Following a medical diagnosis of a physical or mental health problem, or some other kind of personal crisis that destabilises one's ordinary life, an individual will automatically be drawn into an interior process of evaluation. The individual may want to reflect on questions such as:

➤ what went wrong?
➤ when did it happen?
➤ did he or she ignore the signals?
➤ did she or he simply deny that things were going wrong?

Moreover, relationships, values, life choices, regrets and priorities may come up for review.

Negativity and pain may be misunderstood in terms of the purpose they can serve within the greater scheme of life. Maybe we fool ourselves by assuming that all discomfort must be immediately converted into comfort, and that order must be rapidly introduced into all chaotic situations, as if that were even possible.[13] It may be more helpful to label thoughts and feelings as pleasant or unpleasant, rather than as positive or negative. This view that unpleasant feelings can have a useful purpose is often difficult for individuals to grasp. However, the idea that reason and emotions can work in harmony and that you can choose which feelings you stay with can be very helpful.[8]

Case vignette 14.5

Graham had learned to live with his *bipolar disorder* since his twenties. He was acutely aware of the losses of his past even though he had learned to manage the effects of his disorder but, as he stated, 'at a huge cost'. Graham's life had been about trying to hold down jobs in the media sector as he struggled with the unpredictable swings between wellness and illness, while at the same time caring for his mother. When he was in his thirties, Graham became a Christian. He thought he had been 'a good son'. 'In a way, I have coped. Now here I am, 65 years old, still struggling. I feel such sadness for all that's been lost. I missed out on life and now have lost out forever.' He also felt that health professionals who had been at times 'so cold, so harsh' had judged him.

KEY POINT 14.4

The individual experiencing serious and enduring mental health may be particularly challenged by the potential losses brought about by the ageing process.

PROFESSIONAL PRACTICE

When working with individuals who are facing loss, whether in palliative care or serious and enduring mental health, it is necessary to know the usual or 'normal' pattern of the bereavement process in order to identify when this seems to be prolonged, postponed, blocked or even excessively shortened.[18]

KEY POINT 14.5

The individual needs to be supported in grieving for all that has been lost, in her or his own way and at his/her own pace. Each will need to find coping mechanisms specific to their own needs.

As in palliative care, the emphasis is on the quality of the individual's life and on the relationships they have with family and significant friends.

A long-term therapeutic alliance needs to be established with a professional whom the grieving individual can trust. Person-centred, considerate care is needed with the intent to be supportive and encouraging. The helping skills of:
➤ attending
➤ active listening
➤ empathy

. . . help to demonstrate acceptance, care and compassion. By listening attentively while the individual 'tells their story', professionals support the grieving process, helping to break down the barriers of stigma and isolation and thus point towards fresh possibilities. Hope for the future is not an unrealistic promise but a positive, achievable outcome.[18]

The quality of this relationship is dependent on the professionals 'being' as much as on their 'doing'. Many techniques can help us to be present. These all involve ways of calming our emotions and letting go of distractions both from within and from without, enabling us to fully attend to the other.

A safe, nurturing space needs to be created where people can uncover and analyse their own solutions – their unique steps forward. On occasion, this may include the need to take control if an individual is becoming too wild in her or his behaviour or too fantastic in her or his thinking.

SUPPORTIVE CARE

Palliative care and complementary therapies are two movements that have grown almost in parallel. Both are committed to a person-centred approach and recognise that the mind, body and spirit are all connected and that we are each as one connected to the other.

> ### KEY POINT 14.6
>
> Palliative care has the expressed aim of enhancing quality of life, and complementary therapies help to capture something positive about the human spirit's ability to confront difficult issues and painful emotions, and to grow through them.[19]

There are many therapeutic interventions, both physical and cognitive, that may be used to support the individual experiencing serious and enduring mental health, and also family members, and to encourage each to move forward. The availability of these therapies will vary greatly and most will not be available through the Health Service. Such therapies may include:

➤ physical therapies, e.g. massage, aromatherapy, reflexology and movement therapies – help to release deeply held pain
➤ deep relaxation, image-work and meditation practices – help to quieten the mind and bring feelings of peace
➤ creative therapies – help emotional expression and can be uplifting, e.g. art, creative writing, poetry, dance and music
➤ Energy Psychological Therapies, e.g. Emotional Freedom Technique (EFT), Matrix Re-imprinting and other approaches used in Integrated Medicine – help to shift emotional states in mental and physical illness.[20,21]

FAMILY CARERS

Serious and enduring mental health destroys lives and a sense of meaning, not only for the person who is experiencing the concerns and dilemmas, but also for the loved ones around them.

Palliative care is always concerned with the needs of the family caregivers as well as with those of the person who is dying or experiencing serious and enduring mental health. It recognises that the individual and the family together make one unit, with the physical, emotional and spiritual health of each affecting the others. The focus has traditionally been on the anticipatory grief of family members facing the terminal physical illness of a loved one. However, more recently, acknowledgement has been given to the person experiencing serious and enduring mental health.

Recognising anticipatory grief and helping the family to identify their losses and negotiate roles and relationships may help them to feel more validated and supported, thus reducing distress and isolation.[22] Acknowledgement needs to be made of difficult emotions such as frustration, guilt and anger. The potential for practical problems and tiredness, added to sadness at the loss of the person they knew and loved, needs to be comprehensively explored. A safety net of support via carers' groups and the opportunity for respite care may enable the family to continue to care. Moreover, it is important that bereavement support groups are available to offer support after a death, or 'loss' of a family member to a serious and enduring mental health problem.

DEATH EXPERIENCES

Death is the final stage of development in a person's life. It is a time for people to resolve personal conflicts through a process of life review to help find meaning in their lives. It is the time for people to forgive themselves and others, appreciate those they care about, and to be able to say, 'I love you' – and, finally, say goodbye. These processes are just as important and challenging for individuals experiencing serious and enduring mental health as they are for everyone.

SUMMARY

Adjustment to bereavement and loss, like adjustment to serious ill-health, is a process. The time-scale for recovery seems to happen in proportion to the degree of the perceived losses. It is rarely fast, although there is always the possibility of a sudden shift when a new insight, experience, or behaviour brings about a dramatic change of perspective that then leads to new actions and change.

From this it can be seen that principles of palliative care can be applied to mental health care, for example:

➤ symptom management – medication regimes, treatment plans
➤ quality of life – raising self-esteem, building confidence, focusing on enjoyment and new goals and plans
➤ person-centred care – treating with dignity and respect, enabling the exercise of control and moving forward in small, manageable steps
➤ spiritual needs – exploring key values and beliefs, reasons 'to get up in the morning'
➤ physical needs – encouraging exercise, good nutrition, relaxation techniques
➤ support – facilitating a network of supportive people, groups, places, activities
➤ information – providing resources, facilitating meetings, referrals
➤ continuity of care – long-term support, building a therapeutic alliance

➤ care of the family – carers' groups, respite care, bereavement support groups

➤ including the individual as an equal partner – enabling contributions to the process of planning services and facilitating self-help groups.

FINAL WORD

One of life's paradoxes is that an individual may be unable to enjoy life to the full if she or he has never known deep sorrow. The grieving process can be an awakening one, where the person is confronted with the losses that re-order her or his life, often depicted in literature and the arts. Unpleasant, and even devastating experiences *can* have useful purposes. As Rabbi Kushner[23] pointed out when writing about the degenerative illness and early death of his son, the experience made him a more compassionate and aware human being, even though he would rather have remained the man he was and still have his son.[23]

Living with the losses associated with serious illness, whether physical or mental, is about finding ways of overcoming fear and of rejoining life and it needs to be remembered that this is 'not a matter of doubtless certainty but a matter of daring courage'.[24]

The final word goes to a notable pioneer of the palliative care movement, Elisabeth Kubler-Ross,[25] who reminds professionals of what a 'so-called hopeless, chronic *schizophrenic* patient' taught her.

> 'Knowledge alone is not going to help anybody. If you do not use your head and your heart and your soul, you are not going to help a single human being.'[25]

REFERENCES

1 Shakespeare, William (1564–1616). Spoken by Malcolm in *Macbeth*, Act IV, Scene iii. Available at: www.enotes.com/macbeth-text/act-iv-scene-iii (accessed 24 April 2012).

2 Meier DE, Beresford L. Growing the interface between palliative medicine and psychiatry. *Journal of Palliative Medicine.* 2010; **13**: 803–6.

3 Kubler-Ross E. *On Death and Dying.* London: Tavistock; 1970.

4 Kubler-Ross E, Kessler D. *On Grief and Grieving.* London: Simon & Schuster UK; 2005.

5 Parkes CM, Prigerson HG. *Bereavement: studies of grief in adult life.* 3rd ed. London: Penguin; 2010.

6 Worden WJ. *Grief Counselling and Grief Therapy.* 3rd ed. London: Routledge; 2010.

7 Grey R. *Bereavement, Loss and Learning Disabilities: a guide for professionals and carers.* London: Jessica Kingsley; 2010.

8 Griffiths T. *Lost and then Found: turning life's disappointments into hidden treasures.* Carlyle: Paternoster; 2000.

9 Bowman T. Loss of dreams; a special kind of grief. *International Journal of Palliative Nursing.* 1997; **3**: 76–80.

10 Corrigan P, Wassel A. Understanding and influencing the stigma of mental illness. *International Psychosocial Nursing and Mental Health Services.* 2008; **46**: 42–8.

11 Mauritz M, van Meijel B. Loss and grief in patients with schizophrenia: on living in another world. *Archives of Psychiatric Nursing.* 2009; **23**: 251–60.

12 *Survivors of Suicide.* Available at: www.survivorsofsuicide.com (accessed 24 April 2012).

13 Myss C. *Defy Gravity: healing beyond the bounds of reason.* London: Hay House UK; 2009.

14 Yalom I. *Staring at the Sun: overcoming the dread of death.* London: Piatkus; 2008.

15 Steptoe A. *Depression and Physical Illness.* Cambridge: Cambridge University Press; 2007.

16 Hentz P. The body remembers: grieving and a circle of time. *Qualitative Health Research.* 2002; **1**: 161–72.

17 Scott Peck M. *Further Along the Road Less Travelled.* London: Pocket Books, Simon & Schuster; 1997.

18 Penson J. A hope is not a promise: fostering hope in palliative care. *International Journal of Palliative Nursing.* 2001; **6**: 94–8.

19 Penson J, Fisher RA. *Palliative Care for People with Cancer.* 3rd ed. London: Edward Arnold; 2002.

20 Feinstein D, Eden D, Craig G. *The Healing Power of EFT and Energy Psychology.* London: Piatkus; 2007.

21 Edwards G. *Conscious Medicine.* London: Piatkus; 2010.

22 Holley CK, Mast B. The impact of anticipatory grief on caregiver burden in dementia caregivers. *The Gerontologist.* 2009; **49**: 338–96.

23 Kushner Rabbi HS. *When Bad Things Happen to Good People.* London: Pan; 2002.

24 Solari-Twadell PA, Schmidt Bunkers S, Wang C, *et al.* The pinwheel model of bereavement. *Image.* 1995; **27**: 323–6.

25 Kubler-Ross E. *On Life after Death.* California: Celestial Arts; 1991.

TO LEARN MORE

- The Emotional Logic Centre. Available at: www.emotionallogiccentre.org.uk (accessed 24 April 2012).
- Hudson P, Payne S. *Family Carers in Palliative Care.* Oxford: Oxford University Press; 2009.
- Kubler-Ross E, Kessler D. *On Grief and Grieving.* London: Simon & Schuster UK; 2005.
- Kubler-Ross E, Kessler D. *Life Lessons: how our mortality can teach us about life and living.* London: Simon & Schuster; 2001.
- McCasland, L. A. (2007) Providing hospice and palliative care to the seriously and persistently mentally ill. *Journal of Hospice and Palliative Care.* 2007; **9**: 6305–13.
- Payne S, Seymour J, Ingleton C, editors. *Palliative Care Nursing: principles and evidence for practice.* 2nd ed. Maidenhead: Oxford University Press; 2008.

CHAPTER 15

Serious substance use problems and palliative care

Cynthia MA Geppert, April H Volk

PRE-READING EXERCISE 15.1

> **Time: 20 minutes**
>
> Central to the philosophy of palliative and hospice care is that every person deserves to die with dignity in a safe and comfortable setting with their suffering relieved and pain controlled to the extent medically and humanly possible.[1] These goals are seldom reached and often unattainable in our current healthcare system for persons with terminal illness and active substance use and psychotic or dangerous behaviour.
>
> Read Case study 15.1 and identify the primary problems involved in delivering appropriate palliative care to Harry. Try to imagine innovative solutions to these problems both at an individual and at a systems level.

> **Case study 15.1**
>
> Harry is a 49-year-old individual with a long history of intravenous heroin use, serious depression and homelessness. He was admitted to an academic affiliated hospital with end-stage lung cancer that had metastasised to his bones. His performance score was such that his ex-wife had taken him home with hospice services several months earlier. Harry continued to inject heroin and drug dealers were frequently present when the hospice staff arrived for visits while his ex-wife was at work. The hospice team felt it was no longer safe for their workers and discontinued services. Without this assistance, his ex-wife could not manage his care and brought him to the hospital. The palliative care team was consulted. Person-controlled analgesia was recommended. Despite using extremely high doses of opioids, Harry continued to complain of severe and unrelieved pain.

Anaesthesia service was consulted and recommended a peripherally inserted central catheter (PICC) for the direct infusion of narcotics. In a previous admission, Harry had accessed a PICC line, injecting a near fatal dose of opiates. The palliative care team feared this would happen again. Harry's pain was therefore controlled with continuous subcutaneous infusion with return to near prior level of function. Given his history of drug use and aberrant behaviours, community hospices were unwilling to accept him for home hospice. Harry was subsequently admitted to the in-patient palliative care unit where he continued to receive aggressive pain and symptom management with focus on relief of suffering. He was reconciled with his 15-year-old son during this interval. With the support offered to him and his family by interdisciplinary efforts of the palliative care staff, he died peacefully several months after being admitted.

Comment

This case study poignantly depicts many of the interpersonal and institutional struggles that are encountered in attempting to provide palliative and hospice care to an individual with serious physical, mental and substance use problems. The exercise also shows that even in traditional healthcare settings, persons experiencing serious substance use problems who continue to display aberrant behaviours can, with intensive effort and altruistic commitment, die in comfort and peace.

INTRODUCTION

The prevalence of serious substance use problems (SSUP – addiction/dependence) and serious and enduring mental health (SEMH) in palliative care is unknown. In one of the only studies using the CAGE questionnaire[2] for screening, Bruera found 27% of individuals admitted to a tertiary care palliative medicine unit had a diagnosis of alcoholism.[3] There are, however, several epidemiological findings that suggest the cohort may be larger than previously appreciated, and growing. The 2002 National Study of Drug Use and Health found that 4 million American adults had a co-occurring substance use and mental disorder.[4] These co-occurring problems have an adverse effect on illness trajectory and prognosis.[5] This poor outcome is mediated at least in part by failure to seek treatment and non-adherence to therapy, as well as reduced access to medical and psychiatric care. These factors lead to late diagnosis that makes palliative rather than active treatment more likely especially when combined with the recent and laudable emphasis on providing palliative care at an earlier stage of a life-limiting illness.[6] Studies have repeatedly found that individuals experiencing SEMH combined with SSUP have higher mortality rates.[7] Persons experiencing SEMH also lose more years of life and die earlier from the same medical conditions that lead to palliative care in non-SEMH populations such as heart disease, cancer, cerebrovascular and respiratory and lung disease.[8]

Comfort and dignity

Persons like Harry described in the pre-reading exercise embody multiple overlapping vulnerabilities that are among the most stigmatised in human history. Societies and individuals – among them, many healthcare professionals – have frequently feared and often rejected individuals who are experiencing serious substance use problems, experiencing serious and enduring mental health, experiencing a life-limiting illness or are dying. These entrenched cultural attitudes are the greatest barriers to providing competent and compassionate palliative care to individuals experiencing co-occurring SSUPs, SEMH and life-limiting illnesses. The following sections explore the obstacles standing in the way of delivering high-quality palliative and hospice care to persons experiencing SSUPs and SEMH problems at the end-of-life and offer ways in which programmes and professionals can strive to overcome these obstacles in their own practice.

Hospice, hospitals and homelessness

The US Conference of Mayors 2007 *Status Report on Hunger and Homelessness* estimated that 37% of single adults had substance use problems and 22% had serious mental health issues.[9] The majority of persons experiencing co-occurring health problems either die in hospitals or tragically on the streets as opposed to in home hospice or in hospital palliative care units. The reasons are multifactorial and include lack of financing and social support, as well as institutional and programme policies that refuse to provide services, particularly home hospice, to persons who are actively using substances, have disapproved lifestyles or have antisocial behaviour.[10]

SELF-ASSESSMENT EXERCISE 15.1

> **Time: 10 minutes**
> - Before continuing this chapter, had you ever thought about what happened to persons experiencing SEMH and SSUPs when they developed a life-limiting illness?
> - As a professional, what can you do today in your practice setting to improve the experience of these individuals at the end-of-life?

One approach to overcoming obstacles preventing individuals from entering traditional hospice settings is to bring high-quality palliative care to those experiencing SSUPs, SEMH and end-stage disease where they are living and dying with life-limiting illnesses. One innovative programme has successfully done this, providing shelter-based palliative care for the homeless terminally ill. The Ottawa Inner City Health Project was a proof of concept programme to improve healthcare delivery to the homeless. Of the 28 people enrolled in the programme, 82% had either substance use or mental ill-health and the most common physical conditions were liver disease, HIV/AIDS or malignancy, with an average Karnofsky performance score of 40 indicating considerable impairment in function.

KEY POINT 15.1

Two main goals of hospice care – control of pain and reconciliation with families – occurred in more than two-thirds of the individuals.[1]

The expert panel that reviewed the project estimated that without the shelter hospice, 68% of the individuals would either not have received care, or died homeless with no treatment of pain or other symptoms. The cost analysis demonstrated that effective palliative care could be delivered in a shelter setting with a savings, compared with traditional venues, of $1.39 million.[11] Another promising alternative is to try to improve end-of-life care in the hospitals where the homeless most often die, by providing in-patient palliative care services in university, community, government and religious affiliated hospitals, which deliver the majority of care to the underserved.[10]

PAIN AND SERIOUS SUBSTANCE USE PROBLEMS

KEY POINT 15.2

No matter where individuals with substance use problems and life-limiting illnesses receive palliative care, the use of medications with addictive potential will likely be the most difficult clinical and ethical dilemma confronting professionals.

Professionals are truly caught between the rock of regulatory requirements, litigation fears, concerns about inducing or exacerbating addiction and the duty and desire to relieve suffering and treat pain at the end-of-life. What is known is that persons experiencing SSUPs and a life-limiting illness are far more likely to have their pain undertreated than those without these comorbidities. Persons experiencing co-occurring health problems are not only frequently denied adequate pain control, but often stigmatised as 'drug-seeking' in the process of asking for legitimate relief of their suffering. In several influential studies, Breitbart[12] examined the management of pain in persons with one of the most stigmatising diseases: HIV/AIDS. Two hundred and twenty-six of 366 ambulatory individuals experiencing AIDS endorsed persistent or frequent pain over the two weeks prior to being surveyed. Pain control measured with the Brief Pain Inventory showed that nearly 85% of the individuals were receiving inadequate analgesia. In addition, fewer than 10% of the persons experiencing severe pain were prescribed a strong opioid like morphine in accordance with the World Health Organization ladder (available at www.who.int/cancer/palliative/pain ladder/en/ – *see* Chapter 11). Adjunctive medications such as antidepressants lacking addictive potential were also prescribed to only one-tenth of the cohort. Women, those with less education and intravenous drug use as the vector for HIV were among those most likely to receive poor pain management.[12] This finding underscores that healthcare disparities may be risk factors for both inadequate analgesia and social stigmatisation (*see* Chapter 5).

Breitbart in a subsequent study explored SSUPs as a risk factor for poor management of pain in individuals experiencing AIDS. He compared the adequacy of analgesia for pain in persons with and without a history of injection drug use (IDU) among 516 ambulatory HIV persons. Both groups had similar reports of pain prevalence, intensity and interference with functioning. There was also no difference in these parameters among persons continuing to use drugs, those participating in methadone maintenance programmes, and those who denied any current use of drugs. Yet the IDU individuals were much more likely to be given inadequate pain medications, to endorse less relief of pain and more psychological distress. Poor management of pain was not restricted to those actively using drugs, but extended even to those with an IDU history.[13]

KEY POINT 15.3

Breitbart and colleagues emphasise that the individuals' reports of pain were generally valid despite presumptions to the contrary being widespread among professionals and in the literature.[13]

The findings regarding persons in methadone programmes are particularly concerning because there is a mistaken assumption among many professionals that persons receiving methadone maintenance for SSUPs do not require further analgesia for acute or chronic pain. In fact, the methadone merely keeps the individual from withdrawing and craving and does not treat pain.

KEY POINT 15.4

Such persons deserve and require additional opioids – often in high doses, given their tolerance to this class of drugs – to relieve pain.

Similarly, individuals whose opioid dependence is managed with buprenorphine substitution therapy, with a terminal illness, will need the expertise of a substance use and pain specialist for optimal palliative care.

REFLECTIVE PRACTICE EXERCISE 15.2

Time: 10 minutes
- Reflect on your views regarding the use of opioids for individuals experiencing serious substance use problems at the end-of-life.
- Do you think professionals should supply these persons with their drugs of choice as a means of harm reduction?
- Is there any circumstance in which you would feel these persons should not receive pain medications?

On first thought, a compassionate professional may ask why they should be concerned about SSUPs when an individual is terminally ill. This question is aptly captured in the title of a paper examining the issue, 'Managing addiction in advanced cancer patients: why bother?'[14] Passik points out there is a prevalent attitude even among professionals that individuals at the end-of-life should be allowed to use substances of choice at will because they should not be denied one of the only gratifications they can still enjoy and will soon perish.[14] This 'eat, drink and be merry for tomorrow we die' attitude on closer examination is specious, Passik shows.

> Many clinicians perceive that addicts continue in their behaviour because of a desire to 'get high'. Therefore, managing addiction in patients with cancer would be considered tantamount to taking away a source of pleasure. In fact, chemically-dependent patients spent very little time high; the lion's share of their time is spent feeling depressed, being isolated, withdrawing, being obsessed about drug procurement, behaving in a fashion that they themselves consider demeaning or degrading.[14]

It can be humanistically argued that when a person is actively dying, concerns about SSUPs are eclipsed. This may be the only time during the course of a life-limiting illness that this is a convincing claim. At all other points in what may be years of living with an incurable but manageable disease, failure to diagnose and manage SSUPs nearly always has an adverse effect on the individual, family, professionals providing care, community and the course of her or his illnesses of mind and body.

This detrimental impact of uncontrolled or excessive use of substances including alcohol, illicit and prescription drugs is both biopsychosocial and spiritual as reflected in the 2011 American Society of Addiction Medicine definition of addiction.

> Addiction is a primary, chronic disease of brain reward, motivation, memory, and related circuitry. Dysfunction in these circuits leads to characteristic biological, psychological, social and spiritual manifestations.

This is reflected in an individual pathologically pursuing reward and/or relief by substance use and other behaviors.[15]

Untreated SSUPs can biologically interfere with the efficacy of palliative treatment modalities such as chemotherapy through drug interactions and amplification of side effects from treatment (*see* Chapter 11). Psychologically, substances of use, especially when used chronically and compulsively, cause mood lability, impulsivity and erratic behaviour. Poor insight and impaired judgement can lead to missed appointments, non-adherence to therapeutic regimens, and alienation of professionals who become frustrated and demoralised attempting to care for individuals who seem to not care for themselves. Socially, persons experiencing a long history of SSUPs have often alienated family members and friends and thus lack the social support that is essential to cope practically and emotionally with terminal illness and hospice care.[16] When significant others and loved ones learn of the person's life-limiting diagnosis, they will often attempt a reconciliation and offer succour. Repeated relapses, manipulative behaviour and self-sabotage of treatment opportunities may – as in Harry's situation – bring even devoted caregivers to exhaustion and even abandonment.[17] Spiritually, SSUPs enervate the resilience and hope key to positive coping with a terminal diagnosis (*see* Chapter 7 and 8).

KEY POINT 15.5

Adhering to difficult and demanding treatments and making meaning of one's life in the shadow of ineluctable demise is often amplified by isolation.

The moral and emotional resources needed to repair disruptions in interpersonal relationships, attain forgiveness of self and others, and if desired, develop or revitalise spiritual connections with the transcendent will not be available to a person craving substances and pursuing a chemical reward at the expense of other values and needs.[16]

Risk assessment
The treatment of an individual experiencing SEMH alongside a current or historical SSUP and a serious medical illness begins and ends with a sound and thorough risk assessment. (*See* Box 15.1 for a list of common risk factors and domains to be assessed.)

BOX 15.1 Risk factors for serious substance use problems

- Personal history of SSUPs
- Family history of SSUPs
- Legal consequences of SSUPs
- Lack of social support
- Driving while intoxicated or impaired
- Co-occurring psychiatric disorder
- Childhood trauma
- Male gender

Risk assessment is fundamental to early detection and a non-judgemental response to problems controlling either pain or addiction.

KEY POINT 15.6

Screening instruments can be a useful part of a risk assessment, but cannot be a substitute for a good clinical interview.

As Claxton underscores, the most commonly used screening tools have not been validated in palliative care cohorts but have demonstrated their utility in individuals experiencing chronic non-malignant pain.[18] Instruments such as the Screener and Opioids Assessment for Pain Patients (SOAPP) and the Opioid Risk Tool (ORT) are easy to use and readily available on the Internet.[19,20]

Risk assessment enables the professional to correctly distinguish between the related phenomena of:

➤ tolerance
➤ dependence
➤ pseudoaddiction
➤ aberrant behaviour.

Such a distinction is crucial if the professional is to respond with a clinically appropriate and non-judgemental response to the person exhibiting the behaviour. *See* Table 15.1 for definitions of these key concepts and case illustrations.

TABLE 15.1 Key concepts and cases[21]

Concept	Case
Tolerance – is the need to use more of a drug to obtain the same effect. • Does not indicate SSUPs.	A 72-year-old person with prostate cancer has been on high-dose morphine for 2 years when it begins to lose its efficacy. An opioid rotation to methadone is made and the pain is relieved.
Dependence – is the physiological effect in which the body becomes habituated to a substance and exhibits a withdrawal syndrome when the drug is discontinued or decreased. • Does not indicate SSUPs. • Can occur with non-addictive medications.	A 61-year-old man with advanced congestive heart failure visits his grandchildren and forgets to take his morphine. He experiences symptoms of severe withdrawal requiring him to go to a local emergency room to be treated.
Pseudoaddiction – is the display of pain behaviours or drug seeking because of poorly or undertreated pain, NOT SSUPs.[22]	A 25-year-old person hospitalised with bone cancer is placed on oxycodone and acetaminophen every 4 hours and repeatedly pushes the call button asking when he can have another pill.
Medication misuse – intentional or unintentional use of a prescribed medication for a purpose other than as prescribed.[23]	A 32-year-old person with leukaemia uses morphine prescribed for pain to treat associated depression.
Medication abuse – is the intentional use of prescription medication for a non-medical purpose or can also refer to the use of an illegal drug.[18]	A 45-year-old individual experiencing AIDS uses medical marijuana prescribed for wasting syndrome to obtain a high and buys marijuana off the street to supplement his prescription.
SSUPs (addiction) – is compulsive, uncontrolled craving for and continued use of a substance despite harm.[18]	A 57-year-old person with pancreatic cancer crushes a week's worth of OxyContin prescribed for abdominal pain and injects it.
Aberrant behaviour – is a broad academic term with various understandings that clinically encompasses 'mis'-use and 'ab'-use short of dependence.[18]	A 62-year-old woman with breast cancer runs out of her oxycodone a few days before a refill is due and calls the pharmacy for an early refill.

Professionals with palliative care training and expertise will in general lack the knowledge and skills of substance use specialists, and vice versa. A 2011 survey of 57 hospice and palliative medicine fellows asked how frequently persons at risk for opioid abuse were seen in practice and how competent the fellows felt in managing their pain. Over 70% had seen a person experiencing SSUPs and nearly 50% had treated a person they were concerned was misusing opioids in the two weeks prior to the survey. Only half of respondents had a working knowledge of SSUPs, 40% thought their previous training had prepared them to manage opioid misuses and a disappointing 21% were satisfied with their treatment of pain in this group. Training in opioid misuse did increase the satisfaction of fellows and the authors concluded there was a need for more education in this area.[24]

> **KEY POINT 15.7**
>
> Persons experiencing co-occurring health problems, especially those experiencing SEMH, SSUPs and terminal conditions benefit most from intra- and inter-disciplinary approaches delivered in a co-ordinated and integrated fashion.

To offer these individuals competent and compassionate care, palliative care professionals will want to seek out continuing education opportunities and to develop consultative and collaborative relationships with professionals in the professional community serving persons experiencing SSUPs. To assist in this cross-training effort, *see* Box 15.2 for examples of aberrant behaviours that signal a need for further evaluation and intervention. Suggested management techniques for individuals with past or current substance use problems can be found at End-of-Life/Palliative Education Resource Center (EPERC) Online site, www.eperc.mcw.edu/fastFact/ff_127.htm.[23]

BOX 15.2 Aberrant behaviours[26]

- Early refills
- Using multiple doctors and pharmacies to fill prescriptions
- Not informing treatment team of obtaining outside prescriptions
- Taking medications other than as prescribed
- Taking medications for non-medical purposes
- Buying medications off the street
- Trading medications with other persons
- Selling and diverting medications
- Stealing or forging prescriptions

HARM REDUCTION

While the aim of most SSUPs treatment programmes is abstinence, this is often not a realistic objective for individuals with comorbid serious and enduring mental health, SSUPs and life-limiting conditions.[14] Harm reduction

> is a set of practical strategies that reduce negative consequences of drug use, incorporating a spectrum of strategies from safer use, to managed use, to abstinence. Harm reduction strategies meet drug users 'where they're at', addressing conditions of use along with the use itself.[27]

Harm reduction is the philosophy and practice that can provide the most effective and emphatic treatment of SSUPs for individuals experiencing terminal illness and SSUPs. Such strategies (*see* Table 15.2) are most directly applicable to the use of opioids and other medications with addictive potential to manage pain and other symptoms such as anxiety at the end-of-life.

TABLE 15.2 Harm-reduction strategies[16,24,25]

Strategy	Rationale
Adjunctive use of non-opioid analgesics such as antidepressants and anticonvulsants	• Medications lack addiction potential and can reduce use of opioids • May be more effective for some types of pain, such as neuropathic
Use of written opioid agreement or informed consent and education agreement that spells out the rights and responsibilities of the individual and the professional(s)	• Encourages shared decision making • Clarifies expectations of both parties • Offers a measure of choice and control for the person experiencing SSUPs
Consider periodic urine testing but only with informed consent	Identifies potential relapse, diversion and, if sophisticated testing is used, under-treatment
Close monitoring including: • frequent visits • pill counts • prescription of only limited quantities of medication	• A form of relapse prevention • Reduces risk of overdose • Strengthens therapeutic alliance • Helps distinguish if increased pain or decreased function is the result of progression of disease or of substance use
Aggressive treatment of pain • Persons with opioid use disorders often have high tolerance requiring larger doses of opioids to control pain	• Untreated pain is a major cause of relapse as individuals attempt to manage their own distress – physical and mental • Avoids pseudoaddiction
Aggressive treatment of anxiety and depression with psychological and, if necessary, pharmacological methods	• Anxiety causes psychic suffering and reduced quality of life • Leads to overuse of opioids through 'chemical coping'
• Use long- rather than short-acting opioids • Titrate medications and dosing intervals to avoid breakthrough dosing • Use scheduled, not pro re nata (prn – when needed) dosing • Consider subcutaneous methods of delivery (syringe driver)	• Clinical wisdom is that long-acting opioids are less likely to be abused than are short-acting ones • Breakthrough medications may reinforce addiction • Pro re nata (prn – when needed) dosing strengthens the association that the solution to distress is a pill • Pain patches (e.g. fentanyl) can reduce the risk of diversion or accidental overdose
Aberrant behaviour and relapse are the expectation, not the exception	• Compassion and understanding • Increase visits • Closer monitoring • More structure such as residential or inpatient treatment
Self-help and motivational interviewing	For persons who are physically able, recommend Alcoholics and Narcotics Anonymous and other 12-step groups

KEY POINT 15.8

Harm-reduction orientations would not perforce preclude the continued use of alcohol and drugs whether prescribed or illicit while receiving palliative care.

For example, in the shelter-based palliative care programme described above, clean needles, safe syringe disposal, a smoking area, and alcoholic drinks dispensed on demand were provided. Despite this liberal stance, use of substances did not increase.[11] In this programme, and in a true harm-reduction approach, the individual would also continue to be prescribed opioid and anxiolytic medications if needed. For this to be a relatively safe treatment plan, the person must be honest with the professional regarding the frequency and amount of illicit use, and the professional must work alongside the person in a person-centred, matter-of-fact, non-judgemental manner (*see* Chapter 6). In the Ontario programme, there was solidarity among the persons staying in the hospice that functioned as a safeguard; other residents would inform programme staff if they suspected behaviour violating hospice rules and policies.[10,11] These regulations included having all medications under the control of the programme staff, directly observed administration of oral opioids, and the use of patches and pumps less easily diverted or abused whenever clinically possible. Those who breached hospice policies were suspended for 24 hours but not discharged from the programme.

This author shares Kushel's opinion that there are ethical, legal and clinical grounds to suggest that persons with active or past SSUPs resume or continue the use of substances of abuse to relieve suffering associated with life-limiting illness.[10] With the integration of palliative care earlier in the course of life-limiting illnesses, the opportunity for intervention is great.[24]

KEY POINT 15.9

It is the responsibility of professionals and the healthcare system to reach out to the disenfranchised and give them aggressive and high-quality management at the end-of-life so that they are not compelled to turn to the substance of choice (e.g. alcohol) and/or the needle for relief of suffering.

For those persons who are unable or unwilling to reduce or curtail use of substances (e.g. drugs, alcohol or other substances), limit setting to prevent harm to the person and others, and a refusal to abandon the individual no matter what his or her behaviours, are the moral imperatives.

CONCLUSION
The Roman slave Publius Syrus who lived in the first century BC wrote:

> 'As men, we are all equal in the presence of death.'[28]

Those of us alive today cannot know the truth of this ancient maxim until our own passing. What we can say with surety is that the modern experience of dying for the vast majority of those individuals experiencing SSUPs, SEMH and life-limiting illness is often more isolated, anguished and demeaning than it is for those without these co-occurring disorders. Much progress must be made in the flexibility and accessibility of palliative and hospice care delivery for a good death to be equally available to all human beings.

REFERENCES

1 Maxwell TL, Marinez JM, Knight CF, editors. *The Hospice and Palliative Medicine Approach to Life-Limiting Illness*. 3rd ed. Glenview, IL: American Academy of Hospice and Palliative Medicine; 2008.

2 Ewing JA. Detecting alcoholism. The CAGE Questionnaire. *Journal of the American Medical Association*. 1984; **252**: 1905–7.

3 Bruera E, Moyano J, Seifert L, *et al.* The frequency of alcoholism among patients with pain due to terminal cancer. *Journal of Pain and Symptom Management*. 1995; **10**: 599–603.

4 Substance Abuse and Mental Health Services Administration. 2002 National Survey on Drug Use and Health. 2002 [cited 28 March 2004]. Available at: http://oas.samhsa.gov/nhsda.htm (accessed 24 April 2012).

5 Dixon L. Dual diagnosis of substance abuse in schizophrenia: prevalence and impact on outcomes [Review]. *Schizophrenia Research*. 1999; **35**(Suppl): S93–100.

6 Temel JS, Greer JA, Muzikansky A, *et al.* Early palliative care for patients with metastatic non-small-cell lung cancer. *The New England Journal of Medicine*. [Randomized Controlled Trial Research Support, Non-U.S. Gov't]. 2010; **363**: 733–42.

7 Felker B, Yazel JJ, Short D. Mortality and medical comorbidity among psychiatric patients: a review [Review]. *Psychiatric Services*. 1996; **47**: 1356–63.

8 Colton CW, Manderscheid RW. Congruencies in increased mortality rates, years of potential life lost, and causes of death among public mental health clients in eight states. *Preventing Chronic Disease*. [Research Support, U.S. Gov't, P.H.S.]. 2006; **3**: A42.

9 The United States Conference of Mayors. *Hunger and Homelessness Survey: a status report on hunger and homelessness in America's cities: a 23-city survey*. Washington, DC: United States Conference of Mayors; 2007.

10 Kushel MB, Miaskowski C. End-of-life care for homeless patients: "she says she is there to help me in any situation". *Journal of the American Medical Association*. [Case Reports Clinical Conference Research Support, N.I.H., Extramural Research Support, Non-U.S. Gov't Research Support, U.S. Gov't, P.H.S.]. 2006; **296**: 2959–66.

11 Podymow T, Turnbull J, Coyle D. Shelter-based palliative care for the homeless terminally ill. *Palliative Medicine*. [Research Support, Non-U.S. Gov't]. 2006; **20**: 81–6.

12 Breitbart W, Rosenfeld BD, Passik SD, *et al.* The undertreatment of pain in ambulatory AIDS patients. *Pain*. 1996; **65**: 243–9.

13 Breitbart W, Rosenfeld B, Passik S, *et al.* A comparison of pain report and adequacy of analgesic therapy in ambulatory AIDS patients with and without a history of substance abuse. *Pain*. [Clinical Trial Comparative Study Controlled Clinical Trial Research Support, Non-U.S. Gov't Research Support, U.S. Gov't, P.H.S.]. 1997; **72**: 235–43.

14 Passik SD, Theobald DE. Managing addiction in advanced cancer patients: why bother? [Case Reports]. *Journal of Pain and Symptom Management*. 2000; **19**: 229–34.

15 American Society of Addiction Medicine. *Public Policy Statement: definition of addiction*. 2011. Available at: www.asam.org/DefinitionofAddiction-LongVersion.html (accessed 24 April 2012).

16 Kirsh KL, Passik SD. Palliative care of the terminally ill drug addict. [Case Report Review]. *Cancer Investigation*. 2006; **24**: 425–31.

17 Baumrucker SJ. Ethics Roundtable. Hospice and alcoholism. *The American Journal of Hospice and Palliative Care.* 2006; **23**: 153–6.

18 Claxton R, Arnold R. *Screening for Opioid Misuse and Abuse: fast facts and concepts.* End of Life/Palliative Education Resource Center [serial on the Internet]. 2011: Available at: www.eperc.mcw.edu/EPERC/FastFactsIndex/Documents/ff_244.htm (accessed 24 April 2012).

19 Butler SF, Budman SH, Fernandez K, Jamison RN. Validation of a screener and opioid assessment measure for patients with chronic pain. *Pain.* [Comparative Study Research Support, Non-U.S. Gov't Research Support, U.S. Gov't, P.H.S. Validation Studies]. 2004; **112**: 65–75.

20 Webster LR, Webster RM. Predicting aberrant behaviors in opioid-treated patients: preliminary validation of the Opioid Risk Tool. *Pain Medicine.* [Controlled Clinical Trial Validation Studies]. 2005; **6**: 432–42.

21 Weissman DE. *Is it Pain or Addiction? Fast Facts and Concepts.* End of Life/Palliative Education Resource Center [serial on the Internet]. 2006: Available at: www.eperc.mcw.edu/fastFact/ff_68.htm (accessed 24 April 2012).

22 Weissman DE, Haddox JD. Opioid pseudoaddiction – an iatrogenic syndrome. *Pain.* 1989; **36**: 363–6.

23 Reisfeld GM, Paulian GD, Wilson GR. *Susbtance Use Disorders in the Palliative Care Patient: fast facts and concepts.* 2nd ed. End of Life/Palliative Education Resource Center at the Medical College of Wisconsin; 2009. Available at: www.eperc.mcw.edu/fastFact/ff_127.htm (accessed 24 April 2012).

24 Childers JW, Arnold RM. "I feel uncomfortable 'calling a patient out:'" educational needs of palliative medicine fellows in managing opioid misuse. *Journal of Pain and Symptom Management.* 2012; **43**: 253–60.

25 Weissman DE. Understanding pseudoaddiction. *Journal of Pain Symptom Management.* 1994; **9**: 74.

26 Geppert CM. To help and not to harm: ethical issues in the treatment of chronic pain in patients with substance use disorders. *Advances in Psychosomatic Medicine.* 2004; **25**: 151–71.

27 Harm Reduction Coalition. *Principles of Harm Reduction.* New York, NY [cited 4 September 2011]; Available at: www.harmreduction.org/section.php?id=62 (accessed 24 April 2012).

28 Publius Syrus. Available at: www.quotationspage.com/quote/1887.html (accessed 24 April 2012).

TO LEARN MORE

- End of Life/Palliative Education Resource Center (EPERC). Online site with educational materials such as the Fast Facts series on pain and symptom management. Available at: www.eperc.mcw.edu/EPERC (accessed 24 April 2012).
- National Council for Palliative Care (NCPC). Umbrella organisation for all involved in palliative and end-of-life care in England, Wales and Northern Ireland. Available at: www.ncpc.org.uk (accessed 24 April 2012).
- Palliative Care Australia is the national organisation representing the interests of those striving for quality end-of-life care in Australia and New Zealand. Available at: www.palliativecare.org.au/ (accessed 24 April 2012).
- Passik SD, Portenoy RK, Ricketts PL. Substance abuse issues in cancer patients. Part 1: Prevalence and diagnosis. *Oncology.* 1998; **12**: 517–21.
- Passik SD, Portenoy RK, Ricketts PL. Substance abuse issues in cancer patients. Part 2: Evaluation and treatment. *Oncology.* 1998; **12**: 729–34.

CHAPTER 16

Looking after yourself and colleagues

David B Cooper

. . . about courtesy and good manners . . .[1]

PRE-READING EXERCISE 16.1

Time: 30 minutes

Think about the following. Do they relate to you as the person on the receiving end, or are you the person bullying? What would your approach be in each situation?

- A policy that conflicts with the professional's legal obligation is instigated without discussion. When the professional discloses this to colleagues, he is reprimanded and told that he should not have mentioned this at all because he is a manager and therefore should support management.
- You receive a letter stating that during the merger with another social services or health authority, you are among those who might be made redundant but discussion with managers does not seem to clarify your position. This situation of constant worry goes on for over a year before you find out you are to stay in your current post.
- You have been 'slotted in' to your existing post but without consultation, the terms of your contract have changed. When you challenge this, you are told directly that you should shut up . . . that you are 'lucky to have a job'.
- A person in your care has a terminal illness; you know she is going to die within days. The family is told by the senior registrar that, in discussion with the consultant, they have decided that nothing more can be done for their mother and that it is best she be treated palliatively. You are a member of the nursing team on the ward and appreciate the individual's and family's wishes but the junior doctor on call at the weekend dismisses this and tells you the consultant is a strong believer in acute intensive care to the end. You know this will unnecessarily increase the individual's suffering and pain – but do you feel able to say so?

> • A colleague goes off sick often – odd days here and there. You and other members of the team are angry about being let down and the colleague gains a reputation of being lazy and unreliable and she feels uncomfortable on the days she is at work. Several months later she goes on long-term sick leave – she is 'skiving' (being lazy and taking unneeded time off work) as usual – within a few weeks she is diagnosed with late-stage cancer and dies within weeks.

See if this chapter changes your approach.

STRESS AND BURNOUT

Stress is a part of our life and most times it is acceptable. However, stress levels can become excessive and may cause us to feel agitated, tearful and experience sleeplessness.[2] Unacceptable levels of stress can arise when environmental demands exceed our personal and social resources.[2] Davidson[2] suggests that:

> Stress response is multifactorial, including cognitive, affective, behavioural, and physiological components.

➤ **cognitive** – sequelae include excessive worry, racing thoughts, low self-confidence or a sense of hopelessness
➤ **affective** – disturbance may eventually lead to clinically significant anxiety or depression
➤ **behaviours** – e.g. social withdrawal or excessive alcohol, nicotine or drug use can be used to compensate
➤ **physiological** – activity in the sympathetic nervous system increases heart rate and respiration, and diverts blood to the muscles which may be needed for the 'fight or flight' reaction. Constant stress can produce psychosomatic pain, fatigue, or insomnia.[2]

Stress is all-encompassing. Davidson suggests that it is useful to think of *burnout* for a number of reasons.[2]
1 Burnout is limited to sources of stress in the individual's workplace.
2 Burnout among health professionals has been particularly well researched.
3 Burnout is more precisely defined than stress.

The three components and characteristics of burnout are:
1 **emotional exhaustion** – wearing out, depletion of emotional resources, loss of energy, debilitation, fatigue
2 **depersonalisation** – negative, callous, excessively detached towards other people, loss of idealism, irritability
3 **reduced personal accomplishment** – reduction in self-confidence, low productivity, poor morale, inability to cope.[3]

Davidson[2] suggests that:

> Burnout is a chronic condition that can lead to deterioration in the quality of care the individual provides for the patient. This may be a consequence of lowered morale, absenteeism, poor physical health or an increase in marital or family problems.[2]

BURNOUT, STRESS AND WORK

There are several factors that enable us to classify work stressors in our work environment – relationship, task and system management dimensions (*see* Table 16.1).[2]

TABLE 16.1 Job-related stress dimensions

Relationships	<ul><li>communication problems with managers</li><li>lack of teamwork</li><li>conflict with colleagues</li></ul>
Tasks	<ul><li>difficult individuals you care for daily</li><li>role ambiguity</li><li>role adequacy</li><li>role legitimacy</li><li>role conflict</li><li>role support</li><li>low sense of autonomy</li></ul>
System management	<ul><li>inadequate resources</li><li>poor physical environment</li><li>old equipment</li><li>work overload</li></ul>

SELF-ASSESSMENT EXERCISE 16.1 (ANSWERS ON P. 285)

Time: 15 minutes

1 Which of the following are components of 'burnout'?
   a emotional exhaustion
   b reduced appetite
   c loss of libido
   d depersonalisation
   e paranoid ideation

2 Which job factors in healthcare settings contribute to most distress as identified in qualitative research?
   a poor management
   b intimacy and death
   c work overload
   d role ambiguity
   e interpersonal problems

3 Affective signs of work stress include:
   a tremulousness
   b early depression
   c excessive drinking
   d chest pain
   e worry
4 Accumulated Loss Phenomena include which of the following?
   a personal conflict
   b reduced self-esteem
   c social withdrawal
   d agitation
   e aggression
5. Demographic variables that predispose to palliative work stress include:
   a younger age
   b lower social class
   c poor education
   d being single
   e being male[2]

COMMUNICATION

KEY POINT 16.1

Effective communication is a master key . . . it fits all locks and opens all doors . . .[4]

SELF-ASSESSMENT EXERCISE 16.2

Time: 10 minutes
Consider the following:
● When was the last time you wished communication within or outwith your team
  could be improved?
● What steps do you think you could take to improve the communication?

Effective communication can reduce the level of stress and burnout experienced by the professional. Sadly, burnout is no longer rare. There is an increasing level of risk of burnout for the professional in health and social care.

Communication is pivotal when avoiding increased levels of stress and burnout. However, if this is the case – why do we often get it wrong? If effective communication is easy – why do we not practise it? If we are pleased when communication has gone well and angry when it has not – why do we have high expectations of others' effective communication and not pay attention to our own practices? If we are experiencing the effects of stress and burnout ourselves, why are we so unsympathetic to others when they experience the same?

As individuals, we should know *what to do* and *how to do it* – there are no excuses. Yet, we remain ineffective communicators – unless it impacts on us directly. Then we become experts – we notice how ineffective communication damages our day!

Here we provide a foundation for common courtesy and good practice that should be part of our professional and personal lives. We have become too familiar with poor communication and easily oversimplify or underestimate the importance of communication. Consequently, we miss the value it holds for individuals, groups and ourselves.

Table 16.2 offers the definition for key words used in this chapter.

TABLE 16.2 Definitions

Word	Definition
Communicate:	to impart (knowledge) or exchange (thoughts) by speech, writing, gesture, etc.[5]
	to share information with others by speaking, writing, moving your body, using signals[6]
Communication:	the imparting or exchange of information, ideas or feelings[5]
Effective:	productive or capable of producing a result[5]
Intra-	within, inside[5]
Inter-	between, mutually, together, reciprocally[5]

WHAT IS EFFECTIVE COMMUNICATION?

Communication can be subdivided into seven parts:
1 individual, family and carers
2 junior team
3 peers
4 intra-disciplinary team
5 inter-disciplinary team
6 middle management
7 senior management

. . . all are interdependent and interrelated – none stands alone.

KEY POINT 16.2

Integral to, and at the centre of, all our actions is effective communication with the individual, family and carers.

Each person individually experiences the negative consequence of ineffective communication. Therefore, effective communication is like the ripples in a pond, flowing effortlessly between each part.

Communication pond?

Water is made up of millions of individual molecules that collectively give water its fluidity. Individuals within an organisation, or interlinked fields, are like the individual molecules of water. Each is dependent on the other to provide the best possible quality standard of care for the individual, family and carers.

Imagine a stone landing in a pond. The ripples move seamlessly through the water until the pond is smooth, ready for the next stone. In this analogy, you are the stone – represented by **ME** in Figure 16.1. The **ME** is placed anywhere in the organisational structure. Wherever you are in the chart, **ME** is the centre for effective communication. It is your responsibility to ensure your communication flows effectively and effortlessly through the organisation.

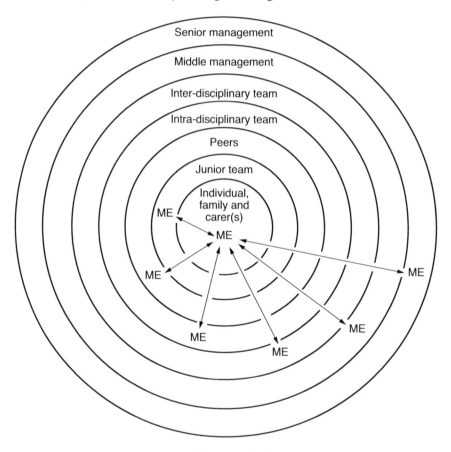

Figure 16.1 Communications pond

Therefore, effective communication emanates like the ripples on a pond, flowing effortlessly. Each professional has an equal responsibility to effectively communicate with the other: each intra- and inter-dependent. Only then can communication . . . and the care of the individual, family and carers . . . be effective.

1 Individual, family and carers

The individual, family and carers are central in any care environment. Every action, act, or omission, from that of the junior member to that of the most senior manager, impacts on these individuals. Ineffective communication makes the treatment and intervention experience devastating and destructive.

The impact of verbal communication between professionals cannot be overemphasised.

KEY POINT 16.3

How professionals share important and routine information related to the individual, family and carers does have a major impact on the successful outcome of any therapeutic intervention.

With the individual's permission, information relating to past and present health or social problems can be discussed with each professional or agency. Just as important is the information available from family/carers relating to the individual's concerns. The individual may forget or be unable to express important facts and information relevant to the presenting problem. Often, individuals and family can feel intimidated by the 'knowledgeable professional'.

The individual, family and carers can become dependent on the professional. This is not a deliberate act. It is easy to feel safe in the hands of a competent professional. The individual comes to depend on immediate access and, consequently, sudden unexpected and unplanned withdrawal is disruptive. The individual, family and carers should be informed at the outset about the level and extent of your involvement in their care. This should be periodically reinforced so the individual is aware of *your* end-date.

Moreover, it is possible for the professional to extend contact with the individual, family and carers beyond that which is therapeutic. We gain subconscious reward from their dependence on us – the professional!

Careful monitoring and clinical supervision will aid awareness of such instances so that effective addressing of the negative aspects can be worked through . . . and overcome.

KEY POINT 16.4

Clinical supervision aids identification of over-involvement and dependence.

Individuals do progress without our watchful eye if appropriate and effective intervention and treatment are managed effectively. We cannot protect them from all ills or dangers. Being aware of our limitations, intervention and the extent of the therapeutic value takes experience. Close monitoring of our actions is essential. A good indicator would be . . . when we come to write the legal records related to the individual and we have little to say about the person's progress – it is time to evaluate one's effectiveness. Ineffective communication is damaging and destructive.

2 Junior team

Students and junior team members often feel isolated from the communication loop. Matters involving the organisation are heard on the grapevine, often half-factual, sometimes totally inaccurate.

> **KEY POINT 16.5**
>
> Effective communication with junior members of the team is just as important as in any other area of the organisation (*see* 'Team trust' below).

Unease and job dissatisfaction arise when the individual feels that he or she is unheard.

New employees are often unsure of the system and reluctant to express ideas and concepts for fear of reprimand or being labelled as troublemakers. Old hands do not always have the best or brightest concepts. Communication *among* and *between* junior team members and senior colleagues should be actively encouraged. Where possible, new ideas and initiatives should be given a fair hearing and encouraged. Yes, it may be that 'it has been tried before and failed' but maybe the time was not right – or indeed the motivation. With supervision, support and encouragement, junior team members bring new ideas to the fore that can improve care and communication.

Why is he or she doing this?

The easiest way to germinate suspicion and misunderstanding is to issue a directive that has no prior or present explanation as to its use. For example, statistics – in any format – are the bane of many. Without careful explanation of the value of new statistic collection (i.e. to ensure that the service is adequately resourced and funded), suspicion can evolve into a negative response. 'Don't they think I am working hard enough?' 'Why are they watching me?' An explanation offsets the misconception, maintains productivity and improves working practice. Explanations of complex or role-changing information should be *face-to-face*. It is *not* acceptable to email or send a memorandum – this is, at the least, bad manners and poor practice.

3 Peers

Communication upwards: managers are not clairvoyant – tell them!

A common complaint from team members is that the manager does not understand them. Like the manager, we, as individuals, have a responsibility to communicate. Managers do not come to the post with a vacuum-packed crystal ball; nor are they clairvoyant – even if the issues seem blatantly obvious to you. Nor do they know everything there is to know about the workforce as a managerial tribal birthright. The manager needs clear and concise feedback. It is no use complaining that the manager does not appreciate the needs of your job, or that one is working in excess of one's designated hours, if this is not explained to him or her. Likewise, it is no use complaining about the excessive workload and yet still work the excess hours for fear that not doing so might jeopardise treatment, care and interventions: *as professionals, we have a responsibility to communicate effectively too!* Moreover, you should support your complaint with statistics!

One cannot place all of the responsibility for ineffective communication on the boss! Each individual is capable of demonstrating how effective communication works. If we remain cognisant of the part each plays in ensuring that we are heard and understood, communication is effective and appreciation of each other's roles develops. In addition, each must exercise the ability to *listen* to others and *analyse* each individual need. Having *listened*, no effective *change* is achieved unless we *act* on the information, and *communicate* it to others.

Peers are an effective means of support, supervision and guidance, yet we are often isolated in our professional practice. Stress and burnout cause ill health. We can all experience it. It is not a weakness.

KEY POINT 16.6

If we truly value one another, and wish to be effective in communication, and to reap its rewards, we would be better placed to support, rather than dismiss, our colleagues. After all, it could be *you* next time!

4 Intra-disciplinary

Communicating information

Some individuals within teams withhold information. To possess information not yet available to others is often misinterpreted as power. Practice and service provision are only effective if information is shared.

KEY POINT 16.7

More power and respect are gained by sharing information and resources with colleagues than from withholding these.

After all, if no one knows you are holding that information – perhaps on a new treatment or approach – how can your influence and knowledge be acknowledged? Moreover, how can your colleagues improve treatment, care and interventions?

> **KEY POINT 16.8**
>
> Regular professional meetings are essential to information sharing.

If you are a hoarder by nature, this will be your opportunity to demonstrate your skill and knowledge, and at the same time, bring the rest of the team up to date.

5 Inter-disciplinary team

The admission process

Whatever your area of work, the admission or acceptance of a planned therapeutic intervention with the individual, family and/or carers is part of your role. To be effective, it is essential that professional communication is co-ordinated. Often, if omitted, the minor considerations have an important impact on creating ineffective communication.

As a result of an individual's emergency hospital admission, other hospital and community appointments can be missed. Other professionals and agencies involved may be unaware of the admission. Even planned admissions cause communication issues. Hospital admission provokes anxiety, in even the calmest individual. People do forget to cancel appointments. Therefore, immediately the individual is engaged in assessment it should be ascertained what other services – directly or indirectly – are involved, and what appointments may be anticipated during admission. Planned appointments that may be missed, proposed community visits and/or clinic appointments need to be noted, and each professional colleague or agency should be informed. With permission, approach the family in case they hold additional information. In addition, direct communication with individuals and agencies by the professional is essential.

It is often easier to share information relating to your involvement with an individual using a multi-copy letter. It is good practice (and will be much appreciated by other colleagues) to give the individual a copy of this letter.

The discharge process

As the needs of the individual change, it may be appropriate to arrange a joint case/family conference to share valuable information relating to the present and future care needs.

The individual, family and carers do feel vulnerable when intensive services are withdrawn. Even though the individual may require no immediate intervention, there is a sense of safety if it is understood that someone will be available to answer any questions they may have should a problem arise. Withdrawal of professional involvement or discharge should not take place until adequate arrangements for the continuation of essential care are agreed and in place. It is bad practice to withdraw a service or discharge the individual without adequate and effective planning. Crises can and do occur. Community services are not always easily accessible at weekends. Ten minutes of pre-withdrawal or discharge preparation will save one or more hours of crisis follow-up contact.

Communication to the primary healthcare team is imperative to progress a smooth transition from hospital to home – even in rapid discharge.

> **KEY POINT 16.9**
>
> It is beneficial if the individual knows the name of the community or clinic professional who is involved in their follow-on care.

This is far more reassuring than being told that 'a letter will be sent to you in a week or so'.

Avoiding unnecessary cost and time-wasting

Our lives are hectic: full of twists, turns and manoeuvres. Consequently, it is easy to become encapsulated within what we do – the task of daily work. It is easy to forget to inform other professionals and agencies about matters that impinge on those professionals' day. If this situation is unmanaged then communication breaks down and ill feeling and rivalry ensue. When one is busy, time is of the essence – it is precious and valued. Visiting the individual at home, only to find that the visit has clashed with a clinic appointment of which the professional was unaware, leaves one feeling frustrated and angry, as if time has been stolen.

For those arguing that this is additional bureaucracy gone mad, the above guidance, if acted on, and carefully followed, is cheaper than the cost of a missed appointment or confusion arising from poor communication. A wasted community visit, or the loss of money due to a missed benefits agency appointment, far outweigh the cost involved in effective communication between busy professionals and agencies.

What can I do to improve personal communication?

> **KEY POINT 16.10**
>
> Common sense, courtesy and good manners form the basis of effective communication.

Allow for a great deal of personal effort, patience, practice and disappointment, but do prevail. We all have an individual responsibility to improve communication. Think . . . *what would I like from others?* **You** are the master key. It is possible for an individual, and team, to effectively improve communication.

6 Middle management
Communicating change

> **KEY POINT 16.11**
>
> The middle manager plays a pivotal role in the communication of change. Change in any organisation is unsettling.

Little encouragement is needed for half-truths and rumours to be disseminated and such rumours can cause dissatisfaction. It is easier to have all your colleagues on board the ship than it is to stop the ship, circle and collect those who have fallen overboard. Change affects all members of the intra-disciplinary team; this in turn impacts on the inter-disciplinary team and *ultimately on individualised care*. To share and be fully conversant with the change and the process involved can and does lead to team support. Involvement and a sense of being part of the change process, rather than excluded from it and unworthy of consideration, are essential for effective communication and ownership of change.

An individual acting as a 'change agent' is beneficial . . . but only if that professional has accurate information, has authority and standing within the organisation and manages his or her communications effectively. Effective communication is not about communicating with senior managers alone . . . it includes all professionals we work with . . . whatever the grade.

7 Senior management
Senior and middle managers need to know the detail of the job each employee undertakes. It is not essential for the manager to be from the same discipline but it is necessary for him or her to be familiar with the exact role of the employee. Only then can respect, mutual understanding and communication be effective. Similarly, the manager needs to share with the employee what his or her own role entails.

One can communicate with a colleague and still encounter misunderstanding. Anyone with a teenage son or daughter will know that even when the benefits of having a clean, tidy room have been explained – for the hundredth time – and a check has been made to ensure understanding of the guidance, numerous reminders administered, and the consequences of lack of action explained, the room remains unclean. Each of us can only try to improve communication – to make communication clear and unambiguous. Human nature dictates that some communications will go unheeded or misinterpreted. However, we are not challenging teenagers – we are adults who would like a good working environment.

Setting an example
During times of pressure and stress, effective communication is the first thing to suffer – yet it reduces pressure and stress. Effective communication frees time to deal with other matters that are important to individualised care. Effective

communication comes from the top. Senior managers lead by example: only then will the employee find the tasks that he or she is set easier to work with and control. However, a lack of such leadership is not an excuse for one's actions, inactions or omissions.

Direction on effective communication comes from senior managers. If the directive is clear, emphasising that effective communication is important, then it is likely that the practice will disseminate throughout the organisation. However, there is little benefit issuing directives, if in personal practice the manager does not lead by example.

The personal touch

Emails and memos have made life easier for the busy manager. The increasing lack of pleasantries within the communication and the formal directness and abbreviation means that it is hard to perceive the literal intention of the message we receive. Managers should be aware of this change and make written communication accessible. Time to include the pleasantries should be spent when developing the communication. Avoid misinterpretation.

Breaking bad news

Never communicate bad news in writing. This should always be undertaken personally. If you wish to speak to someone about an issue, this should be undertaken immediately. It is poor and ineffective communication to leave an employee waiting overnight or over a weekend wondering if there is a problem. If the matter involves discipline or reprimand, wait until you are able to see the person. If you have to send a written communication, include information about the anticipated nature of the topic. Likewise, if the meeting is set up verbally, involves a routine matter, and is to take place in a few days, give some indication as to the topic. This avoids rumour, speculation and anxiety. After all, a happy workforce is more effective than an unhappy one. Moreover, they are often willing to give in excess of their hours to the organisation – so why disrupt it!

KEY POINT 16.12

Personal face-to-face communication is far more productive and fruitful in terms of manager and employee relationship than any other form of communication, e.g. telephone or email.

It cannot be overemphasised that if the employee you wish to speak to is in the next room or same building and is immediately available – stand up, walk out the door and speak to him or her. This will be better received than an email or memo from someone who is only feet away. It establishes and earns respect.

Communicating with a colleague

It is frustrating to feel that one's professional communications and the important issues you wish to raise within and outwith the team at junior, peer, intra-disciplinary, inter-disciplinary, middle and senior management levels are disregarded, unheard or dismissed. It is essential to remember that effective communication is a two-way process. Often information needs reinforcement and clarification. All parties need to understand what is:

➤ required of them
➤ said
➤ not said.

To keep interaction effective, and the inevitable knock-on effect on the individual, family and carers' interventions running smoothly, do:

➤ write
➤ meet personally
➤ telephone
➤ email
➤ fax
➤ thank colleagues
➤ respect colleagues
➤ acknowledge your limitations
➤ seek help when needed
➤ understand the demands on others
➤ be aware of others' feelings
➤ assume that you need to clarify your actions
➤ keep communicating effectively – even if others give up.

This is basic good manners; sadly, it is often forgotten!

TEAM TRUST

There is a need to seek and receive support and accept our own feelings. Being able to trust colleagues – be that a person of the same standing, junior or senior – and to talk openly of our own feelings and experiences are essential.[7] Building trust is crucial to any team, and can only be achieved when each person feels a sense of security.

KEY POINT 16.13

Each individual has the right to be treated with respect, as an intelligent, capable and equal human being.

Examples would be that the:
> health or social carer should be acknowledged for skills, knowledge and experience in areas such as manual handling
> medical officers should be able to question, in a safe environment, without feeling that they should have all the answers.

Organisational attitude is crucial to the success of the team. The team needs to be aware of the organisation's acceptance of the effect of stress. Each individual should be encouraged to express his or her concerns without fear of stigma or reprisal. The principles of the therapeutic relations with the individual and family (*see* Chapter 6) *do* extend to those we work alongside.

It is important to demonstrate that teamwork is valued. That is, each individual has to feel valued. A work team can be compared to a football team – illustrating the need for different roles to work together, each reliant on the others to produce a positive result.[8] In nursing, the charge nurse could be the captain or coach, the staff nurse being the shaper or forward, and so on. The team captain plays in any position and may fill many over a period, leading by example and acting as a role model. He or she must be prepared to pass the ball (hand over leadership) to the best player who can advance the team advantage and achieve the (person's or family's) chosen goal. This model of teamwork is demonstrated in this comparison of teamwork to a formation of flying geese.[9]

> As each goose flaps its wings, it creates uplift for the following birds. By flying in a V formation the whole flock adds 71% greater range than if they flew alone. When the lead goose tires he falls back and another takes over. The geese at the back 'honk' to encourage those ahead. When a goose gets sick or wounded two geese drop out and follow it down to help protect it. They stay with it until the goose dies or is able to fly again.[9]

Evidence of outcomes
Evidence suggests that the best treatment outcomes are achieved by contact with a team that is least hierarchal and shows the greatest collegiality.[10] There is less duplication and fragmentation of care when the team works effectively, and the individual and family we care for benefit from greater co-operation, co-ordination and collaboration.

Eleven values of good-quality teamwork
1   Humour
There is a defined link between humour and good health, reduction of stress and creativity. Humour in the workplace:
> improves productivity, person-centred service and morale
> reduces sickness and stress
> increases creativity

➤ strengthens teamwork
➤ enhances communication.

The power of humour:
➤ teaches
➤ inspires
➤ motivates.

Humour is effective as a:
➤ **best medicine** – laughing for the health of it
➤ **stress buster** – smiling to reduce stress
➤ **creative spark** – stimulates brain power
➤ **teaching aid** – use humour to reach your audience more effectively.

However, there is a need to manage inappropriate humour by setting limits to what is not funny.

2 Approachability

It is important that colleagues feel another colleague is approachable. The freedom to discuss not only service and team development but concerns and problems, and openly ask for help, is essential.

3 Identifying the needs of others

Individually, team members need to be open minded and to realise that others might not have the same expertise or coping skills. Offering help, guidance and support *before they are requested* is pivotal to skilled teamwork.

4 Confidence and trust

Confidence and trust are hard earned, but essential, individual characteristics of the successful team. All participants must be inclusive of this team principle.

5 Enjoyment of work

It is 'okay' to enjoy your work, even when dealing with serious and enduring mental health problems, death and dying. There is much satisfaction in making someone more comfortable, or relieving physical, psychological, emotional and spiritual pain. Acknowledging that work is enjoyable, and sharing that with others is okay.

6 Practice sessions

It is advantageous to hold formal practice meetings, at least monthly, at which the team and individuals within the team can openly reflect on the quality of care and practice. The aim is to constructively develop good practice and to learn from experience without destructive criticism.

7 Debriefing

While debriefing is time consuming, there are benefits to spending a few minutes ensuring that, at the start and end of each shift, each individual feels all right, and can freely discuss issues of concern, and not carry such concerns home or into the workplace.

8 Team building

The annual 'away-days' have a strong place in effective teamwork. The team meets, off-site, unencumbered by the demands and expectations of the workplace. The aim is to review how the team works together and how this could be improved and developed and to strengthen workplace relationships.

9 Gossip and self-discipline

It is destructive and bad practice for the team or individuals to talk about a colleague outwith his or her presence. This should not be encouraged or accepted. Each individual should hold his or her own court.

10 Respect

Feelings of team respect is essential. Each individual should feel valued and cared for. Sadly, while great emphasis is correctly placed on the value and care of the individual and family, we are often destructive in valuing and caring for our colleagues. Respect is earned by maintaining the values and practices outlined here.

11 Time out

No matter how dedicated one is, sometimes we need to take 10 minutes for ourselves during the working day. It permits the gathering of thoughts and emotions, and/or puts into perspective something that has impinged upon us during the shift. It clears one's head. Colleagues should expect, respect, accept and reciprocate this individual need. There should be no shame or guilt attached to taking 10 minutes to oneself.

Developing teamwork

Developing a team is hard work. Weaknesses at times can be difficult to accept and individual strength can sometimes appear overwhelming. Overcoming perceived professional differences and hierarchy is essential. These can be overpowering and destructive. Ensuring problems are discussed openly, without issues becoming personal, requires patience and skill on the part of the team and the appointed team leader. Leading an effective team does not negate the need for team management and compromise has to be truly acceptable to each individual. With the will of each individual, teamwork is effective and successful as long as each remembers that it is the individual and family we care for who truly lead the team.

CONCLUSION

> Some managers feel that what we do is easy . . . straightforward . . . but it isn't easy and straightforward for the individual and family . . . we have to help them untangle the web of dis-ease they find themselves facing . . .
>
> A community psychiatric nurse in clinical supervision.

This chapter reflects on a small number of examples of *poor* communication and of *effective* communication, and on ways to improve communication, thus reducing the level of stress and burnout within our own work environment.

When we learn to look after ourselves we must not forget to learn to look after our colleagues . . . no matter what their roles are within the organisation.

KEY POINT 16.14

It is about looking after each other and ourselves.

There is a plethora of ineffective communication examples that one could describe: each one of us has our own personal story! This chapter aims to demonstrate that, with a little work from *you*, as an integral individual, effective communication can happen within and outwith *your* organisation: *you* just have to give it brain space and effort. It is not a *thing* to do later but an instrument to use constantly – always at the forefront of everyday activities.

Effective communication is cost-effective and saves time. Misunderstanding, anger, frustration, complaints and worry . . . for the individual, family and carers, other professionals and oneself . . . can be avoided provided we communicate effectively.

Why keep walking into doors? Life is difficult enough! Each individual within and across an organisation has a responsibility to communicate effectively. Not just for oneself but for others whose lives we touch in one way or another and who are unable to care directly or indirectly for themselves. Effective communication is the master key . . . it fits all locks and opens the way to therapeutic treatment and interventions.[1]

Having said all the above, none of this is of any importance if the receiver of communication does not listen. This two-way process is imperative if communication is to be effective.

No professional wants the individual, family, or carers to suffer as a consequence of his or her inaction – yet, we risk this every day through poor communication. It is not *their* responsibility – it is *our* responsibility to make communication effective and meaningful to the best of our ability and understanding. If there were just seven words of wisdom in professional practice and effective communication, these would be:

Never assume people know . . . they do not![1]

POST-READING EXERCISE 16.1

Time: 15 minutes

Consider each of the following statements. How do they fit your experience of your workplace? Answer 'yes' or 'no' to each as honestly as you can; a maybe is a 'no'. It is probably best to put down the first answer that comes to you. These are simple indictors of your work experience; there is no need to get too analytical about them.

Taking care of yourself at work

Y N

❑ ❑ I get a good night's sleep.

❑ ❑ I eat a healthy, well-balanced diet.

❑ ❑ I take plenty of exercise.

❑ ❑ I can talk through work problems with my partner/a close friend.

❑ ❑ Work does not interfere with my personal time.

❑ ❑ Other people's problems at work do not get to me.

❑ ❑ I practise some form of meditation or relaxation regularly.

❑ ❑ I can withdraw appropriately if a situation at work gets too stressful.

❑ ❑ I have a day a month when I do exactly as I please.

❑ ❑ I allow myself a good read, or something similar, every day, for at least half an hour, that takes all of my attention and is nothing to do with work.

❑ ❑ I make sure I get my proper breaks for meals and refreshments at work.

❑ ❑ I know my limits and boundaries and keep to them.

Scoring

The above explores whether some of the conditions for burnout are present in your life. Count your responses to each question and total the 'yes' responses. The higher your 'yes' response, the less is the likelihood of burnout occurring. If you score 100%, you are probably kidding yourself, or you are in denial. Most people who are okay in their lives and work will get around 75 per cent. The lower your score the more a problem is indicated. In general, a score of 50% or less should be a warning sign of a real problem that will provide seedbed for burnout. The risks would be incrementally greater if the score was below 50%.

Conversely, each question has an implicit solution. It is important not to get into trying to get a high score on all of them at once if there is a problem. Putting that degree of energy in to it will probably make things worse. Be gentle on yourself. If there are problem areas, set one or two realistic goals rather than trying to sort the whole lot out.

Remember, it is the overall picture, rather than individual responses, that count. The intention of the whole is to raise awareness of the situation so that things can change if necessary.

Post-Reading Exercise 16.1 is reproduced with the kind permission of Rev.

Prof. Stephen Wright. © Wright S, Sayre-Adams J. *Sacred Space – right relationship and spirituality in health care.* Cumbria: SSP; 2010. Wright S, Sayre-Adams J. 'Burnout – a spiritual crisis' essential guide booklet. *Nursing Standard.* **27**: 2005.

REFERENCES

1 Cooper DB. Communication: the essence of good practice, management and leadership. In: Cooper DB. *Developing Services in Mental Health–Substance Use.* 2011. pp. 161–70.

2 Davidson R. Stress issues in palliative care. In: Cooper J. *Stepping into Palliative Care 1: relationships and responses.* 2006. pp. 135–45.

3 Maslach C, Jackson SE, Leiter MP. *The Maslach Burnout Inventory.* 3rd ed. Palo Alto, CA: Consulting Psychologists Press; 1996.

4 Cooper DB. The standard guide to . . . communication. *Nursing Standard.* 1994; **8**: 42–3.

5 McLeod WT, managing editor. *Collins Dictionary and Thesaurus,* in one volume. Glasgow: HarperCollins; 1991. Reprint.

6 *Cambridge Dictionary* online. Available at: http://dictionary.cambridge.org/ (accessed 25 April 2012).

7 Nichols K, Jenkinson J. *Leading a Support Group.* London: Chapman & Hall; 1991.

8 Powell H, Kwiatek E, Murray G. The ward manager's premier league nursing management. 2005; **12**: 12–5.

9 Anon. Lesson from geese. Available at: www.agiftofinspiration.com.au/stories/inspirational/geese.shtml (accessed 25 April 2012).

10 Feigel SM, Schmitt MH. Interdisciplinary health teams: its measurement and its effect. *Social Science on Medicine.* 1979; **31**a: 217–29.

TO LEARN MORE

• Maguire P. Psychological barriers to the care of the dying. *British Medical Journal.* 1985; **291**: 1711–13.

• Riordan RJ, Saltzer SK. Burnout prevention among healthcare providers working with the terminally ill: a literature review. *Omega.* 1992; **25**: 17–24.

• Harris PE. The Nurse Stress Index. *Work and Stress.* 1989; **3**: 335–46.

• Hipwell AE, Tyler PA, Wilson C. Sources of stress and dissatisfaction among nurses in four hospital environments. *British Journal of Medical Psychology.* 1989; **62**: 71–9.

• Vachon MLS. Staff stress in hospice/palliative care; a review. *Palliative Medicine.* 1995; **9**: 91–122.

ACKNOWLEDGEMENT

The author is grateful to the editors and Radcliffe Publishing for permitting adaptation of this chapter: © In: Cooper J, editor. *Stepping into Palliative Care 1: relationships and responses.* 2nd ed. Oxford: Radcliffe Publishing; 2006. pp. 69–80, 128–31 and 135–43. Thank you.

ANSWERS TO SELF-ASSESSMENT EXERCISE 16.1 (P. 267)

1. a & d
2. b & e
3. b
4. a & b
5. a & d

Index

Entries in **bold** refer to tables, figures and boxes.